I0100951

I Survived Cancer and Here Is How I Did It

35 Cancer Survivors Share Their Journey

By Savio P. Clemente, NBC-HWC

Copyright © 2022 Savio P. Clemente, NBC-HWC

The Human Resolve LLC

All rights reserved. No part of this publication may be reproduced, distributed, or transmitted in any form or by any means, including photocopying, recording, or other electronic or mechanical methods, without the prior written permission of the publisher, except in the case of brief quotations embodied in critical reviews and certain other noncommercial uses permitted by copyright law. For permission requests, write to the publisher, addressed "Attention: Permissions Coordinator," at the address below.

First printing edition 2022

Published by Authority Magazine Press
3903 Labyrinth Rd
Baltimore, MD, 21215
www.authoritymag.co

Printed in the United States of America

10 9 8 7 6 5 4 3 2 1

Library of Congress Control Number: 2022902840

ISBN 979-8-9857595-0-1
ISBN 979-8-9857595-1-8 (ebook)
ISBN 979-8-9857595-2-5 (audiobook)

Dedication

None of us are promised a bed of roses in this life, but it's my honor to shower you with flowers.

Mom & Dad — thank you for always believing in me.

Yitzi Weiner — this book would have never come to fruition without your support.

And to those unseen forces who have guided me along the way — the path illuminates with hope.

About the Author

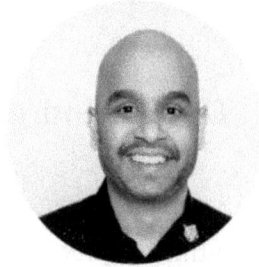

Savio P. Clemente coaches cancer survivors to overcome the confusion and gain the clarity needed to get busy living in mind, body, and spirit. He inspires health and wellness seekers to find meaning in the "why" and to cultivate resilience in their mindset. Savio is a Board Certified wellness coach (NBC-HWC, ACC), syndicated columnist, podcaster, stage 3 cancer survivor, and founder of The Human Resolve LLC.

Savio has interviewed notable TV personalities, and is featured in prominent publications from Authority Magazine, Thrive Global to BuzzFeed. He has covered numerous wellness, technology, and travel industry events in the United States and abroad. His mission is to offer clients, listeners, and viewers alike tangible takeaways in living a truly healthy, wealthy, and wise lifestyle.

Savio pens a weekly newsletter where he delves into secrets from living smarter to feeding your "three brains" — head, heart, and gut — in hopes of connecting the dots to those sticky parts in our nature that matter. He lives in the suburbs of Westchester County, New York and continues to follow his boundless curiosity. Savio hopes to one day live out a childhood fantasy and explore outer space.

For more information: www.isurvivedcancer.co
Accelerated Path Coaching: www.thehumanresolve.com
Instagram & Twitter: @thehumanresolve
LinkedIn: @saviopclemente

Table of Contents

Introduction

I was born in Mumbai, India, but my ancestral heritage is from Goa, India, a former Portuguese colony located on the southwestern coast. My family and I moved to the United States in the late '70s when I was only three years old. Throughout my elementary and high school years in the suburbs of Westchester County, New York, I was a sensitive child who was plagued by social anxiety and a stuttering impediment. I went to a Catholic elementary school and served as an altar boy, but there were always these lingering questions about life that kept me up at night. While in college at Fordham University in New York City, I faced several challenges from sexual identity to speaking my mind and expressing my individuality. Needless to say, I spent most of my formative years searching for meaning.

In July of 2014, I was visiting London and Amsterdam with a friend and noticed that my bed sheets the next morning were completely drenched with sweat. Fast forward a week later, my stomach eventually grew distended. At the insistence of my naturopath, I received a sonogram and was informed that I should visit the nearest hospital. An hour later, I was admitted to the 5th floor. After a bone marrow aspiration and nephrostomy procedure, I was given the grim diagnosis of Stage 3 Diffuse Large B-cell Non-Hodgkin's Lymphoma (DLBCL), a blood cancer affecting 70,000 plus individuals yearly.

I couldn't help thinking the road to recovery would be paved with much burden to family and friends. Strangely enough, a sense of calm enveloped me. My fifteen day stay at the hospital included a thoracentesis which drained over five liters of peritoneal fluid in the space between my lungs and chest, a handful of CT scans throughout my upper and lower cavity, and a recommendation from the Medical Director that I should start first my round of R-CHOP chemotherapy.

Cancer is not something which magically appears without the furtherance of a cause. Even if it cannot be fully understood by medical science, it is something that unfortunately manifests due to variables beyond our human comprehension.

There is great purpose in the darkness that we must "learn to sit with" asserts author and theologian Barbara Brown Taylor. This was just my particular challenge. I needed to rise above and find a way to meet my higher self. My physical body was dis-eased, but my mind certainly wasn't, and neither was my spirit. This is the kind of "grit" psychologist and educator Angela Lee Duckworth speaks of in her TED Talk presentation. It is available to all, but requires sticking with it — "living life like it's a marathon, not a sprint."

As the tears flowed down my cheeks waiting to hear if I would be yet another victim of the big C, I made a decision to choose life. Deep within my thoughts all I kept hearing was: *find the middle way; to know thyself is to heal thyself.* Scenes from the movie *Little Buddha* flashed before my eyes, "If you tighten the string too much it will snap, and if you leave it too slack, it won't play."

An integrative path is what I eventually chose to follow and was cancer-free four months later in December of 2014. I focused all my energies like a laser beam on the healing process and left no stone unturned. I scoured through medical journals, incorporated biohacking techniques, setup Google news alerts, joined Facebook groups, found passages in the Christian Bible, read Buddhist texts, and even searched for wisdom in the Quran.

When you start your journey with cancer the goal is remission, but I am also wise enough to know the experience came into my life for a reason. Where it would eventually lead was still a mystery.

I once heard Brendon Burchard, New York Times best-selling author and personal development coach say, "It is okay you don't have all the answers but you better have the ambition to grow." Up until that point I felt that I needed to figure everything out before I could ever facilitate a meaningful conversation with someone. What I learned is that you can still help someone because your life path and your struggles can illuminate where they sit today. It wasn't until I hit my five year remission mark that I had the courage to pursue my Board Certification and thus establish my coaching career. Up until that point, it seemed too far-fetched of an idea.

Despite my remission status, the experience left me with more questions than answers — from the fear of recurrence to the anxiety of future side effects, and the emotional toll of survivor's guilt. I quickly learned it was not only about dealing with the physical aspect of cancer, but about the totality of the human experience; connecting to all 7 energy centers. I am now free of cancer for seven years and coach cancer survivors. I help them overcome the confusion and gain the clarity needed to get busy living in mind, body, and spirit.

Here is an interesting story that taught me a lot. Early in my career, I was in such a hurry to facilitate a transformation for my client that I created a mind map in advance and plotted key areas to explore. I was so eager to dig into my creation that I wasn't truly listening to their needs. My client just wanted to be accepted where they were on that journey. They were seeking the true meaning of empathy; understanding what the other person is experiencing and feeling. It was a course correction because even though my intentions were noble, I realized that I can't control where they will ultimately land. Sometimes a person just needs to be heard. All I can do is hold space for that request.

And this leads me to why I felt this book was needed. After interviewing nearly 175 cancer survivors for my series with Authority Magazine and its syndication in Thrive Global, I felt the urge to give voice in book form to their inspiring stories. I wanted to highlight what they learned physically, mentally, emotionally, and spiritually from this very difficult experience which has forever shaped their worldview. My intention is to spread hope for second chances — that there is life after cancer and we are here to support each other through each and every battle.

Seeing my name printed on the cover lights me because I am able to tell the story of those who have faced the ultimate fight and are still here to pick up the broken pieces.

This book was written with a purpose, and here are the main lessons that I hope readers take away after finishing this book.

Physical

Live fully the human experience. For many decades, I was so caught up in living a spiritually fulfilling life, that I neglected the things that made me human. I would scoff and think that my spiritual awareness was far greater than anything else. But through my cancer recovery, I have come to learn that we are meant to embody all that life sends our way, and in order for us to be truly grateful, we must therefore fully immerse ourselves in both extremes.

Resource the right energy. Food can be satisfying as it can be harmful. Know what you are putting into your body and what you want to get out of it. A little indulgence is a good thing and food prep can be a lifesaver, but I've often found that when I have slowed down enough to figure out what my body is actually yearning for, have I been able to make the right decisions. In the book *Women Food and God*, Geneen Roth states, "Food is only the middleman, the means to the end. Of altering your emotions. Of making yourself numb. Of creating a secondary problem when the original problem becomes too uncomfortable." This quote was an eye-opener in how I viewed my relationship with food and the emotions linked to them. It allowed me to separate the biological need for eating versus the want for indulgence. It helped me see that the automaticity of choice and action are intertwined. It wasn't until that moment that my outlook on food changed from sabotage to healing.

Check in with the three brains. Documented studies in neuroscience have proven that we indeed have more than one brain. Known in embodiment circles as multiple brain integration — the head, heart, and gut holds deep inner wisdom that can help us connect the dots to those sticky parts in our nature that matter. Like a detective with their magnifying glass, we can examine our bodies like instruments looking for clues. As the saying goes, *the body knows*.

View your body as a stranger. Try the simple tactic of tuning into your heart. What words, images, and feelings are coming up for you? If your heart could talk, what would it say? What wisdom does it have to share with you? The heart holds not only painful memories from our past, but through the lived experience it collates those significant moments for greater understanding.

Mental

The benefits of meditation have been quite profound in my life. Meditation supports the practice of surrendering. Meditation aided in my ability to successfully process my stage 3 cancer diagnosis. Contrary to popular belief, meditation is not about blissing out, but about finding the bliss inward. Meditation requires effort that never ceases because living is the only choice we have.

Make to-do, will-do. I love flipping the script from the dreaded to-do which I sometimes never even get to completing, to will-do; a few simple but important tasks that need our attention stat. Doing so not only eliminates the clutter in and around your environment, but it helps strengthen your will in getting it done no matter the excuses.

Create a gratitude journal. This is my favorite ritual for mental wellness — the ability to check in with yourself at the end of the day and figure out why those things you are grateful for actually took shape and form. It helps you savor the feeling so it can continue long after.

A quote which resonates deeply is, "Your playing small doesn't serve the world. There's nothing enlightened about shrinking so that other people won't feel insecure around you," spoken by author and spiritual leader Marianne Williamson. This was a powerful reminder to always put my best foot forward even when failure might be lurking around the corner. It has helped me follow paths that many in my social circle have feared to tread. It continues to inspire me to keep moving forward despite the insistence of some to stand still. It is central to what I believe to be true—life is what you make of it...there must be equal amounts of sorrow, so you can truly appreciate the joy.

Emotional

Emotions as a divining rod. Explore your emotions like a treasure map. Where is the emotion pulling you? What are you fixated on that needs letting go of? What emotions are being suppressed? What do you really want? I use breath as a way to channel my emotions, even the unresolved ones. Conscious breathing is about energizing those frozen feelings that are often trapped.

I've had many people come in and out of my life, and sometimes not by choice. The person who gave me the most encouragement was a good friend who I built a close relationship with for nearly twenty years. She taught me to always seek the deeper meaning and to confront myself continuously. It is the only way to "polish the facets of your character," she would say. Although we are no longer in contact, I will always cherish the time spent. Sometimes loss teaches you to not only let go, but to acknowledge that the love you did let in changed you for the better.

Spiritual

Detach from your triggers. Those who think spiritual wellness is all about meditating, breathing, chanting, and performing elaborate yoga poses are clueless. Spiritual wellness is a daily practice and requires work as it challenges the basis for our understanding of the human condition. If you can view life from a slightly detached perspective, it can give you greater clarity in how to proceed no matter what obstacle lies in your path.

Spirituality is connecting to something greater than ourselves. When out in nature, we can appreciate the beauty and share in its infinite glow. It is a reminder that although our lives here are fleeting, nature always finds a way.

Seek the truth in everything. It's been said that truth is like a gemstone. There are slivers of truth in every facet of the stone. When it comes to our spiritual life, we must cultivate an understanding of acceptance. Although some may be misguided and differ from our perspective, spiritual wellness teaches us compassion for all things seen and unseen.

There are so many books about cancer out there. Why is this one important and unique? A singular thread that runs through each of the 35 cancer survivor stories highlighted in this book is that true transformation is not granted through *wishful thinking, but through willful action.* None of us truly knows why cancer came into our lives. But we have a choice, and that choice is for us to honor the pain, but not live by its shackles.

There is a concept in coaching called "The Transtheoretical Model." It posits that true lasting change is based on a series of steps. It suggests that people are not resistant to change; they just don't know how to successfully move through these stages. Implementing change behavior is tricky. It requires discipline, focus, and restriction at times. In order to get comfortable in the uncomfortable we must move through our feelings and motives into deliberate action.

Here is a broader impact that I hope that this book can help bring about — a movement around bartering. I believe all of us have innate gifts and talents but are often caught up in receiving monetary gain for our time and energy which often separates us from our why. It would be wonderful if we could spend just one day helping, aiding, and consoling one another without expecting anything in return. I am curious how this simple shift in mindset could alter things in our world.

Allen Chankowsky: I Survived (Carcinoma) Cancer and Here Is How I Did It

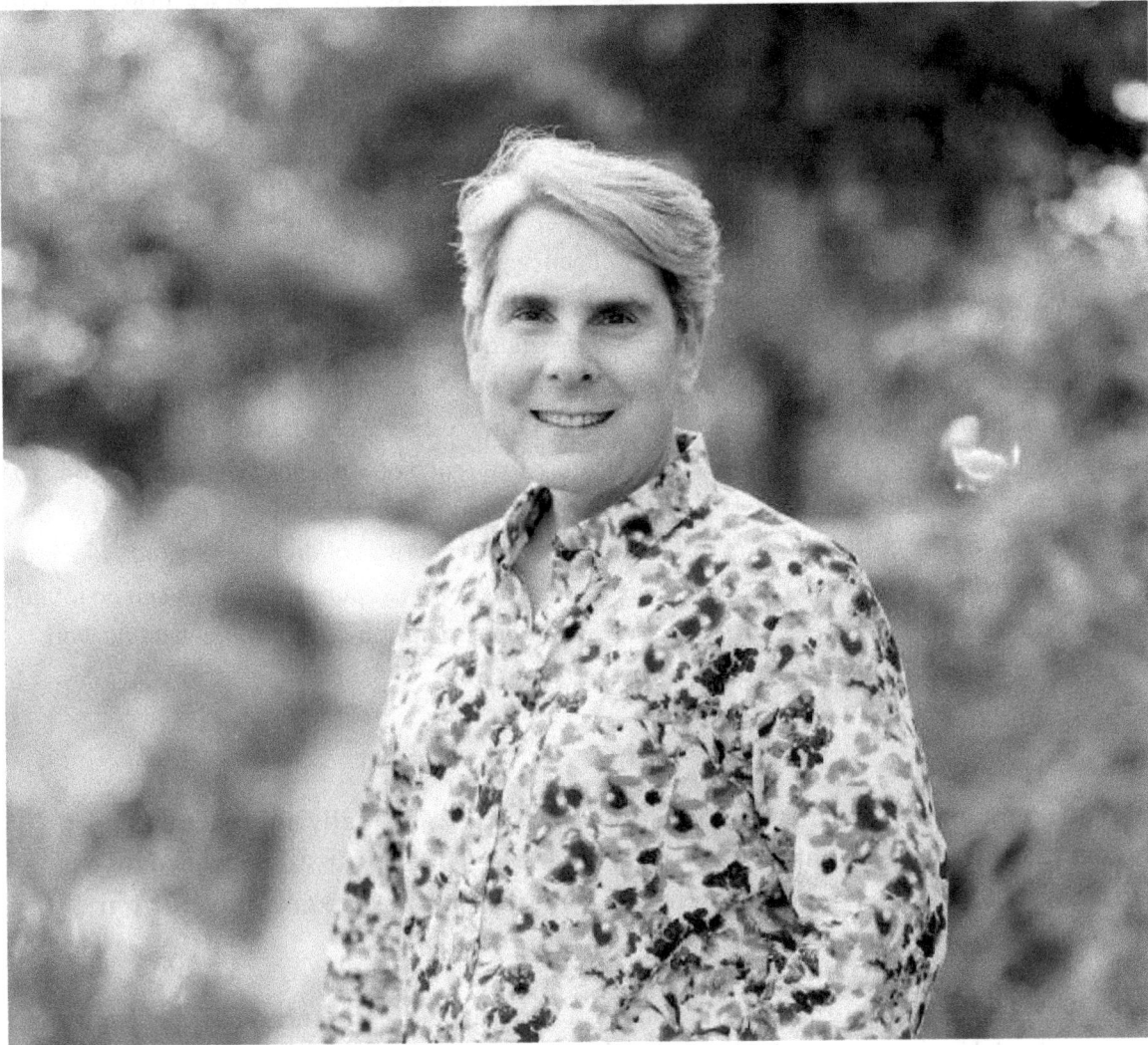

Photo Credits: Eric Benchimol Photography

Appreciate your caregivers and show them that they matter too. I know this one well, because I fell into the trap of becoming overwhelmingly consumed with my awful prognosis that I neglected the emotional needs my girlfriend Cynthia. Think about it—if your caregivers aren't coping well, how can they be expected to take care of you? By acknowledging and appreciating them, you're not only being sensitive to their needs but you're also investing back into your own care by helping them cope better. Yes—you can help them in simple ways. Maybe they need to speak to a mental health professional.

Cancer is a horrible and terrifying disease. Yet millions of people have beaten the odds. Authority Magazine created a series called "I Survived Cancer and Here Is How I Did It." In this interview series, we spoke to cancer survivors to share their stories, in order to offer hope and provide strength to people who are being impacted by cancer today.

As a part of this interview series, I had the pleasure of interviewing Allen Chankowsky. Allen is a sales promotion marketing expert specializing in contest promotion strategy and execution. He is celebrating his 30-year survivorship of two types of cancer, including his stage 4 terminal diagnosis in 2016 where the chances of him surviving five years were less than 20%. Against all odds, through Allen's hands-on approach fueled by the love of his life Cynthia, they actively researched and managed his cancer resulting in him outliving his diagnosis and becoming an exceptional cancer survivor. In his highly anticipated book release, On the Other Side of TERMINAL, Allen shares his incredible 30-year story of survival that serves to inspire and teach others about the steps he took to achieve the state of radical remission. His goal is to help as many people as possible to do the same. Originally from Montreal, Allen lives in Toronto, Canada with his two children, Ethan and Hila and his girlfriend Cynthia and her two children, Elena and Hayden. In his spare time, Allen can be found winning backgammon tournaments at the United States Backgammon Federation, where he won the Intermediate Division at the 2021 US Open.

Thank you so much for joining us in this interview series! We really appreciate the courage it takes to publicly share your story. Before we start, our readers would love to "get to know you" a bit better. Can you tell us a bit about your background and your childhood backstory?

Thank you Savio. Congratulations on your own survival of stage 3 cancer. I applaud you and the editorial team at Authority Magazine for taking the bold step in publishing this series. I also congratulate every contributor for their decision to share their own vulnerability through difficult emotions and intimate details of their cancer journey.

I was born in Montreal, Quebec, Canada in 1969, joining my family as the youngest sibling to my two older brothers. My parents, who we are blessed to still have with us today, are practical (Mom) and very sociable (Dad) people with a very healthy sense of humor. A typical day growing up would often include several off-colour jokes at the dinner table from my Dad who continues to be a quintessential showman at the age of 84. The content of his jokes together with their delivery usually resulted in contagious giggling and sometimes full-on belly laughs lasting several minutes and often requiring some recovery before resuming dinner. Good times!!

From an early age, I embraced the friendships I developed as a schoolboy and to this day, I'm so incredibly proud of the fact that at 52, I remain close with the vast majority of them. These friends are people of great character, each with their own unique sense of humor and individuality. The mixture of our personalities when together is infectious and have us all coming back for more at any opportunity. The group is so devoutly loyal to one another that we would literally do anything to help each other, no matter the consequences. They say that one can be judged by the company one keeps and I am honored to be judged by anyone, anywhere, based on the people I call friends. To me, they are brothers, and as a family we all count on each other.

The parental modeling I had was generally one where the seriousness of life was often blunted by comedic relief. This taught me that difficult life events are often easier to accept if they are received and then approached in a way that is less about negativity and more about the life lessons that are imbedded within the event. For example, when a particular societal issue would be news-of-the-day, the jokes that would inevitability ensue would serve to highlight the issues by examining them through laughter rather than addressing them directly through more traditional conversation. This mostly worked; however, there was one life event that occurred in 1988 that could not, under any circumstance, lend itself to examination through a comedic lens. On July 14th of that year, one of my siblings, at the age of 23, died in a car accident and my family was thrust into the depths of exquisite pain that was to last a lifetime. I was 19, and short of grieving the loss of my paternal grandfather 8 years earlier, I never had exposure to such intense emotional turmoil. Never had I seen my parents brought to their knees and express unimaginable emotions of loss that they themselves never knew possible. Until that day, my privileged childhood shielded me from situations that involved untenable emotional destruction. The bubble of my childhood innocence had been pierced and I was forced to grow up quickly. I not only lost one of my brothers, I also lost part of my parents and they in turn lost pieces of themselves and of each other. Still, we as a family soldiered on together and moved forward with our individual lives best we could. I moved on to higher education, first pursuing a path in Life Sciences and then out of necessity (more on that below), I changed my focus of study to Environmental Sciences, receiving my Bachelor of Arts from Concordia University in Montreal in 1994.

Can you please give us your favorite "Life Lesson Quote?" Can you share how that was relevant to you in your life?

"You can never cross the ocean until you have the courage to lose sight of the shore."
— Christopher Columbus

I knew from an early age that my fears must be directly addressed if I was to have the best opportunity of overcoming them. Life has knocked me down continuously, however, rather than take the easy way out by allowing myself to be anchored down by the fear of getting up, I gathered myself together, stood up, looked the fear straight in its eyes and didn't back down. The alternative was simply non-negotiable. Never looking back, I have paved many paths for myself because I pushed myself to move forward. The conscious act of not looking back and not allowing the shackles of emotional and physical turmoil to define who I am is deeply satisfying. The elation of self-empowerment by removing the shackles of fear and freeing yourself to move forward is something that I hope we can all achieve.

Let's now shift to the main part of our discussion about surviving cancer. Do you feel comfortable sharing with us the story surrounding how you found out that you had cancer?

Yes, and thank you for asking. I first met cancer in 1991 when I was 21 and in the throes of achieving my undergraduate degree. This version of cancer was dressed as stage 2 Hodgkin's Disease, a blood cancer. It first revealed part of itself as a lump above my left clavicle. This was a sign to look deeper into my chest via an array of imaging scans that exposed the bulk of a massive tumor sitting smack in the middle of my chest. Over the course of two agonizing months, I was successfully treated with radiation therapy targeted to the chest, head/neck and abdomen. In 1991, the use of ABVD chemotherapy (Adriamycin, Bleomycin, Vinblastine and Dacarbazine) was usually reserved for stage 3 and 4 Hodgkin's Disease. While there was some debate as to its utility in my case, my oncology team in Montreal decided that radiation alone should be used as the approach of choice for eliminating this malignant threat to my life. The thinking at the time was that by doing so, damage caused by the radiation to collateral tissue would be limited to the periphery of the radiation field rather than damage done to my whole body with systemic chemotherapy. Spoiler alert: radiation probably wasn't the best choice...

During the course of my radiation treatment and in my quest to seek and learn everything about Hodgkin's Disease and radiation therapy, I came across a book from Dr. Mortimer J. Lacher and Dr. John R. Redman titled *Hodgkin's Disease: The Consequences of Survival*. I thought the title to be intriguing and foretelling. The major theme of their work revolved around the long-term effects of surviving Hodgkin's Disease. Reading the book etched a permanent stain on my brain because I wanted so desperately to be a long-term survivor and, if I was lucky enough to become one, I also needed to be prepared for the possible consequences.

In the two decades that followed, I was in the best physical shape of my life — or so I thought. I ran 4 times a week and completed my first half-marathon in 2012. Then, in 2013 at the age of 43, I suffered a heart attack after a training run and required two cardiac stents be installed to open the blockages. The underlying heart disease was a direct consequence of the radiation from 1991. It turns out that the body doesn't forget what happened to it. Ever so slowly, the tissues of my cardiovascular system were reacting to the insult of the repeated radiation to my chest from 1991. But my cardiovascular system wasn't the only area of my body that didn't forget...

Three years after my 2013 heart attack, I discovered a lump on the right side of my neck in July of 2016. A fine needle biopsy of that lump confirmed cancer; however, it was unclear what type of cancer. A head/neck oncology surgeon from The Princess Margaret Cancer Centre in Toronto was asked to perform what is known as a neck dissection to assess for the type of cancer and the extent of its spread. I remember the day of surgery very well. The extent of the neck dissection was as invasive as the cancer itself. Most of the removed lymph nodes (and there were more than 20) were positive for cancer. A bad cancer. A very, very bad cancer. This time the cancer had dressed itself up as salivary duct carcinoma, and it made its presence known in an extremely aggressive way by spreading to neck muscles and surrounding tissue. This "second cancer" developed as another direct consequence of the radiation I had received 25 years earlier. The lymph nodes affected in my neck were now pregnant and swelling with one of the worst head/neck cancers that one could suffer, and the story only gets worse. It was stage 4, otherwise known to be the worst of the worst stages of cancer known to humanity. Despite the skilled hands of an amazing surgeon, the cancer ensured that I would always know of its presence by the resulting hole that followed the removal of half of my right neck. As if that wasn't bad enough, I was also left with a slash across the underside of my throat like a victim of a knife fight. I had effectively been maimed for all to see and gawk at in public. That used to bother me, a lot. But now, I wear my maimed neck proudly as it reflects part of my survivorship. How can't I be proud of that? It's normal human behavior to be drawn to the unusual. It's like a moth that can't help itself when it's drawn to the flame. So I understand how my neck attracts looks in public. I accept it just as I accept other types of behavior traits as being part of the human condition. Rarely do I engage, however, it's oddly satisfying when on occasion, I catch someone looking and I ask them if they want to get a closer look. Most react by quickly turning away without saying a word. Some apologize. But one thing is certain, they could all line up in single file to kiss my ass because I'm alive!!!

What was the scariest part of that event? What did you think was the worst thing that could happen to you?

1991—Stage 2 Hodgkin's Disease:

It's never an easy thing to receive a diagnosis of cancer; however, it's particularly difficult as a young adult given that this first diagnosis occurred less than three years after my brother's fatal car accident. My sense of profound concern was shared equally between my own mortality at the tender age of 20 and the further impact on my parents and extended family, regardless of if I lived or died. I've seen, felt and continue to feel the devastation that a loss of a child does to a family and the thought that my death could be the trigger of another major loss was all but paralyzing. Make no mistake; the extent of the emotional impact was straight up trauma. Once one experiences trauma, it never fully goes away but rather becomes an ongoing situation requiring active emotional regulation. Dealing with this trauma, however, cut both ways. On the one hand, the ongoing nature of the threat to my life and to my family was excruciating. On the other hand, living was a good thing, but it came at the cost of learning how to manage the ongoing threat. My fear was that I would be cursed by having the trauma haunt me if I wasn't able to control the emotional impact and that I would not be able to fully enjoy life under the weight of the pressure to live. I wanted to hastily advance my life—to begin working and be self-sufficient like my friends. I wanted to marry, to have children and grandchildren. To have a partner to enjoy life's wonders with and to help each other cope with its inevitable difficulties. But my greatest fear of all wasn't for me, it was (and is) that I would die before one or both of my parents.

In my upcoming book, *On the Other Side of TERMINAL*, I describe the circumstances, effects, and the detailed story around my first cancer diagnosis in 1991.

2016—Stage 4 Salivary Duct Carcinoma: This will be the focus for the balance of the interview.

Twenty-five years later, life had changed, and this was mostly good—very good. I was still alive. Alive and kicking. Surviving cancer for 25 years isn't just about surviving, particularly as a young adult. It's about developing the emotional wherewithal to weather the inevitable difficult moments that are certain to come along in life. However, if there's one event that takes the wind out of one's sails, it's the diagnosis of another cancer. While I am grateful for the 25 years of life, nothing can prepare one to receive a diagnosis that can only be described as a singular word:

Generally, once the initial shock of a cancer diagnosis subsides, it's often met with feelings of hope through the reliance on modern medicine. However, no matter the type of cancer, when doctors designate the stage of cancer to be terminal, for many, it usually signifies certain and imminent death. How could it possibly mean anything else?

My life had changed markedly from 25 years earlier in that I had two children who were dependent on me. Ethan was 12 and Hila 9. Cynthia and I finally found each other three years earlier in 2013. Imagine my elation of finally finding the love of my life, the one who had been holding the key to my heart all along and then this. The diagnosis was akin to the explosion of a nuclear bomb. The utter devastation made it difficult to breathe. The stakes were higher now. Much higher than in 1991. I couldn't die. Not now. It didn't matter that the second hospital in New York and the third hospital in Houston confirmed this awful diagnosis; it wasn't my time to die. It couldn't be my time.

My greatest fears were that I wouldn't be able to fulfill my obligations as a father, as a son, as a life-partner, as a member of my family and as a friend to so many. I feared that I wasn't going to able to fulfill the obligation I made to myself in 1991 to live a complete life. A life in which I was able to experience what most people experience in a "normal" lifetime—school graduations and weddings of my children, the satisfaction of watching them develop into well-grounded and functioning adults, witnessing with pride as they do what they love in life and helping them through difficult life transitions with the emotional tools I helped them to acquire. But those dreamy possibilities that every parent hopes for were disintegrating right in front of me.

How did you react in the short term?

My initial reaction was one of shock and awe because I had been feeling great prior to the neck surgery. Then panic set in because eliminating the cancer was no longer an option. The cancer had freed itself from the confines of my head and neck and migrated to my lungs. If I didn't find a solution to extend my life beyond the hopelessness found in the dismal statistics, it was game over. I couldn't bring myself to the point where I was able to have frank discussions with my family and my friends about the dire seriousness and urgency of my medical problems. I had to protect my parents at all cost for as long as possible. The only person I let in was Cynthia. My fearless cheerleader—she had been with me every step of the way. Despite the statistics, she was overflowing with positivity and hope. But like so many before me, the thought of impending death forced me into my shell and I asked Cynthia to come in with me. I asked that she please not reveal the details or gravity of my medical and emotional emergency to family and friends until I was ready. This meant that Cynthia herself carried with her the weight of impossible news and worse still, she couldn't get the support that she needed. I hated myself for burdening her with my request. Cynthia lovingly obliged and honored my request and told no one of the bleakness that was all but certain to unfold.

After the dust settled, what coping mechanisms did you use? What did you do to cope physically, mentally, emotionally, and spiritually?

According to the statistics, my chances of surviving 5 years with my stage and grade of cancer was at best, 20%. However, Cynthia didn't want to talk about the overwhelming probability being 4 in 5 that I would die within 5 years and most likely sooner. She instead wanted to focus on the 1 in 5 chance that I would live. She would ask, "Why can't YOU be that 1 person out of 5 who lives?" Her point was a good one. The challenge was how to become that 1 in 5 person. So we got to work.

I promised myself that if I became that 1 in 5 person who outlived a terminal diagnosis, I would write a book and share the story of how I did it. That was my private goal that I made for myself, and it helped fuel my desire to live. In my book, I expand on what Cynthia and I did and how we did it so that others may benefit from this knowledge and live longer and better lives despite cancer—even a really bad cancer.

Is there a particular person you are grateful towards who helped you learn to cope and heal? Can you share a story about that?

To fully appreciate what it takes to care for a cancer patient, one must understand that the care is comprehensive. I sat down and wrote out the key doctors, residents, nurses, technicians, pharmacists, clerks, students and counted more than 30 people who cared for me. Then my friends and family who, despite my need to step out of the limelight and become unavailable, continued to offer me their support in any way they could. I owe them all a debt of gratitude, particularly my parents, Mona and Marvin Chankowsky.

Many of my relationships have suffered on account of my need to turn inward. While I won't apologize for needing to focus exclusively on surviving and thereby becoming unavailable to family and friends, they all need to know that their love and support were key factors in helping me see the light. These people know who they are, and they know how grateful I am. I hope to make up for lost time.

There are, however, two people that must be singled out and acknowledged because if not for them, I truly believe that my life would have ended over the course of the last 5 years.

When it became clear that I was deathly ill in 2016, Cynthia stopped working to be available to me. From stoically sitting with me at every hospital appointment, travelling with me to New York and Houston for second and third opinions, to having to listen to my initial and then repeated negativity, her love and support was as reliable as one could hope for. Despite the overwhelming sense of dread, Cynthia would not give up being positive every day and that proved to be one of best aspects of this story. When I couldn't guide myself through the flames of certain death, she took control and led me to a clearing where I could escape the scorching heat. It was an impossible task but she did it out of love. I am the luckiest person alive to have met Cynthia.

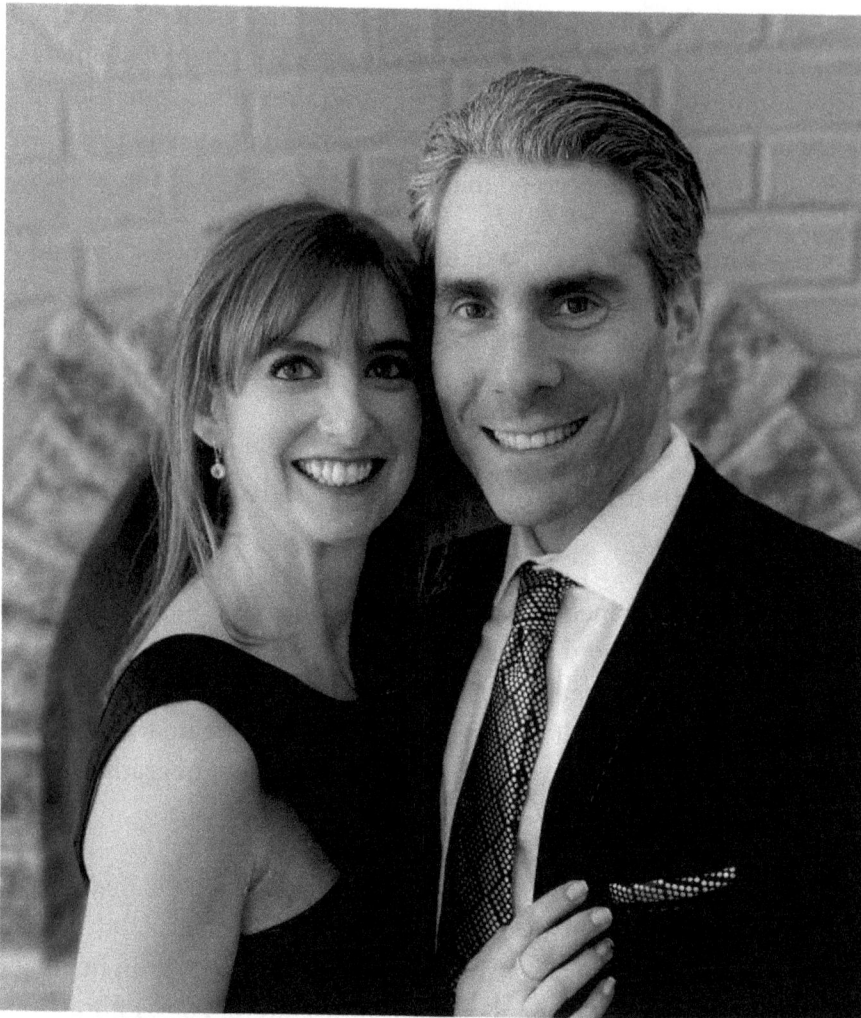

As part of my circle of care at The Princess Margarete Cancer Centre in Toronto and given my dire circumstances, I was referred to the Psychosocial Oncology Clinic for the purpose of receiving psychological supportive care. Over the course of the last 5 years, I had the good fortune of working closely with Dr. Madeline Li, who took me under her capable wing and helped me through a very dark and deep depression. At our first meeting, she indicated that she saw the potential in me, saying at the end of the meeting, "I think we can do some really good work together." Her statement, even in the context of my awful diagnosis, made me feel that all wasn't lost. Perhaps there may be a glimmer of hope. While my book expands further on the value of Dr. Li's contribution to my emotional healing, I would be remiss if I did not single her out here as being a central figure and significantly instrumental to my emotional healing. Always professional in her demeanor, Dr. Li is kind, understanding, approachable, non-judgmental, and always willing to go that extra step if she feels it can help.

In my own cancer struggle, I sometimes used the idea of embodiment to help me cope. Let's take a minute to look at cancer from an embodiment perspective. If your cancer had a message for you, what do you think it would want or say?

My cancers did and do have similar messages for me. Like reading the same work of poetry across many years, the messages held in the words take on different meaning depending on when in life you read them. For example, at age 20 when my 1991 Hodgkin's Disease told me that there was urgency for me to change my study plans and advance my life, I heeded the call and decided not to continue with my goal of advancing to medical school. I preferred to achieve a Bachelor of Arts degree and head straight into the workforce. Pursuing higher education beyond an undergraduate degree was viewed as an obstacle to me realizing the privilege of marrying and the honor and responsibility of having children. But even the best-laid plans often go awry because the bonus experience was a messy divorce. While my 2016 cancer had a similar message, having had 25 years of life experience under my belt offered me a different point of view as to how to live. I have two children and they keep showing me every day that I was born to be a Dad and I intend to live that dream for as long as I can.

What did you learn about yourself from this very difficult experience? How has cancer shaped your worldview? What has it taught you that you might never have considered before? Can you please explain with a story or example?

There is one other very important message that my 2016 cancer had for me. And that was to pursue my other love for the game of backgammon. For those who don't know, backgammon is a mind game where one uses skill to move 15 checkers around a board as directed by the luck of throwing a pair of six-sided dice. The goal is to bear off your checkers before your opponent does. At any given state of the game, there is only one best move to choose from after you roll your set of dice. Choose the wrong move and the likelihood of losing the game increases. To compete at the highest levels, modern players train with software that calculates the percentage of winning (or losing) at every stage of the game. One day I was participating in a backgammon tournament, playing a final game in a match, and I was losing the game by a very large margin. In fact, I thought that the chances for me to survive the game and win the match were zero. The game turned around and I made an improbable comeback and ultimately won the game and the match. I took the game file and imported it into the software, and it calculated that my chance of winning the game at my worst possible position was 2.3%. And there was the message. It was the same message that Cynthia had been telling me all along but this time in a different form. Even if it seems that you don't have a chance to survive, think again because you do. Fight hard. Make wise decisions and never give up hope.

How have you used your experience to bring goodness to the world?

Unfortunately, I'm late to the sharing party because it's taken me time to finally come to terms with the reality of my situation. While it's true that my cancer is indeed terminal and that won't change, it's also true that the durability of my status of being an exceptional survivor persists. So, after realizing my lofty goal of living 5 years, I'm trying to make up for lost time by self-publishing my upcoming book, *On the Other Side of TERMINAL*, which will soon be available. I take readers through the emotional journey of my life and the steps I took to achieve the state of radical remission that I continue to enjoy. For cancer patients and caregivers alike, the book is for anyone who wants to be inspired about how terminal isn't about that final destination, rather, it's about the journey. Through publishing *On the Other Side of TERMINAL*, I look forward to sharing my journey with everyone who wants to join me and benefit from the experience.

What are a few of the biggest misconceptions and myths out there about fighting cancer that you would like to dispel?

Myth: Cancer is a death sentence

Look, it's 2021 (almost 2022) and I'm alive AND kicking. It's possible that new growth of my cancer could be identified tomorrow or next week, next month, next year or in 10, 20, 30 years from now. Who knows? The important part is that, despite all odds, I'm alive today because of the deliberate steps Cynthia and I took to create the opportunity for me to achieve a state of radical remission.

According to the American Cancer Society's *National Cancer Institute's Annual Report to the Nation on the Status of Cancer*, from the years 2014 to 2018, overall, cancer death rates decreased 2.2% per year (on average) among males and 1.7% per year (on average) among females. Cancer death rates decreased an average of 0.9% per year among adolescents and young adults, and an average of 1.4% per year among children. And overall cancer incidence rates are leveling off among males after earlier declines and increasing slightly among the female and adolescents/young adult cohorts.

What does all that mean? While cancer is being diagnosed at the same or slightly higher rates, the overall death rate is decreasing year over year. There are several good reasons for this including but not limited to the fact that cancer screening is being done earlier and by more people. The sooner cancer is detected; the chances are lower that the patient will die from their disease. And if the cancer needs to be treated, we can rely on an amazing number of medical and therapeutic advances to aid in the management and cure rates. So, while some advanced cancers are strongly associated with death, the data overwhelmingly supports that when looked at from a global point of view, people are generally living longer and better lives after a cancer diagnosis. And I am a prime example of this.

Fantastic. Here is the main question of our interview. Based on your experiences and knowledge, what advice would you give to others who have recently been diagnosed with cancer? What are your "5 Things" You Need To Beat Cancer? Please share a story or example for each.

Even if your cancer is labeled as "terminal," you may have an opportunity to outlive your diagnosis. I hope these "5 Things" help make that dream a reality for you, just as it did for me:

1. It is critical to know the genetic and biomarker profile of your cancer. If you only remember one of these "5 Things," this is the one. To have the best chances of surviving your cancer, you absolutely need to know all you can about your disease—all its strengths and all its weaknesses. You do this by working with your doctor to organize the DNA sequencing of your tumor. This is also known as Biomarker Sequencing, Whole Genome Sequencing or Next Generation Sequencing (NGS.) The sequencing process unlocks the critical information about what drives your cancer to grow. Knowing that information is the first step in identifying treatment options such as targeted therapies with new and emerging drugs or even older drugs that are now being re-purposed for cancer types that were never even considered when the drug was originally developed. We have this technology and it's readily available. In fact, I had my tumor sequenced back in 2016 and that was 5 years ago. While tumor DNA sequencing isn't new technology, many people still don't know about it or if they do, many still don't understand the power of its value. Not knowing the mutations, pathways and checkpoints that drive the growth of your cancer can lead to incorrect treatment selection, potentially affecting how long you have to live. But there's a simple way to make the best available treatment choice for your

cancer—and it's to get your own tumor's DNA sequenced. Ultimately, your choice of lab to sequence the DNA of your tumor is a personal choice and only you, together with your doctor, can make the decision as to which lab you want to work with. That said, I recognize that tumor biomarker sequencing is new to many patients and because of this, I wanted to share the links of two sequencing labs in North America, strictly for information purposes. These two are reputable and well known within the oncology community but there are others. I do not have any business relationship with these companies and will not financially benefit if you choose to use them: Foundation Medicine (USA): www.foundationmedicine.com, Foundation Medicine (Canada): www.foundationmedicine.ca

2. Use your smart phone or computer as a research tool to unlock access to treatment information. While this seems obvious, you would be amazed how many people don't view their connected devices as excellent tools to research their cancer. Some say, *yeah, that's my doctor's job, or that's what they went to medical school for.* The fact is there's never been a better time in history where cancer patients themselves have direct access to information related to their disease and treatment options. We have never before had this level of access to medical information. Back in 2016, I was researching the mutations of my cancer and found research journals from all corners of the world that were in support of a novel and not well-known treatment for my cancer type. I brought those peer reviewed journals into several meetings with my oncologist. She had not yet come across the research that supported my choice of treatment that I thought had the best chance at extending my life. That meant that while my oncologist was ready to prescribe the standard chemo that results in 4 out 5 people dying within 5 years, it was my iPhone that facilitated my access to a better treatment option that would ultimately help me outlive my best before date. It wasn't my oncologist's fault that she wasn't yet aware of the research I brought in, nor is it any doctor's fault. The sheer volume of medical journals being published every day around the world is incredible and the rate of publication is increasing rapidly. With physician workloads, it's impossible for any doctor to keep up with the pace of research publications. But you are the person closest to your cancer. You have the ability to be laser focused on your cancer. A connected computer or smart phone is one of the best keys to unlock vital information and access to new and emerging treatment options. Who knows, perhaps you'll discover a treatment option of your own to help you to live longer and better.

3. Develop excellent communication and follow up skills. When you have a serious disease posing a direct threat to your life, having access to a cooperative oncologist or primary care provider with whom you have a good working relationship is critical. Like myself and so many others, your disease may have been diagnosed at an advanced stage, so to address the threat properly and expertly, you need to have excellent and sustained communication with your medical team. If your doctor is one of those people who thinks they know everything and isn't open to learning from educated patients who are being proactive about saving their own life, I suggest finding a new doctor who is. In some cases, it's not possible or reasonable to expect that a patient can have these conversations with their team. Chemo brain fog or sedation from any number of drugs are but a few reasons why it can be challenging. If this is the case, ask one of your caregivers to speak and advocate on your behalf.

4. Look outside of cancer and find something you love doing. Life doesn't and shouldn't stop because you have cancer. Surviving cancer involves other things outside of the medical realm and it's important to understand why. Having cancer is hard. Really hard. Particularly having cancer at an advanced stage like me. It's normal to need a temporary reprieve from the intensity of your cancer experience. There's a whole range of activities from faith-based programs to fundraising or reading books, to watching movies or even throwing yourself deeper into your work or a personal project. For my dear friend Lara, who successfully battled invasive ductal breast cancer 5 years ago, she maintained her demanding physical training while on chemotherapy, radiation and Herceptin and went on to complete a full Iron Man competition 12 months later. For me, of all the things to choose from, it was playing backgammon that did it for me. By re-engaging in a game that I used to love playing, it helped me take my mind off my disease. Not only do I enjoy playing the game for the pure experience of playing a competitive game, but backgammon also reinforces that no matter how bad you are losing, there is always a chance that the game can turn around. In my upcoming book, *On the Other Side Of TERMINAL*, I talk more about the significance of backgammon and its contribution to my own cancer experience. While avidly enjoying playing, I also won the Intermediate Division at the 2021 US Open through the United States Backgammon Federation and then went on to be crowned the best backgammon player in the city of Toronto through the Canadian Backgammon Federation. I don't say this to toot my own horn. Rather, it's to identify that if you temporarily turn your mind to something other than cancer — to something that you enjoy doing, something that you can excel at or accomplish — you're enhancing your life. Studies show that cancer patients do better when they engage in personal enjoyment and a sense of accomplishment. So find something that you like, or even better, something you love — something from your past that you once enjoyed or perhaps something that you've always wanted to do but never had the chance. Set a goal for yourself. Mine was to self-publish a book and I'm only weeks away from checking that one off my bucket list.

5. Appreciate your caregivers and show them that they matter too. I know this one well, because I fell into the trap of becoming overwhelmingly consumed with my awful prognosis that I neglected the emotional needs of my girlfriend Cynthia. Think about it — if your caregivers aren't coping well, how can they be expected to take care of you? By acknowledging and appreciating them, you're not only being sensitive to their needs but you're also investing back into your own care by helping them cope better. Yes — you can help them in simple ways. Maybe they need to speak to a mental health professional. Perhaps they would benefit from speaking with a friend or another member of the family about their fears, concerns, and emotional needs or maybe they just want to spend a few hours doing absolutely nothing. And if they do want to do something, perhaps it will have nothing to do with you or your cancer — and that's ok. I didn't understand this at the beginning of my journey because I was too wrapped up in my own despair. It prevented me from seeing that Cynthia, the love of my life, also needed help and her own space to process these impossible emotions. So be mindful of the emotional impact on your caregivers. And if you get it right or even close to right, you will both benefit because your relationship will be stronger for it.

You are a person of great influence. If you could inspire a movement that would bring the most amount of good to the greatest amount of people, what would that be?

Thank you for the compliment, Savio.

The primary reason I sought to publish my book, *On the Other Side of TERMINAL*, was to share the steps I took to outlive my terminal diagnosis with as many people as possible. It is my hope that the book will serve to educate, inspire and ultimately help as many cancer patients and their families as possible. I also hope my book could help physicians better understand what radical remission is. Understanding that for many patients, achieving a state of remission may be attainable if they take the proper steps according to their patient's individual medical circumstances.

Rare cancers are those cancers that occur much less frequently in a given population as compared to common cancers. For example, the prevalence of breast cancer is far more common as compared to salivary duct carcinoma. Research and fundraising efforts are mostly driven by common cancers because there are more patients and families affected by these cancers. Rare cancers, on the other hand, don't generate the research dollars needed because there are not enough patients and families to generate enough money for researchers to recuperate their research and development investment. Since researchers are usually granted their allotment of research money in relation to the most common cancers, this leaves a huge void in the research needed to address patients with rare cancers, like me. The movement that I would like to inspire is to recognize those cancer patients who have rare cancers by motivating governments to incentivize multi-national pharmaceutical giants to establish more significant R&D budgets to address these rare diseases. This is important because while one rare cancer type may represent a small amount of people, the combined amount of people across all rare cancer types is very large.

The rare cancer population is severely underserved, leaving them to fall through the cracks. The mystery of their rare disease is buried with these patients when they die and that needs to change. Look at how the world mobilized to come up with an answer to COVID. Just imagine what would happen if cancer became infectious and how the world would mobilize to address the threat.

We are very blessed that some very prominent names in Business, VC funding, Sports, and Entertainment read this column. Is there a person in the world, or in the US with whom you would love to have a private breakfast or lunch, and why?

Ben Stiller. There are a few common experiences that we share. First, it would seem that we both benefited from the big comedic personalities afforded us through our respective dads. With parental personalities that large, it would have been impossible for each of us to not have been positively affected. We were both diagnosed with cancer at age 47. We both kept the details of our cancer private for a significant length of time. Like me, I assume Ben had to do some significant introspection before he fully came to terms with his cancer. We both have two kids roughly the same ages. We both played the drums. We are both big Howard Stern fans. In fact, Ben first revealed that he had prostate cancer on the Howard Stern Show. My cancer has many similarities to prostate cancer in terms of its genetic mutations and my ongoing cancer treatment is managed by an oncologist who specializes in prostate cancer. This means that at age 47, I found myself in the prostate clinic for regular follow ups. I'm fairly certain that Ben had a similar set of prostate clinic experiences. Few 47-year-old men have the experience of sitting in a waiting room full of elderly men with prostate cancer. It's surreal, bordering on comical, and among other things, I'd love to chat with him about that. But most important is that he has a great sense of humor that I am certain helped him navigate his cancer experience in a novel way, as it did mine (and continues to do so...).

How can our readers further follow your work online?

Please visit my website for more information and to get notified when *On the Other Side of TERMINAL* becomes available. I also encourage you to please send this interview to anyone you feel may benefit from it. I look forward toward connecting with you soon.

www.AllenChankowsky.com or www.OnTheOtherSideOfTERMINAL.com

Scan the QR code to view my "5 Things" To Survive Cancer YouTube video:

Amanda Rice of The Chick Mission: I Survived (Breast) Cancer and Here Is How I Did It

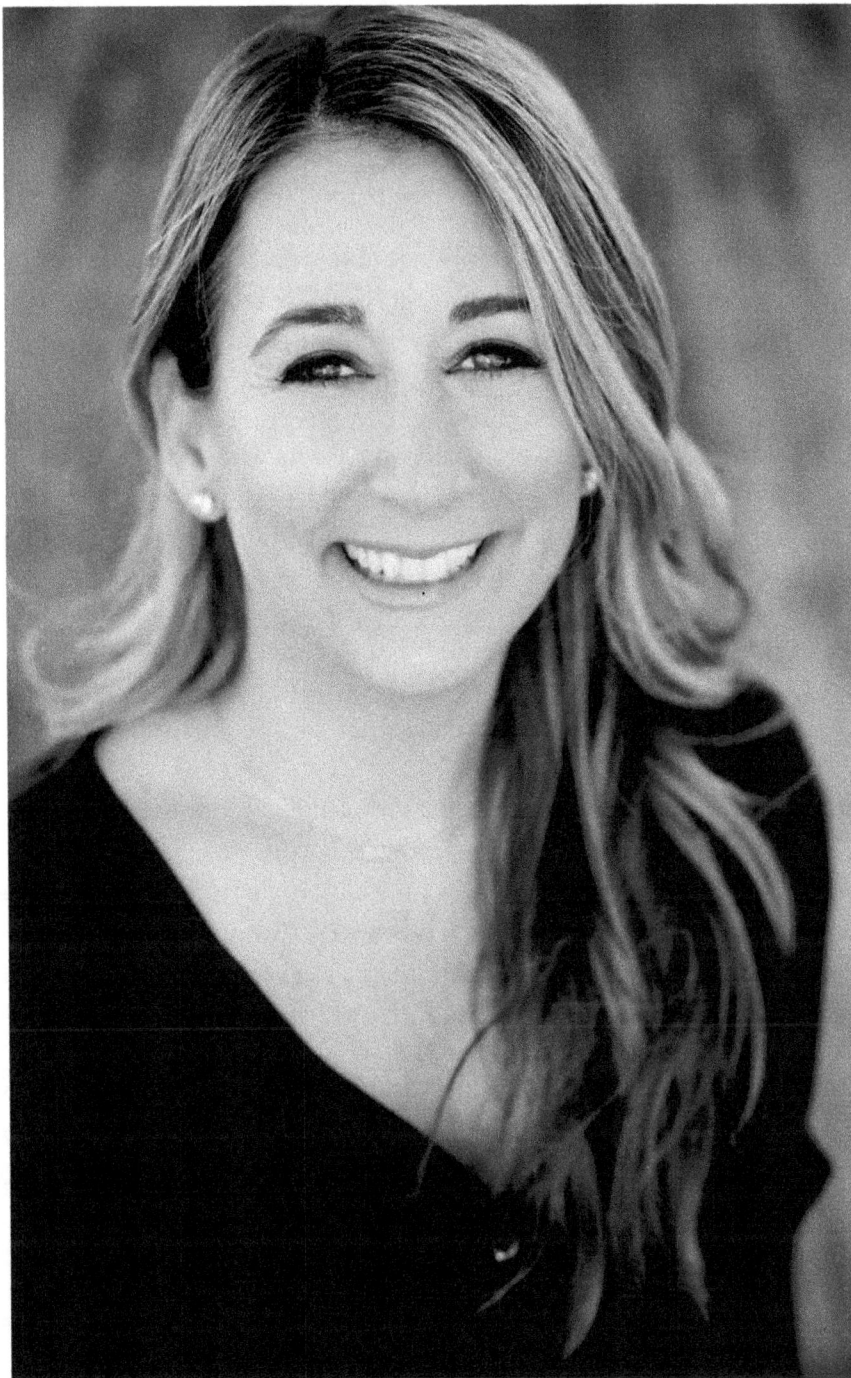

Everything hurts during treatment, but the less talked about side effects for young adults include depression, anxiety, infertility and/or early menopause.

I had the pleasure of interviewing Amanda Rice. Amanda is a three-time cancer survivor (all before the age of 40). She is the founder of nonprofit, The Chick Mission, which advocates for fertility benefits for cancer patients, and provides resources where the system has failed through Hope Scholarships, educational resources and community-building events. Amanda works on Wall Street by day, splitting her time between New York and Texas, and is almost always seen with her adorable pup, Nola, by her side.

Thank you so much for joining us in this interview series! We really appreciate the courage it takes to publicly share your story. Before we start, our readers would love to "get to know you" a bit better. Can you tell us a bit about your background and your childhood backstory?

I was born and raised in White Plains, NY with two parents who were dedicated to their two daughters, but also to their careers. Growing up with a working mother allowed me a strong motivated female role model that has set the tone for my own career goals. We, unfortunately, lost my father the year I turned 18, which created a sort of tenacity that carried me through all three of my cancer experiences and pushed me to create The Chick Mission.

Can you please give us your favorite "Life Lesson Quote?" Can you share how that was relevant to you in your life?

"If you found out you were dying, would you be nicer, would you love more, try something new?" Cancer shifts your perspective on everything—particularly your own mortality, as you're abruptly faced with it. While this motto seems a bit grim, the reality is we're all dying, whether there's a specific timeline or not—our time here on Earth is limited. Through this lens, it only makes sense to lead each day with a little more forgiveness, kindness, and empathy—and to not be afraid to take bold action. Who knows what the next day will bring, so why wait?

Let's now shift to the main part of our discussion about surviving cancer. Do you feel comfortable sharing with us the story surrounding how you found out that you had cancer?

Yes, it's important to talk about; the only way we learn and heal is through sharing our stories—and I feel so grateful to have shared mine with fellow cancer patients and supporters like Sterling K. Brown through Bristol Myers Squibb's Survivorship Today, which is a great initiative that's helping to illuminate the realities of living with cancer. For many people cancer doesn't end on the last day of treatment, it's something that you carry with you for life. That's a big part of my story, actually. The first time I was diagnosed with cancer (breast), I was hitting my stride in my career in NYC. I had an active social life and was healthy—I'd never had an extended stay at the hospital, not even for a broken bone. When I found out I had breast cancer, I was shocked, to say the least, and overwhelmed with emotions and decisions to make. What ended up being one of the most challenging aspects was being told that if I wanted any chance of having a biological family one day, then I needed to freeze my eggs immediately. But this is something insurance wouldn't cover—despite my not electing to have cancer. I was baffled and overwhelmed; as I was facing my mortality I also had to think about the potential of producing another life. This experience is in large part what led me to go on and create The Chick Mission. I saw there was a gap and a lack of information out there around the topic. There needed to be more resources out there and conversations held so that as the number of people who are surviving cancer continues to grow, people are able to live the lives they've dreamt of.

What was the scariest part of that event? What did you think was the worst thing that could happen to you?

Being overwhelmed with so many decisions to make—and feeling like I didn't have the answers to the problems I was being faced with. I'm very action oriented, so as I tried to dig for answers, I was frustrated that more wasn't laid out for me, despite the staggering number of cancer diagnoses per year and the growing number of cancer survivors. I not only worried about my own condition but my friends and family's—you need a team to get through cancer, and as much as I knew their support was unwavering, it's hard to see those you love being put through this pain, too—particularly, with something like cancer, which no one chooses to have.

How did you react in the short term?

I got to work, trying to create a plan. I caught my friends and family up to speed and we committed to be by each other's sides, through all the ups and downs.

After the dust settled, what coping mechanisms did you use? What did you do to cope physically, mentally, emotionally, and spiritually?

I feel compelled to share the deep, dark points of cancer that often come after treatment is done. This is part of the reason I agreed to be part of Survivorship Today. You should be celebrating because you "beat" cancer, yet I found myself lost and depressed. I wasn't actively treating the cancer after I "rang the bell," and I didn't feel like myself. I was overwhelmed and felt alone, and I needed to seek treatment for my anxiety and depression, and ultimately used medication to help me through this dark time. This is often something I mention to those in treatment, so that they aren't shocked by it.

Is there a particular person you are grateful towards who helped you learn to cope and heal? Can you share a story about that?

When I was first diagnosed, a friend connected me with a friend who had gone through cancer a few years before. She was so kind and forthcoming, and put my mind at ease from the very start. Shoshana had no idea how helpful this was for me and that this conversation would lead to hundreds more of those types of conversations to follow. I have spoken to friends, friends of friends, colleagues of friends and complete strangers who reach out through The Chick Mission or my personal Instagram. These types of conversations are incredibly important. Breaking down the opaqueness of a cancer diagnosis can help ease some of the fear.

In my own cancer struggle, I sometimes used the idea of embodiment to help me cope. Let's take a minute to look at cancer from an embodiment perspective. If your cancer had

a message for you, what do you think it would want or say?

I think this goes back to the quote I stand by—cancer amplifies everything, particularly how short life can be. It simultaneously speeds things up and slows them down; it really shows you all of the roller coaster emotions of life.

What did you learn about yourself from this very difficult experience? How has cancer shaped your worldview? What has it taught you that you might never have considered before? Can you please explain with a story or example?

I've learned a lot throughout my cancer journey, but the biggest lesson has been empathy. Many people in this world are suffering, whether it be cancer, infertility, depression, you name it...we have to be more kind to each other. I was being treated in NYC with its hustle and bustle, and I remember looking into these strangers' eyes and just feeling very drawn to those that were suffering.

How have you used your experience to bring goodness to the world?

Through creating The Chick Mission! Over the past few years, we've been able to provide over 170 cancer patients with full coverage of their fertility treatment; giving them the option to create a future family if they so choose. We've been able to touch thousands more cancer survivors and supporters through speaking opportunities and community events and fundraisers. We're slowly chipping away at shifting the conversation around fertility/cancer treatment from taboo to more mainstream.

What are a few of the biggest misconceptions and myths out there about fighting cancer that you would like to dispel?

As brilliant as doctors are, nobody knows your body like you do. Your body shares things with you every day, through symptoms, signs or signals and you MUST listen. In my case it was blood coming from my breast, a dark spot on my arm that popped up out of nowhere and a small lump. Each time I saw a change, I sought out a doctor to do further testing. Regular screening and testing are important, but monitoring your body is the MOST important.

As I touched on before, a common misconception is that life goes back to normal once treatment ends. It doesn't. This is often the most challenging part. You come out of your cancer journey with different views on the world and your own mortality; you may feel anxious or depressed, not jubilant. This is all very normal.

Fantastic. Here is the main question of our interview. Based on your experiences and knowledge, what advice would you give to others who have recently been diagnosed with cancer? What are your "5 Things" You Need To Beat Cancer? Please share a story or example for each.

1. It's a marathon, not a sprint.
2. Scars are awesome...and something to be proud of.

3. No one knows your body like yourself. Your body communicates with you. Listen to it and speak up!
4. Everything hurts during treatment, but the less talked about side effects for young adults include depression, anxiety, infertility and/or early menopause.
5. Emotional healing is ongoing; I continue it every day through my work at The Chick Mission helping others through their own journey.

You are a person of great influence. If you could inspire a movement that would bring the most amount of good to the greatest amount of people, what would that be?

I feel pleased that I've already started to do some great work with The Chick Mission. Being able to tell people yes, they can have their fertility treatment covered, after the system has told them no, remains incredibly empowering. But as much as we're doing good work and it's fulfilling; The Chick Mission's ultimate mission is to go out of business—for there to be changes at a legal level. Right now, 40 states do not have it mandated that they need to provide fertility benefits for cancer patients. And in the 10 states that have passed mandates, there are countless loopholes patients fall through. My team and I won't stop rallying around legislation, like House Bill 293 in Texas, until all cancer patients are granted fertility benefits. We're going to keep up our fight, and hope others join us in the process on both a state-by-state and national level.

We are very blessed that some very prominent names in Business, VC funding, Sports, and Entertainment read this column. Is there a person in the world, or in the US with whom you would love to have a private breakfast or lunch, and why?

I am a huge fan of the power breakfast—if I'm dreaming big, I would pack mine with a fearless foursome.

Kate Ryder—Maven

Natalie Maines—The Chicks

MacKenzie Scott—Philanthropist

How can our readers further follow your work online?

Give us a follow on Instagram: @chickmission—where we share the latest in the cancer/fertility space, inspiring stories from survivors, and exciting upcoming initiatives we're working on. Also, visit our website: www.thechickmission.org and sign up for our newsletter!

Chloe Harrouche of The Lanby: I Survived (Breast) Cancer and Here Is How I Did It

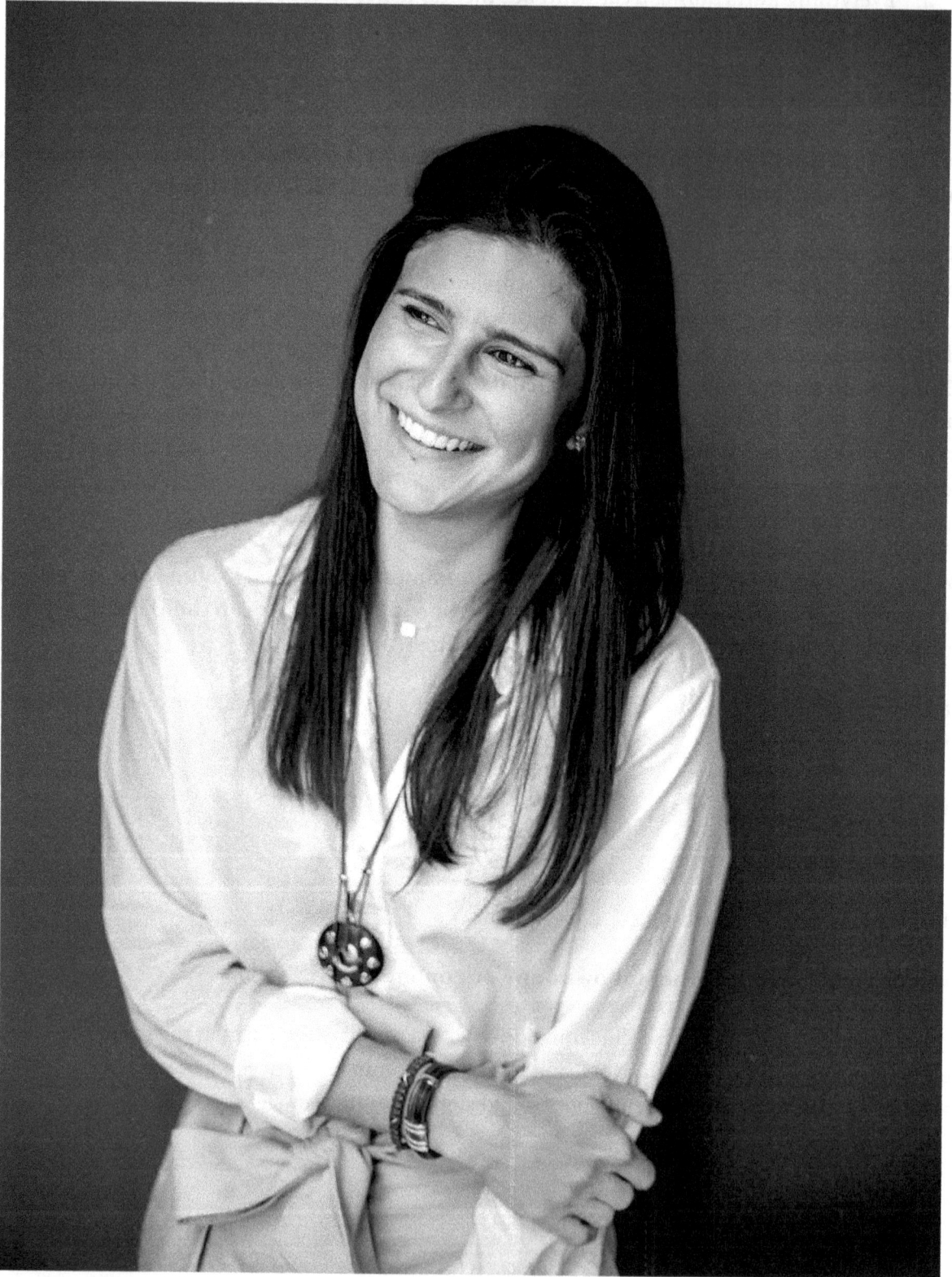

*Stay active and hydrated: push yourself to go on a short walk every day —
the increased circulation will dramatically speed up your recovery post*

treatment. A very dear family friend told me early on that staying hydrated was the most important chemo hack, and he was right. On the days surrounding treatment, you want to make sure you're drinking at least 2-3L of water/day to make sure the toxins don't stay in your bladder for too long, which can cause irritation.

I had the pleasure of interviewing Chloe Harrouche. Chloe is a Co-Founder of The Lanby, a hospitality-forward primary care members club. A skilled healthcare growth strategist, with experience spanning multiple touchpoints within the industry, Chloe's personal experience as a young survivor of breast cancer shaped her firsthand perspective of what patients want and need to feel supported in the primary care system. With the patient perspective at its core, The Lanby is reimagining concierge medicine for the modern generation.

Thank you so much for joining us in this interview series! We really appreciate the courage it takes to publicly share your story. Before we start, our readers would love to "get to know you" a bit better. Can you tell us a bit about your background and your childhood backstory?

I was born and raised in NYC. My parents are both originally from Iran, but my mom grew up in Paris. My childhood was filled with love. I'm incredibly close with my two sisters (I'm the middle child) and I've always felt lucky to have the family I have.

I wasn't always the best student, but I was super competitive, and that ultimately fueled my desire to get good grades and excel in sports. It was definitely in high school where I first learned to be disciplined and resilient.

Can you please give us your favorite "Life Lesson Quote?" Can you share how that was relevant to you in your life?

When I was first diagnosed with breast cancer, my first instinct was to question what this all meant. Not in a self-deprecating "why me?" kind of way (because I've always believed everything happens for a reason). I wanted to understand what this diagnosis meant in the greater context of my life—I wanted answers as to how this would influence me and those around me moving forward. When I asked my Rabbi, he said, "You may never know the answer, but what you should always remember is that God only gives us what we can handle." Those of us given difficult challenges have the most potential. That message has stayed with me through every struggle I've faced since. It has helped me see the bigger picture and look at challenges as opportunities to pivot and grow, to gain perspective and derive new meaning out of life. I'll probably never say I'm glad I had breast cancer, but I will say with confidence that I've gained a lot from the experience and I'm a better person for it.

Let's now shift to the main part of our discussion about surviving cancer. Do you feel comfortable sharing with us the story surrounding how you found out that you had cancer?

I was one year out of college—23 years old. I had felt a bump in my breast for a while, but never thought it was abnormal. The next time I went in for my annual gyno appointment, I brought it up with my doctor, who felt it and said it was just dense tissue (a fair assumption given my age and family history). Over the next 6 months, I didn't think twice about it. I was a healthcare consultant, traveling every week to North Carolina. I'm not exactly sure what prompted it, but as I was drying myself after a shower, I felt the same lump I had always felt, but much harder than it ever was. I called my gynecologist and she suggested that I get a sonogram. The radiologists agreed that it was probably nothing, but decided to do a biopsy in case. I would get the results the following Monday. I went back to North Carolina assuming they were right, that it was nothing. Shortly after arriving at my client's office, I got a call from my parents. They told me the doctor had called and that I needed to come back to New York for more tests. Still assuming it was nothing, I told them I would be back on Friday and would do the tests then. After a lot of back and forth, they finally blurted out that the biopsy came back positive for cancer cells. I studied bioengineering in college, but I had no idea what "having cancer cells" meant. It sounded serious enough that I knew I had to fly home, so I told my team I would be back the following week (of course, I didn't go back but instead took a leave of absence for 8 months). I was terrified, but I still didn't understand what the diagnosis was. I remember finally breaking down as I arrived at the check in counter, begging the airline attendant to let me change my flight because I had just been diagnosed with cancer. I remember calling my boyfriend, who I had been with since freshman year of college, to share the news. I didn't even know what to say. I can't imagine what must have gone through his mind. I also vividly remember my dad's reaction. Always cool, calm and collected, he proceeded to call me every ten minutes while I waited in the airport to make sure I too stayed calm. I knew how sad he would be to hear me sad, so I hid any fear from my voice. From that moment on, I promised myself that I would never let myself break down in front of the people I cared about.

What was the scariest part of that event? What did you think was the worst thing that could happen to you?

The scariest part was not knowing how serious the diagnosis was. I didn't know if cancer cells meant full blown cancer, or to what extent the treatment would affect the rest of my life. I learned after the MRI that I was at least Stage 2, possibly Stage 3, which meant I needed chemotherapy on top of a mastectomy. The mastectomy didn't scare me at all; in fact I opted for double instead of a single because I wanted to be as aggressive as I could be. But the thought of being a chemo patient really threw me. You see in the movies people losing their hair and becoming so frail and sick. I couldn't imagine that happening to me. The first oncologist I met with was also so matter of fact—zero emotional intelligence. She bluntly warned that my ovaries would most likely age from the chemo and that I wouldn't be able to have kids for ten years while I was on tamoxifen, no if's, and's or but's. I don't think I ever feared I was going to die, but perhaps superficially, I worried that this would change the course of my life and no one would ever look at me the same.

How did you react in the short term?

I really tried not to show emotion. I was committed to putting my head down and plowing forward. I didn't want to show weakness, mostly because I didn't want my family, boyfriend (now husband), or friends to worry about me. I sort of laughed it off, like no big deal. My sisters were instrumental in that respect. They never pitied me, but somehow made the whole thing one big joke. My little sister named my tumor Ellen, which was so random and hilarious, I remember cracking up in the hospital room screaming "F*** Ellen!" We went to Ricky's to try on costume wigs in every crazy color imaginable (pink, purple, and blue). We somehow found a way to turn everything that could be sad into something silly.

After the dust settled, what coping mechanisms did you use? What did you do to cope physically, mentally, emotionally, and spiritually?

I think the hardest part for me psychologically was the moment "the dust settled." I had my surgery, finished chemo and radiation, and I was ready to get back to the real world. But I was still bald, no eyebrows. It is hard to re-emerge as a healthy 24-year-old when you look like that. That's when all the emotions I had suppressed through the course of my treatment came piling on. I became depressed and frustrated, and I struggled to find the right outlet to cope. Ultimately, what has helped me the most is taking control of my health. I've taught myself so much about nutrition and various other wellness modalities to optimize my health and focus my efforts on prevention. I know so much of our health is up to chance, but there's so much we can do to minimize our risks. Giving myself that opportunity has made me feel a sense of ownership over my future, which is probably what I craved the most coming out of treatment.

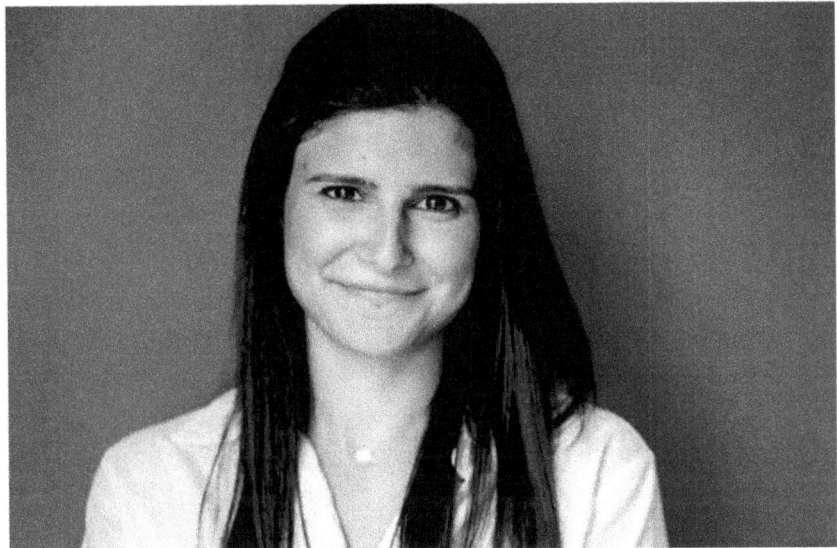

Is there a particular person you are grateful towards who helped you learn to cope and heal? Can you share a story about that?

I take a Jewish learning class once a week with a woman who I've known since college. She is so spiritual and resilient, and her glass is always full, no matter what life throws at her. My classes with her have given me more mental health than any therapist I have ever worked with. She inspires me to lead with gratitude. My sessions with her are completely unrelated to my cancer journey, but they've taught me what it means to have humility, to appreciate the blessings in my life, and to take on challenges as opportunities for growth.

In my own cancer struggle, I sometimes used the idea of embodiment to help me cope. Let's take a minute to look at cancer from an embodiment perspective. If your cancer had a message for you, what do you think it would want or say?

Given how much we hated Ellen, it's hard to imagine my cancer offering a positive message. But I guess I would hope that Ellen would want me to know that she was just a nuisance, not a death sentence. I've always had faith that my cancer was not meant to completely derail the rest of my life. Rather, I believe it was put in my path as a small bump in the road to wake me up, broaden my worldview, and live a deeper and more meaningful life. I'm not sure if Ellen would have warned me of this, but I'm glad I got rid of her sooner than later!

What did you learn about yourself from this very difficult experience? How has cancer shaped your worldview? What has it taught you that you might never have considered before? Can you please explain with a story or example?

It's shown me that life is fragile and we have to savor every moment of it. It's taught me the importance of having family and friends that can turn a sad moment into a happy one.

Life is full of ups and downs, and we all have our own unique battles. I used to worry that cancer would define me. I now can see that it has shaped me, but it by no means defines me. It has given me the perspective to appreciate the good and enjoy my life. I've faced many challenges since my diagnosis, and some hit me even harder than my diagnosis. But what eventually brought me back was regaining that perspective, knowing how blessed I am in so many other ways and taking advantage of those opportunities instead of dwelling on the imperfections.

How have you used your experience to bring goodness to the world?

The most helpful thing I think I can do is be totally available to anyone who's been newly diagnosed. I try to be as open and honest as I can to prepare them for what's to come. Most importantly, I try to empower them and give them the confidence that they'll come out of this stronger than they could have ever imagined. That this is just a bump in the road and won't define them, unless they let it. I encourage them to be kind to themselves, but also push themselves to stay active to accelerate their path to recovery.

Through my own experience, I also learned firsthand what patients struggle with the most—and not just cancer patients, any patient dealing with an acute health crisis or looking for support to optimize their health. I founded The Lanby alongside my co-founder, Tandice, because we felt primary care needed to be overhauled. We drew lessons from our own patient journeys to create a service that was patient-centric and comprehensive. The Lanby has just opened in New York City as the first patient-developed primary care practice with an integrative approach to health. Tandice and I believe The Lanby is leading primary care into the 21st century and we couldn't be more proud watching our vision come to life.

What are a few of the biggest misconceptions and myths out there about fighting cancer that you would like to dispel?

I think the biggest misconception about chemo is that you're basically bed-ridden the whole time. I definitely experienced all of the well-known symptoms (i.e. nausea and fatigue) in the first few days following my treatments, but I made a conscious effort every day to go for a walk even if it was just around the block to get my blood circulating and boost my energy. Starting on Day 5, I felt myself again and I would take complete advantage by going on runs in the park, having dinner with friends, whatever I wanted.

Fantastic. Here is the main question of our interview. Based on your experiences and knowledge, what advice would you give to others who have recently been diagnosed with cancer? What are your "5 Things" You Need To Beat Cancer? Please share a story or example for each.

1. Have a positive attitude: anyone who asks "why me?" is doomed. There will always be someone who's been dealt a worse hand than you. Be grateful for what you do have and focus your energy on getting healthy.
2. Laughing heals, crying paralyzes: surround yourself with people who will make you laugh and keep you light. You don't need anyone's pity, you need a good laugh.
3. Be kind to yourself: It's okay to have days where you let yourself be sad. As my friend would tell me, wallowing is part of the healing process. If you're sad, accept it, treat yourself to some ice cream, and re-start tomorrow.
4. Stay active and hydrated: push yourself to go on a short walk every day—the increased circulation will dramatically speed up your recovery post-treatment. A very dear family friend told me early on that staying hydrated was the most important chemo-hack, and he was right. On the days surrounding treatment, you want to make sure you're drinking at least 2–3L of water/day to make sure the toxins don't stay in your bladder for too long, which can cause irritation.
5. Medicinal marijuana was the only thing that alleviated my nausea, masked my joint pain, and gave me the appetite I needed to avoid losing too much weight. I'm not sure to what extent doctors are recommending it today, but based on my experience; I believe it should be in every cancer patient's care package.

You are a person of great influence. If you could inspire a movement that would bring the most amount of good to the greatest amount of people, what would that be?

In a nutshell, The Lanby. By providing people with better support and guidance, I hope to inspire others to treat their bodies with the utmost respect and kindness. We only get one, so we better take care of it and do whatever we can to minimize its aging. Yes, there's a lot in life we can't control, but there's so much we can do to improve our odds and extend our youth. I want to give people the resources they need to be the healthiest, happiest, and most fulfilled versions of themselves.

We are very blessed that some very prominent names in Business, VC funding, Sports, and Entertainment read this column. Is there a person in the world, or in the US with whom you would love to have a private breakfast or lunch, and why?

Before we started hiring, I read Reed Hastings' *No Rules Rules* book and became obsessed with his philosophy around maximizing talent density, which allows organizations to rid themselves of rules, thereby fostering a culture of innovation and continuous growth. If I could have a private lunch with anyone right now, it would be Reed. I'd love to pick his brain as we think about setting the tone for The Lanby and creating a culture that attracts and retains the best talent in healthcare.

How can our readers further follow your work online?

Sign up for our newsletter on our website: www.thelanby.com and follow us on Instagram: @the.lanby

Author Christine Handy: I Survived (Breast) Cancer and Here Is How I Did It

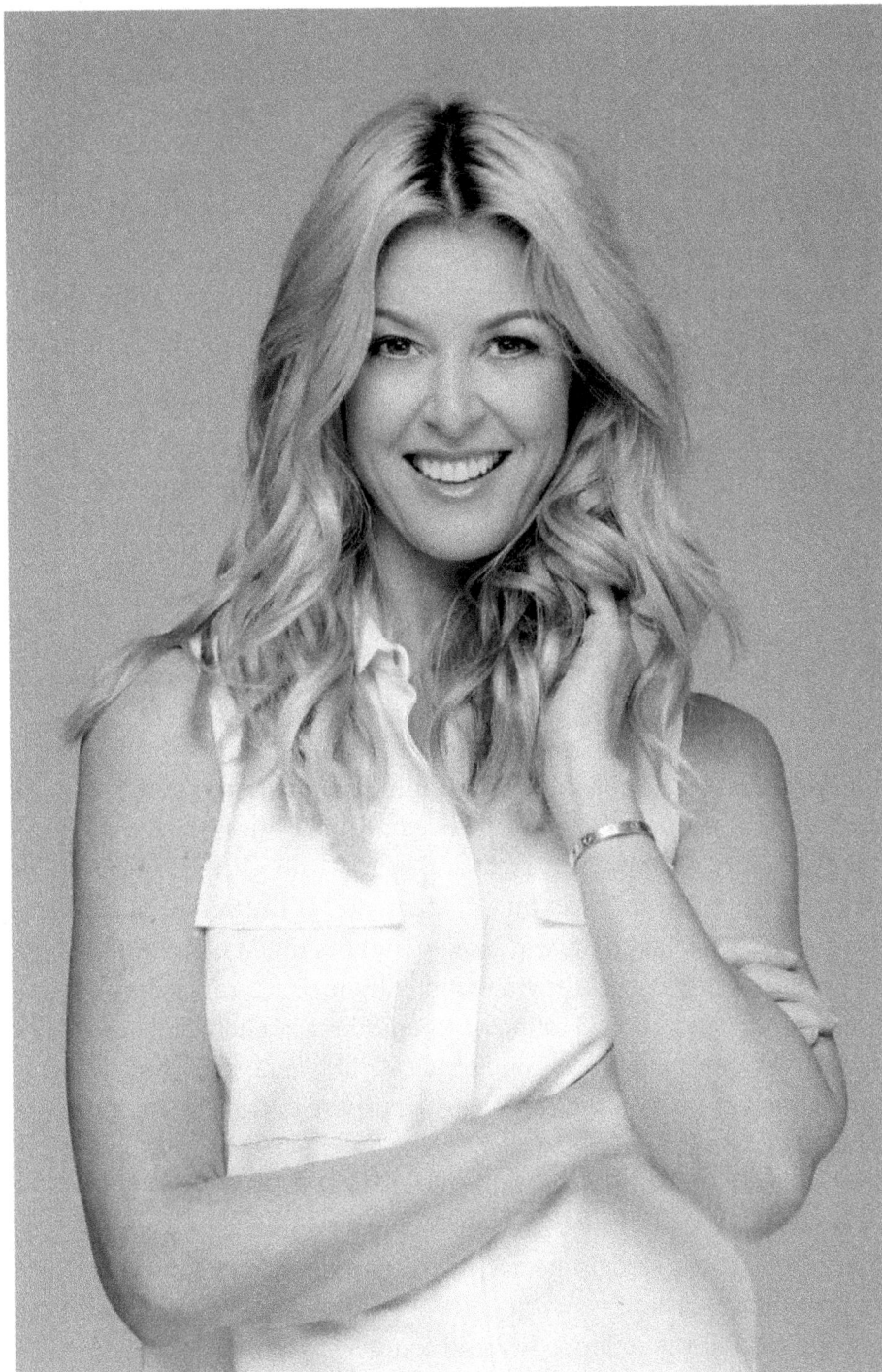

I needed to serve others. Because I knew that my pain had purpose, I wanted to teach that to others in order to lighten their load.

I had the pleasure of interviewing Christine Handy. Christine is an Author, Model, Breast Cancer Survivor, Motivational Speaker and Humanitarian. Christine published her first book 'Walk Beside Me' in 2016—it is in the works to becoming a film. Recently, Christine collaborated with a bathing suit brand to manufacture a line of swimwear for women who have lost their breasts to cancer. Christine is also on the Board of two Nonprofits: Ebeauty and People of Purpose.

Thank you so much for joining us in this interview series! We really appreciate the courage it takes to publicly share your story. Before we start, our readers would love to "get to know you" a bit better. Can you tell us a bit about your background and your childhood backstory?

With pleasure. I was raised by my parents in St. Louis, Mo with my three other sisters. We even had a female dog so my father was definitely outnumbered. I have always been close to my family, but even more so after my cancer diagnosis. I left the Midwest to go to SMU in Dallas for my undergraduate degree. I stayed in Dallas for more than 20 years but recently relocated to Miami, Florida. Currently, I am getting a master's degree from Harvard University.

Can you please give us your favorite "Life Lesson Quote?" Can you share how that was relevant to you in your life?

My "Life Lesson Quote" is one I made up at the beginning of my cancer battle. There is always purpose in pain. It is a quote I have clung to and lived my life by over the last ten years of life and illness. Pain is inevitable, but how we react to it and what we do with it, is our responsibility. When I was diagnosed with breast cancer on October 1, 2012, I had young children I was trying to love and parent. I also just had my right arm fused. From the time I had turned 40 years old to my 41st birthday, I had gone from being a thriving mother, model, self-proclaimed athlete and wife to a sickly, handicapped woman facing 28 rounds of chemotherapy and who knew how many surgeries. Pain consumed me, emotionally and physically. I had no choice but to give myself a lifeline and that lifeline was my new motto, "There is purpose in pain." Whether I was going to survive breast cancer or not was out of my control, but I had to believe that all the pain I was enduring had meaning for my life and hopefully for others as well. One of my friends said to me in the early days of my diagnosis, "People are watching you." I didn't fully understand it at the time, but she was right. I could model what survival or fighting illness looked like in any way I chose. I could show courage or fear, worry or faith, grace or anger and on and on. I chose to be vulnerable and honest about the suffering but also courageous and hopeful in the fight.

Let's now shift to the main part of our discussion about surviving cancer. Do you feel comfortable sharing with us the story surrounding how you found out that you had cancer?

I was actually traveling to New York City for an orthopedic doctor's appointment when I felt the lump on my left breast. I lived in Dallas at the time, but my arm surgeon was at Hospital for Special Surgery in NYC. I was in a hotel room trying to take a shower with a cast on my right arm that covered my fingertips to my shoulder. For months, I had poured liquid soap over my shoulder instead of struggling with a bar of soap and a casted arm. On this day, I held the bar of soap while suspending my casted arm out of the shower, and as I gently passed the soap over my left breast, I immediately felt a large, tough lump. My first reaction was panic. I had just been through an enormous health trial that ended in a full wrist fusion in my dominant arm. I was trying to figure out how I was going to be a mom and drive a car with a full fusion. With no family history of breast cancer, it never occurred to me that this could happen, especially at 41 years old. I was diagnosed with cancer five days later over the phone.

What was the scariest part of that event? What did you think was the worst thing that could happen to you?

The scariest part was the fear that I could or would die and leave my sons behind. I wanted to be their mom; I couldn't imagine someone else having the privilege of raising them. That haunted me and to some extent, still does.

How did you react in the short term?

In the short-term I had terrible thoughts and anxiety. One moment I was all in for fighting the disease and the next minute I was too overwhelmed and exhausted to even try. Some days, I told friends and family I was quitting. It was a horrendous roller coaster that pillaged my emotions in many different ways. Fortunately, I quickly started to believe enough in myself and in my faith that I started to really fight the fight.

After the dust settled, what coping mechanisms did you use? What did you do to cope physically, mentally, emotionally, and spiritually?

I depended heavily on family and friends during treatment. My friends often sent me pictures of them out living when I was too sick to leave my house. They would remind me that someday I would be well again too, and to keep looking at the pictures to see what I could look forward to. My father also gave me an island to swim to so to speak. He promised me a trip when chemotherapy and the surgeries were completed. There are so many hours of waiting when you have cancer. Waiting for various doctors, for surgery, for chemotherapy and even during chemotherapy the time passes slowly. I often focused on that trip, day dreaming of where I might like to go and looking on my phone for places to visit. What my father was doing was giving me another lifeline. Also during this confusing and frightening time, I poured into learning more about faith. I listened to podcasts on faith and spirituality which readjusted my own self-pity into trust and confidence in God.

Is there a particular person you are grateful towards who helped you learn to cope and heal? Can you share a story about that?

I had an enormous group of strong, dedicated women who gave up much of their time to help me and my family throughout my battle. The unity of the group really taught me what it looks like when women become champions together. It goes back to what my friend told me in the beginning of my treatment, that people were watching. My group of friends showing up for me, in turn showed our community that spirit of alignment and self-sacrifice. The more they showed up for me, the more courage I had. And the more courage I showed, the more I was helping my family and the community learn to be brave.

In my own cancer struggle, I sometimes used the idea of embodiment to help me cope. Let's take a minute to look at cancer from an embodiment perspective. If your cancer had a message for you, what do you think it would want or say?

You matter. I had been insecure for so long, cancer showed me that I mattered. Not the disease, but the willingness of family and friends to carry me until I could carry myself. I began to believe in myself again. My community of women embodied that I mattered enough to show up for.

What did you learn about yourself from this very difficult experience? How has cancer shaped your worldview? What has it taught you that you might never have considered before? Can you please explain with a story or example? I

I learned who I was most importantly. Cancer brought me to my knees, and when I was down there I learned that I had grit and grace, I learned that I didn't need to rely on my physical appearance for others to give me love or attention, I was whole even with no hair, no external beauty. I was a model. I started very young and my career continued throughout my twenties and thirties. Being faced with cancer and enduring chemotherapy, the loss of my hair and then breasts was traumatic enough without that external value that I measured my self-worth on. I had not considered myself worthy of great love and affection without the beauty I had. The good news was that my beauty had nothing to do with why my friends and family loved me. I started to see things, stuff differently. Faith, myself, and relationships became more important than the designer bags or my beautiful long blonde hair.

How have you used your experience to bring goodness to the world?

I try every single day to bring goodness to the world out of my tragedies. Whether it be on social media, by people reading my book, or my speaking engagements, my message is consistent, there is always hope and purpose in pain.

What are a few of the biggest misconceptions and myths out there about fighting cancer that you would like to dispel?

I love answering this very important question. Once patients have completed chemotherapy, and or radiation, surgeries, oftentimes the side effects of the solution linger for years. I endured tremendous chemotherapy which left lasting side effects. I am 7 years out from my diagnosis and I have other health issues. The specific chemotherapy regimen I was on "could" affect my heart and it did. Just last year I had my third and fourth mastectomies because of implant complications. I often speak to other cancer patients who share my frustration in the misconception that once treatment is over, complications are behind you too. Being cancer-free does not equate to being problem-free emotionally or physically after cancer.

Fantastic. Here is the main question of our interview. Based on your experiences and

knowledge, what advice would you give to others who have recently been diagnosed with cancer? What are your "5 Things" I wish I knew about living with cancer? Please share a story or example for each.

The "5 Things" I needed to get through cancer were faith in God and a hope for a future. I needed to repeat "Let Go and Let God" instead of I am scared and have no hope. Secondly, I needed people. I needed family, friends, even strangers to encourage me, cheer me on and show me that I mattered. The simplest asks of kindness went a long way. Sending a text or a letter, even a phone call helped encourage me. It doesn't require money to help others, often; it only takes a few seconds to send a text. Third, I needed something to look forward to. A place to visit, something that got me out of my head and helped me mediate on a positive and uplifting future experience. That could be a trip to see family or a party at the end of treatment. Fourth, I needed to work on myself. I needed to change the voice in my head to be more encouraging. The old insecure mindset had to shift. And lastly, I needed to serve others. Because I knew that my pain had purpose, I wanted to teach that to others in order to lighten their load.

You are a person of great influence. If you could inspire a movement that would bring the most amount of good to the greatest amount of people, what would that be?

I would shout from the rooftops how important self-talk is to the well-being of our lives. I would teach others how to nurture their self-esteem and that it takes time, it's a daily practice. Just like going to the gym to work on your muscles or going to school to work on your brain, we need daily work to nurture and elevate our self-esteem so the world can't tear it apart.

We are very blessed that some very prominent names in Business, VC funding, Sports, and Entertainment read this column. Is there a person in the world, or in the US with whom you would love to have a private breakfast or lunch, and why?

I would like to speak to Oprah, sit down and have an intimate chat. She got knocked around as a child and climbed many a ladder to use her voice. One of the greatest voices of all time. I know my story helps people, if I had a bigger voice more and more could learn from my story, my pain. It would not be for my glory at all, but for the opportunity to reach more cancer patients in a collaborative effort with Oprah and in the end we would spread great hope.

How can our readers further follow your work online?

www.christinehandy.com

Instagram: @christinehandy1

Twitter: @handychristine1

Pinterest: @1christinehandy

Scan the QR code to view my "5 Things" To Beat Cancer YouTube video:

Dr. De Vida Gill: I Survived (Breast) Cancer and Here Is How I Did It

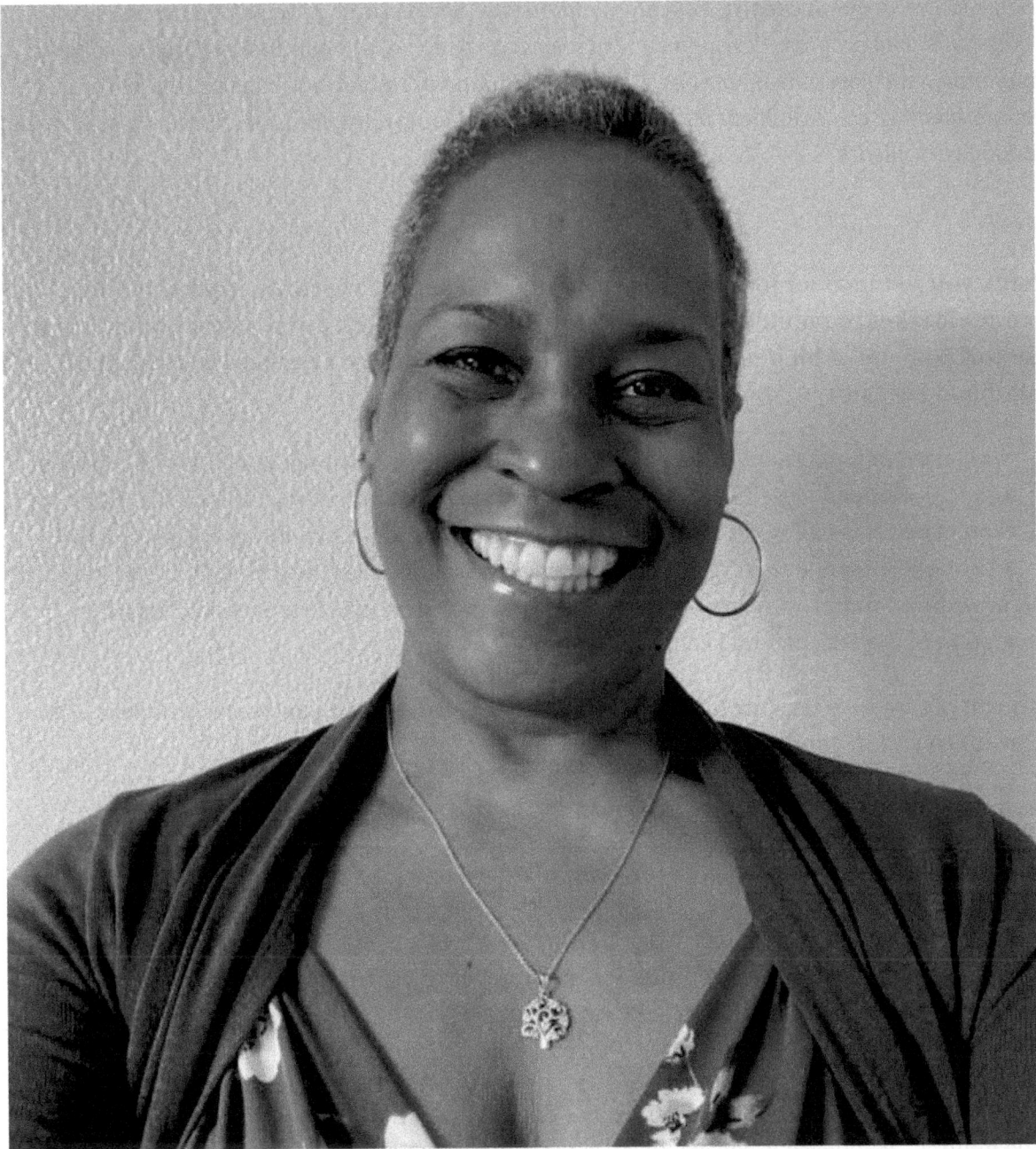

Cancer has opened my eyes to life through a different lens—the lens of showing how I see myself and the world around me. There were times my allergic reaction to treatments made me question how I saw life and how precious it was; how life can change in an instant without notice, and to live life and be happy. That peace of mind is everything!

I had the pleasure of interviewing Dr. De Vida Gill. De Vida is a Licensed Clinical Social Worker, Certified Life Coach/ Strategist, Educator, and Author. She has over 25 years of personal, professional, and program development experience working with nonprofits, for-profits, schools, community, and government entities. With a background in the performing arts, she has incorporated her creative talent into her daily work, developing programs, facilitating training, and working with clients.

Thank you so much for joining us in this interview series! We really appreciate the courage it takes to publicly share your story. Before we start, our readers would love to "get to know you" a bit better. Can you tell us a bit about your background and your childhood backstory?

I was raised in California, where I found my love for the performing, visual, and literary arts. As a child, I wrapped myself in theater, dance, and music and found my calling in artistic expression...stage, film, teaching, and mentoring. As an adult, I continue my passion for artistic expression, integrating it into my practice as a therapist, coaching practices, teaching, and in writing children's literature. My mission is to provide social awareness through the integration of the arts, mental health, and education.

Can you please give us your favorite "Life Lesson Quote?" Can you share how that was relevant to you in your life?

I have several, but the two I use most often are:

(1) I AM a creative person, and I can solve any problem, and (2) For every one problem, there are ten solutions.

During my cancer treatment, I consulted with several doctors in western and eastern medicine. I was determined to find a treatment solution that was best for me. After talking with them, it seems there are many. You just have to keep looking.

Life is full of both successes and character building days. With the most challenging days, I have to be mindful, acknowledge the craziness, assess the situation, lean into my emotions through creativity, and pivot when needed. In short, the thought of cancer is crazy. Moving through it, I needed to acknowledge the reality. As the treatment plan and side effects continued to change, in the early days, I had to pivot almost every time I had an appointment.

Let's now shift to the main part of our discussion about surviving cancer. Do you feel comfortable sharing with us the story surrounding how you found out that you had cancer?

Sure. One night I woke up in pain and felt a big knot on my breast. I initially thought it was just a cyst and would go away, but after a day or two, the pain was still there, and it didn't feel right, so I contacted my doctor.

What was the scariest part of that event? What did you think was the worst thing that could happen to you?

The scariest part was finding out how I would tell my two daughters and the rest of my immediate family. I had more questions than answers myself and was trying to process it all myself. I was not ready for all the emotions that would come from EVERYONE! The worst thing that I felt could happen is dying and not being here for my family. We had just lost my father a year ago. So this, on top of THAT loss, was too much!

How did you react in the short term?

I cried nonstop and then leaned into my emotions and fears. I decided to jot down my feelings, which led to writing my children's book, *I AM NOT My Cancer*. I kept it on my phone during my entire treatment and read it almost daily as a fuel source to get through each day. In my book, the feelings I recorded (through artistic expression) of my positive side reminded me during those lonely and challenging days that it (positive side) was still here!

After the dust settled, what coping mechanisms did you use? What did you do to cope physically, mentally, emotionally, and spiritually?

Honestly, I'm not quite sure that the emotional dust has totally settled. Like school, it is an experience you never forget as there are always reminders, but as a graduate, often you are glad it is over.

Physically, I didn't do much because I was under very aggressive treatment where there were days I could barely walk. I had a lot of unbearable pain, so I constantly shifted my body and moved, even if it was only rolling my shoulders and head. It was challenging to find comfort in the pain.

Mentally, I practiced meditation and relaxation techniques. To aid in the process, I lit candles, recited positive affirmations, read fun books, watched movies that made me happy, spent a lot of time with my family, played music, and talked to my friends on the phone. I wrote in my gratitude journal and did a lot of self-reflection work. During treatment, since no one could join me due to COVID, I always Facetimed my family on a group call to feel like they were with me. That helped tremendously during chemo treatments. I looked for peaceful places that took me away from the physical pain and the reoccurring "what if" mindset.

Emotionally, I monitored my emotions, was mindful of negative thoughts that came up, gave myself grace, and didn't allow anyone to entertain any negative thoughts in my space. This process was challenging due to being diagnosed during COVID. I was completing my second doctoral degree, teaching, working with the local high schools, and running my private practice. Many people tried to tell me to quit, that it was too much stress, and I couldn't do it. I knew stopping what I was doing would be the worst thing I could do for ME, and I wasn't ready to buy into the limitations of others on MY journey. So, I pivoted and modified as needed, eliminated outside distractions, and did what was best for me. I realized that not everyone was going to be on this journey with me and that although I had a lot of initial support; ultimately, I would be going through it alone. I practiced a lot of grounding work to center me, such as deep breathing and meditation.

Spiritually, I prayed A LOT and leaned on my faith.

Is there a particular person you are grateful towards who helped you learn to cope and heal? Can you share a story about that?

I would say my family and a few of my close friends. They were my rock and still are as I continue with treatment. My youngest daughter moved home from college during COVID in March to finish her education, and in September 2020, I was diagnosed. She was my taxi, my receptionist notetaker, my medication manager, and everything else in between. My family would attend all my appointments via FaceTime to hear what my treatment team had to say and ask questions. My oldest arranged with her boss to drive down from the San Francisco Bay Area every other week to help.

In my own cancer struggle, I sometimes used the idea of embodiment to help me cope. Let's take a minute to look at cancer from an embodiment perspective. If your cancer had a message for you, what do you think it would want or say?

You are stronger than you think you are. I keep trying to beat you, even brought in more of my cancer friends to join in the attack, but you keep knocking us down as if to say—not today. LOL

What did you learn about yourself from this very difficult experience? How has cancer shaped your worldview? What has it taught you that you might never have considered before? Can you please explain with a story or example?

I learned that not everyone would go on my life's journey, and that's okay. The people who were/are there for me were meant to be there. It reminded me of the power of thought(s) and mindset and reaffirmed that what people think of me is none of my business. It is more important to know yourself and do what's BEST for you.

Cancer has opened my eyes to life through a different lens—the lens of showing how I see myself and the world around me. There were times my allergic reaction to treatments made me question how I saw life and how precious it was, how life can change in an instant without notice, and to live life and be happy. That peace of mind is everything!

It taught me that everything happens for a reason and it's up to me to self-reflect and identify what is important in life. For me, it was to slow down, not compromise my happiness, and listen to my body. I never really listened to my body as I listen to it now.

I remember days when I was trying to finish my doctoral courses, projects, dissertation, etc.— exhausted from treatment. I had to plan my life around my naps and pain and adjust as needed. I realized how important flexibility was and how giving myself grace was imperative.

How have you used your experience to bring goodness to the world?

I think the biggest plunge for me was when I went public with my diagnosis on social media. I'm a very private person, but I felt I should tell my story if I can help one person. My story has many twists and turns in it that most people are unaware of, but I feel if I can break the cycle of isolation during character-building days, it might bring a glimmer of light to a darkened day.

What are a few of the biggest misconceptions and myths out there about fighting cancer that you would like to dispel?

To only use western medicine. I had a lot of allergic reactions to my treatments as my body didn't do well. I was fortunate to have two people on my treatment team who had the knowledge and practiced both eastern and western treatment modalities. I think consulting with both types of treatment teams helped me not only in understanding my treatment, side effects, and possible remedies, but it left me feeling like I wasn't alone.

That everyone's cancer journey is the same. This is a HUGE misconception. I had side effects that weren't in the books, and my body did not like the treatments. Not everything is black and white, so it is imperative to talk to your treatment team about everything and ask questions.

Fantastic. Here is the main question of our interview. Based on your experiences and knowledge, what advice would you give to others who have recently been diagnosed with cancer? What are your "5 Things" You Need To Beat Cancer? Please share a story or example for each.

1. An excellent treatment team—Make sure you and your family like your treatment team.
2. Positive mindset (what you say to yourself and about yourself)—stay positive as much as you can.
3. At least 1–3 people who are your accountability partners and will check in on you—be honest with them about how you are doing. These people should also be your "in case of an emergency contact" if you need to go to the hospital. They should also be honest with you. Everything is not okay all the time. This is a fight, don't believe otherwise!
4. A treatment toolbox (fuzzy socks, warm blanket, ginger tea, nausea gum, scriptures, aloe vera plant, warm heating pads, journal, list of hobbies you can do that don't require energy, music, etc.).
5. Schedule 10–30 minute virtual get-togethers consistently, via phone, FaceTime, or in person. Human contact is important, even if it's virtual.

You are a person of great influence. If you could inspire a movement that would bring the most amount of good to the greatest amount of people, what would that be?

As I said before, integrating the arts, mental health, and education. These three fields of study are in everything we do, say, and be. We interact with each of them every day, yet we don't recognize them in their natural form.

We are very blessed that some very prominent names in Business, VC funding, Sports, and Entertainment read this column. Is there a person in the world, or in the US with whom you would love to have a private breakfast or lunch, and why?

Ms. Oprah Winfrey or Mrs. Michelle Obama. I believe they understand the power of thinking and how one significant life-changing event (even if just for a moment) can change a person. They each used that power to pivot and help others.

How can our readers further follow your work online?

You can find my children's books at www.diversechild.com and some of the other things I do at www.mahoganyvida.com

Google's Eve McDavid: I Survived (Cervical) Cancer and Here Is How I Did It

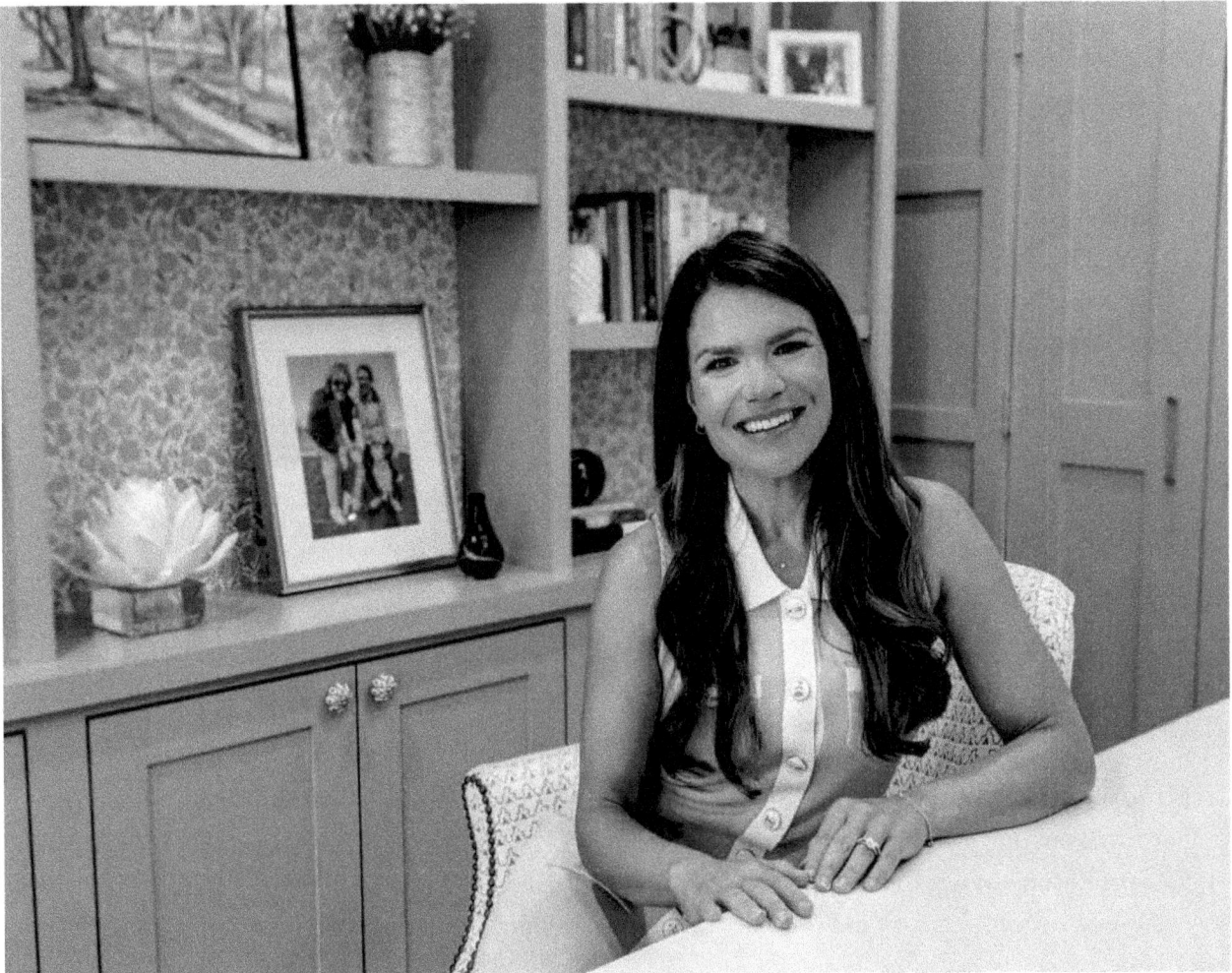

Prepare to celebrate EVERY. SINGLE. WIN! Staying positive all the time is hard, so find ways to recognize the good and raise it up. Had an easy time getting the IV in for an infusion? Ring the bell to cheer you on! Made it through your first brachytherapy procedure? That's cause for a balloon drop! Every milestone is one closer to the rest of your hard-fought, hard-earned life so be sure to recognize your incredible accomplishments as you go!

I had the pleasure of interviewing Eve McDavid. FemTech entrepreneur, Eve, is a Google strategy executive and stage IIB cervical cancer survivor. Forever transformed by her diagnosis, Eve is a passionate advocate for women's healthcare access and equity. As a woman in tech who specializes in complex problem solving, she's joined the World Health Organization's fight to eradicate Cervical Cancer by 2030 and is collaborating with Weill Cornell Medicine to redesign treatment devices to improve women's care, outcomes and access.

Thank you so much for joining us in this interview series! We really appreciate the courage it takes to publicly share your story. Before we start, our readers would love to "get to know you" a bit better. Can you tell us a bit about your background and your childhood backstory?

Thank you so much for having me. It's an honor to be here to discuss such a meaningful topic. I'm a proud wife, mama of two kiddies and a strategy executive at Google. Most recently, I'm a cervical cancer survivor who's drawing from all parts of my life to support the global movement to eradicate cervical cancer.

I grew up in a suburb of Washington, D.C. Being so close to the nation's capital; I always felt I was part of something greater than myself. From a very young age I understood I had a gift to lead and connect with people in an emotionally intelligent capacity. I've tapped into this talent to navigate challenging and high performing environments throughout my lifetime.

My grandmother, Ann, a fierce, hardworking business owner, was my role model. I grew up on her stories of our Jewish ancestors' persecution and high-stakes journeys to immigrate from Eastern Europe to America, instilling in me the worth and strength through her I'd inherited. She too, was a cancer survivor and became my vision of a hard-working woman with a big life.

Can you please give us your favorite "Life Lesson Quote?" Can you share how that was relevant to you in your life?

"Real change, enduring change, happens one step at a time." — Justice Ruth Bader Ginsburg

I have tremendous gratitude for all the work the late Justice Ginsburg did to advance women's equality. I've learned that great leaders are capable of both setting vision and methodical execution to make the dream a reality. The spirit of her words reminds me to continue the hard work every day in service of a better future for all women and families.

Let's now shift to the main part of our discussion about surviving cancer. Do you feel comfortable sharing with us the story surrounding how you found out that you had cancer?

I'm comfortable sharing, thank you for asking. I was 35-weeks pregnant with my son, Arthur, and went to see my OB/GYN for a routine prenatal visit. My OB/GYN checked my cervix and commented that it felt "irregular." She then performed a Pap Test, which is a cervical cancer screening diagnostic. There was a lot of blood, which was not typical. The next morning, she called to let me know she believed I had cervical cancer and needed to plan for Arthur's early delivery and determine a treatment plan immediately.

The following day, I met with my oncologist and she described my diagnosis as best as could be determined from the scans. Since I was pregnant, clear and definitive results were difficult to make. She explained that my case was likely stage IIB, that it grew extremely rapidly to seven centimeters in just a few months and that I would need to start chemotherapy and radiation very quickly.

I had a C-section the next day and I wept when I met Arthur, praying I would wake up again after I went under anesthesia for the biopsy. I did, dazed and woozy in the recovery room, holding Arthur for the first time and learning the good news that the cancer didn't appear to have spread, though I'd have further scans to confirm. By the weekend, my diagnosis was confirmed at stage IIB and because pathology returned better than anticipated results, I went home with Arthur, my husband and two-year-old daughter, Ruby Ann, for two weeks before treatment began.

What was the scariest part of that event? What did you think was the worst thing that could happen to you?

The scariest realization was understanding how grave my case truly was, and the fact that all of a sudden, both my life and Arthur's were in danger. At that moment, there was a lot to fear: there was no margin of error for either of us, and while we were in the incredibly capable hands of a world-class care team, their alarm was palpable—cervical cancer is typically slow growing and so my case was highly unusual. It was clear that every minute I remained pregnant, the greater the danger for me, but less time for Arthur's in utero development—this was the beginning of, very rapidly, making tremendously difficult decisions.

How did you react in the short term?

I experienced overwhelming shock and grief trying to grasp the weight of so much happening all at once. To see clearly, I made a list of all the questions about Arthur's delivery and treatment's consequences I needed answered so I could eventually feel prepared for the loss of each experience: a vaginal delivery, breastfeeding, the ability to freeze my eggs to have more children, whether surgery could replace chemotherapy and radiation, whether I could avoid early menopause.

It was devastating, but for the chance to survive, I had to give them all up, all at once. I'd never felt more out of control and that led to incredibly dark moments of pain, grief, and most curiously but most profoundly, an undertow of shame. It took me well into recovery to understand, address and begin healing from each, and then collectively.

After the dust settled, what coping mechanisms did you use? What did you do to cope physically, mentally, emotionally, and spiritually?

My husband, Matt, my partner in the truest sense of the word, sprang into action as soon as I was diagnosed, organizing my patient record and test results for additional consults and second opinions throughout the city. After we came home from the hospital with Arthur, I tapped in and this boosted my confidence. Here's what else I did:

Physically: As soon as I could bear weight, I bundled Arthur into a baby carrier and wore him on my chest for walks in Prospect Park, almost daily. Walking in nature, the cold was an escape for me and it gave me precious time back with Arthur.

Emotionally: Matt is a clinical psychotherapist and quickly found a therapist with whom I clicked. Therapy was the safe place I needed to access the feelings of fear, shame, loss and guilt. I'd been in therapy before and I understood its importance while in the eye of the storm; I've continued ever since.

Spiritually: Cancer deepened my and my family's faith in Judaism. Matt converted to Judaism while I was pregnant with my daughter, Ruby Ann, and I could see how deeply he was drawing on our family's shared faith to get through. His faith re-inspired mine: we began celebrating Shabbat every Friday night, which has been particularly restorative during the pandemic. We also sing a prayer called the "Mi Shebeirach," a blessing for healing to help us honor all we've endured.

Mentally: Moments before my diagnosis, I ran YouTube's public sector business. For me, treatment was like showing up to a new job: an aggressive, intellectually stimulating environment, learning new people, products and processes. It lit up my curiosity. I kept track of the answers to questions that puzzled me, the limitations of present technology and tools, and how women's experience at the center of preventable, treatable, curable cancer suffered. This kept me sharp and ready to act once I reached remission.

Is there a particular person you are grateful towards who helped you learn to cope and heal? Can you share a story about that?

There is no one more important to my experience than Matt. We were partners before, but no effort is greater than what Matt did for me in treatment. He put his therapy practice on hold to become my primary caregiver. Before I could face my diagnosis and get involved in care decisions, Matt ran point on all medical communications, running on foot throughout the city, begging doctors to see me.

He drove me to every treatment and when I asked that he be strong so I may be weak, he processed his fear and grief privately to not burden me. He put everything on the line to ensure a successful outcome. I know, today, that I experienced my extraordinary outcome due to his unwavering commitment. Only later, would I understand the enormous toll it took on him; throughout, he absorbed everything for me so I could focus and just get through.

In my own cancer struggle, I sometimes used the idea of embodiment to help me cope. Let's take a minute to look at cancer from an embodiment perspective. If your cancer had a message for you, what do you think it would want or say?

My cancer brought with it a blaring message: "pay attention." During my pregnancy, I had bleeding and was tremendously drained. I voiced my concerns at prenatal visits, though because I was pregnant, with a demanding job, a toddler at home, and have a blood type that explained the bleeding, I didn't present any differently from a healthy pregnant woman. And of course, I was anything but that.

It's well documented that women are conditioned to minimize pain and discomfort. Cancer showed me how risky this truly is. We only get so much time and we have but one body—and so I learned to listen to my body and mind together to protect, take care of and restore my being. I'm now much more thoughtful, intuitive and trusting of myself before making a choice or booking the next commitment.

What did you learn about yourself from this very difficult experience? How has cancer shaped your worldview? What has it taught you that you might never have considered before? Can you please explain with a story or example?

Cancer is a life-changing mirror. It's well understood that humans constantly face moments where everything forever is different. The only question is how much time in the aftermath do we have to make something of the moment?

Feeling the shame and stigma of HPV-related cancer, and learning that many women with the same diagnosis experience the same, was a wake-up call. Shame creates an extraordinary barrier to accessing quality care and it's something that we can use our voices to change. Before cancer I never would have considered speaking publicly about my HPV diagnosis or Abnormal Pap Test results—now I want to encourage all women to talk about cervical health so we can see how truly common our experiences are and destigmatize the diagnosis.

How have you used your experience to bring goodness to the world?

I feel honored to use my experience to now make a contribution to the conversation. I've become a women's health advocate with a goal of destigmatizing HPV and cervical cancer, joining the many women who've paved the way to speak up and speak out before me. I'm also using my expertise in tech to modernize the technology used in today's cervical healthcare system and to expand access to women's healthcare. I have recently become a part of the World Health Organization's initiative to eliminate cervical cancer by 2030 and am collaborating with my treating physician to redesign treatment tools to offer women safer, more humane procedures while also improving physical and mental health outcomes.

What are a few of the biggest misconceptions and myths out there about fighting cancer that you would like to dispel?

1. Myth 1: I should be strong enough to "get through" without extra help. I learned to use my voice in every way during cancer—asking for anxiety medication when I needed it, increasing my dosage of anti-nausea medication, requesting the "special forces" nursing team every week at chemo to make IV placement easier. I learned to let others accommodate me, not the other way around. There's no better time to be vocal than when you're fighting for your life.
2. Myth 2: You have to take risks to give yourself the greatest chance for survival. I passed on

a clinical trial recommended by a number of physicians because I was young and healthy, so I "could take more chemo." I had enough concerns on the trial to pass, and looking back, I'm glad I did—it recently wound down after having shown no greater efficacy. Trust your judgment and vet your decisions with your care team, you know more than you realize as you evaluate decisions.

3. Myth 3: Cancer is time-bound to treatment. Recovery is just as important as treatment. Recovery is a long journey and it happens in time. Be patient with yourself and set boundaries to preserve your time in recovery. Take as much time as you need to heal; only you can set that for yourself.

Fantastic. Here is the main question of our interview. Based on your experiences and knowledge, what advice would you give to others who have recently been diagnosed with cancer? What are your "5 Things" You Need To Beat Cancer? Please share a story or example for each.

1. A badass care team in which you see yourself: Find the providers who will fight for you because they understand and care about you as a person. I sensed and trusted the approach and care I received by two female physicians for gynecological cancer. I was confident my doctors looked out for me both as a patient and a woman. This made all the difference in my care and post-treatment quality of life.

2. A small inner circle: "Your circle may get smaller as you go through this" was wisdom I received early on. Holding close a select few trusted loved ones will be your mirrors when you can't see your way through and your railings when you need someone to hold onto to steady yourself. Cancer is horrific. It's as ugly as you think, and then so much worse. It's okay that not everyone has the stomach to join you for the journey and it's helpful to be prepared to watch your relationships transition and change as you go.

3. A self-preservation mindset: Believe you deserve the freedom to put yourself first and ask for everything you need. You can hit pause on the demands of life as best as possible as you go through this. Outsource as much as you can without fear of judgment (errands, meals, childcare, etc.) You'll both need and use the time, space and energy, so carve it out from the jump.

4. Safe processing tools: This looks different for everyone, but the important thing is to identify and try them to see what works for you. A few that comes to mind: therapy, acupuncture, massage, CBD, and cannabis products.

5. Prepare to celebrate EVERY. SINGLE. WIN: Staying positive all the time is hard, so find ways to recognize the good and raise it up. Had an easy time getting the IV in for an infusion? Ring the bell to cheer you on! Made it through your first brachytherapy procedure? That's cause for a balloon drop! Every milestone is one closer to the rest of your hard-fought, hard-earned life so be sure to recognize your incredible accomplishments as you go!

You are a person of great influence. If you could inspire a movement that would bring the most amount of good to the greatest amount of people, what would that be?

To destigmatize and raise our level of awareness and understanding of HPV and cervical cancer screening. When we're uncomfortable and under informed, we're less likely to recognize a problem or voice a concern; this can be life-threatening. My hope is to bring these conversations out of the shadows and whisper networks so every woman feels comfortable advocating for herself to prevent cervical cancer.

We are very blessed that some very prominent names in Business, VC funding, Sports, and Entertainment read this column. Is there a person in the world, or in the US with whom you would love to have a private breakfast or lunch, and why?

I would love to share a meal with @kamalaharris and @melindagates and—please let me know when we're scheduled! :) I'm so inspired by each woman's extraordinary work: Vice President Harris' commitment to fighting cancer and Melinda's work to lift girls and women in some of the dangerous environments globally. Their dedication to women's health, domestically and internationally, is powerful confirmation that using my voice to do this work is so very important.

How can our readers further follow your work online?

Please visit www.EveMcDavid.com to stay close to my journey to transform cervical healthcare, connect with me on LinkedIn and follow me on Twitter: @evemcdavid

Flora Migyanka of The Dynami Foundation: I Survived (Breast) Cancer and Here Is How I Did It

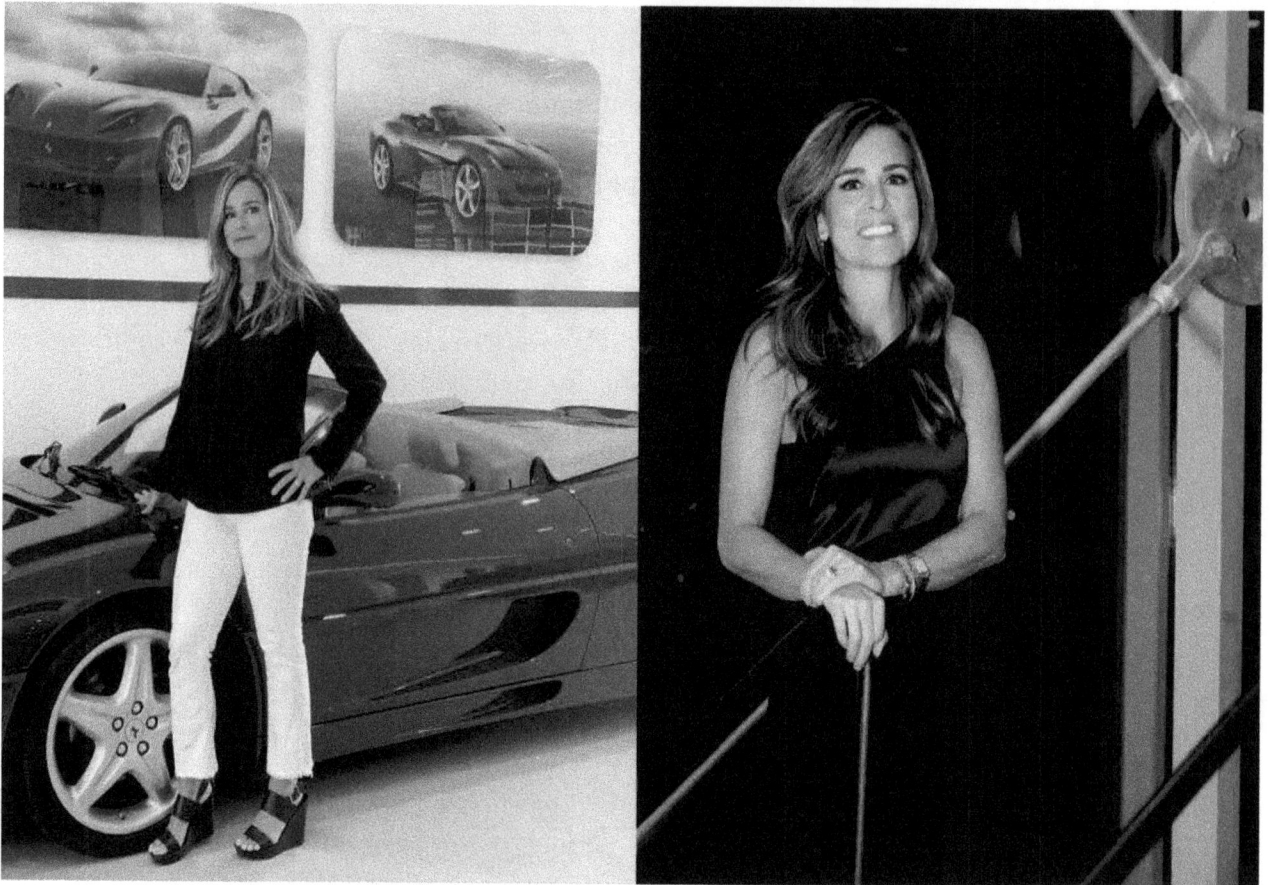

Gratefulness makes you happy. Happiness does not make you grateful. Learning to see the beauty in any situation and not react. Stress is also a very important factor in managing not only your physical health but mental health. Take up a yoga class or some form of release. Learn to breathe and let go of situations that you have no control over. We must let go of certain things in life that may bother us. Lowering our stress level is easier said than done but it is important to find that outlet to find your inner peace. It is a daily practice and journey.

I had the pleasure of interviewing Flora Migyanka. Flora is the Founder and President of The Dynami Foundation. Most importantly, she is a mother of two children, breast cancer survivor and patient advocate.

After she went for her first mammogram screening at age 40, Flora was diagnosed with Stage 1 Invasive Lobular Carcinoma and treated at the University of Michigan Rogel Cancer Center, one of the nation's leading centers for breast cancer care. After a long road which involved a bilateral mastectomy, reconstruction, and ongoing tamoxifen therapy, Flora came out on the other side healthy and cancer-free.

Flora felt healthy and inspired to spread her story to increase funds and awareness surrounding breast cancer, which affects one in eight women in the U.S., by creating The Dynami Foundation. The foundation's key fundraiser, Uncork for a Cure was launched six years ago in a suburb in Michigan as a fundraiser for breast cancer research. Since then, the annual event has grown tenfold, incorporating the city's award-winning chefs, sommeliers, and artists all uniting for one cause: breast cancer research and awareness. To date, over one million dollars have been raised.

Aside from hosting Uncork for a Cure, Flora volunteers her time teaching yoga to cancer survivors for the Cancer Support Community. She is on the Breast Cancer Patient Advisory Board at University of Michigan, and the National Steering Committee for the Lobular Breast Cancer Alliance.

Flora has a passion for her Greek roots (Dynami is the Greek word for 'strength') and resides in Plymouth Michigan with her family. Besides advocating for breast cancer, Flora is an account executive at a global biotech company.

Thank you so much for joining us in this interview series! We really appreciate the courage it takes to publicly share your story. Before we start, our readers would love to "get to know you" a bit better. Can you tell us a bit about your background and your childhood backstory?

I grew up in New London Connecticut, a small coastal New England town also known as the whaling city. I grew up at the "beach" and the sea is my happy place. My family is from Greece and owned a produce business, specifically bananas. My mom helped with the business bookkeeping, managed me and my siblings and loved to cook. I have one older sister and older brother. I was the third child. They were both a bit older than me so I was very much independent at a very young age. I had to figure out a lot on my own at a very young age. I started my first job in 4th grade as a paper route delivery person. I would get on my bike after school each day and deliver the newspapers to all my customers. My father instilled in me at a young age that we work hard, have grit, a bit of tough love, and that life sometimes is not fair. I most likely got my work ethic from him. As I got older, I held 2–3 jobs working in restaurants as a server, bus girl, bartender you name it. I loved working in the hospitality industry. I started my post college career at Johnson and Johnson as an account rep. It was great extensive training and mentorship to better articulate, communicate and learn to work with people. I have now been with a biotech company focusing on new cancer therapies for over 10 years as an account manager and in the industry over 25 years. I love helping people and making a difference.

Can you please give us your favorite "Life Lesson Quote?" Can you share how that was relevant to you in your life?

"You get strength, courage and confidence by every experience in which you really stop to look fear in the face...do the thing you think you cannot do." —Eleanor Roosevelt

It takes a lot of courage to be vulnerable and face fear and being dealt with a deck of cards you did not ask for. I learned this at a young age as my father had Parkinson's disease and suffered for a very long time and tragically died. I watched first hand suffering, courage and being vulnerable. As I move through my own health journey, I find through sharing my story and connecting with other women and knowing I can provide a sense of calm and help work through this fear together, is an incredibly healing process for me and the women I have met along this path.

Let's now shift to the main part of our discussion about surviving cancer. Do you feel comfortable sharing with us the story surrounding how you found out that you had cancer?

For me, the clock stopped on April 21, 2012 at 4:03 pm. I answered the phone while en route to the bus to pick up my daughter from kindergarten. My thee-year-old son was still napping. I had my first routine mammogram just weeks earlier, and mostly it had just been an annoyance to schedule. I was a busy working mom, and why should I be thinking about cancer? I was only 40 and I was healthy. I practiced yoga, ate well, did not smoke, and a small family history. People who are in good health don't get cancer, or so I thought. After my first images, radiology called back, but I didn't think much of it. We were away on a ski trip and I thought I would deal with that when I get back. I had to get more images, then immediately two biopsies, and then four days of waiting. And then the call. "YOU HAVE BREAST CANCER." You never want to hear those words. It literally took my breath away. I was diagnosed with Stage 1 Invasive Lobular Breast Cancer.

I knew I wanted the best care I could possibly get. Every case is different and unique. The University of Michigan Breast Center was the absolute best choice for my case. Even through the terror of the diagnosis, I had a sense of peace when I met my doctors. When you're diagnosed with a disease like cancer, you quickly become an expert on things you never thought you would want or need to know like how many doctors' appointments you can fit into a day while juggling being a mom and keeping that brave face for your children. You will experience a new form of tiredness you never thought possible. The day you are diagnosed is the day you will see life from a different lens.

After a Bilateral Mastectomy reconstruction, I had a long road of rehabbing with complications from my surgery. I was unlucky and developed lymphedema, seromas, and post mastectomy pain syndrome. I was in occupational therapy and physical therapy for two years. It was a full-time job to get well. I had my family and an army of good friends and neighbors who helped me and felt very fortunate. I am now in my 9th year of taking tamoxifen, a type of anti-estrogen therapy that is recommended to decrease the chance of a type of breast cancer that needs estrogen to return. These therapies have shown to increase the chance of survival in women but must be taken for long periods of time—at least 5 years maybe 10 or longer and they come with their own set of side effects to manage. I have had many bumps on my journey, but I am VERY fortunate today.

What was the scariest part of that event? What did you think was the worst thing that could happen to you?

How my cancer diagnosis would affect my children and my husband, John. Our children were so young at the time -3 and 5 years old. They needed their mom. I was so worried about my family and so determined to get well to be present for all the milestones.

After the dust settled, what coping mechanisms did you use? What did you do to cope physically, mentally, emotionally, and spiritually?

I worked through the stress by diving deep into the practice of yoga to ease my mind, body and spirit—an act so critical to my healing process that I became a certified yoga instructor and volunteered my time teaching yoga to cancer survivors through the Cancer Support Community of Greater Ann Arbor. I find great peace in yoga and it's a daily practice to stay grounded. It is life changing.

Is there a particular person you are grateful towards who helped you learn to cope and heal? Can you share a story about that?

My husband John, my children and my friends who are so incredibly dear to me. I cherish every one of them.

In my own cancer struggle, I sometimes used the idea of embodiment to help me cope. Let's take a minute to look at cancer from an embodiment perspective. If your cancer had a message for you, what do you think it would want or say?

Being grateful. Gratefulness makes you happy. Happiness does not make you grateful. Learning to see the beauty in any situation and not react. Stress is also a very important factor in managing not only your physical health but mental health. Take up a yoga class or form of release. Learn to breathe and let go of situations that you have no control over. We must let go of certain things in life that may bother us. Lowering our stress level is easier said than done but it is important to find that outlet to find your inner peace. It is a daily practice and journey.

What did you learn about yourself from this very difficult experience? How has cancer shaped your worldview? What has it taught you that you might never have considered before? Can you please explain with a story or example?

Patients should become experts on their disease and feel empowered to ask many questions to their cancer team. Be bold. You need to be CEO of yourself, build your team of experts, research the best care and clinical trials and generate a strategic plan that best suits you. I feel the more engaged you are the more control you have—mentally and physically—over your care. You must not let the fear of the unknown paralyze you. It is very important to learn all of your family history. Whatever disease it is. Having a family history of early onset breast cancer in close relatives may be a reason to investigate genetic testing. Women with close relatives who've been diagnosed with breast cancer have a higher risk of developing the disease. So, for you, it is important to be proactive and have the conversation with your doctor and be followed closely.

Maybe that is a closer screening plan which would be tailored to your situation.

Research is also critical. I have worked in the biotech industry for over 25 years and know firsthand the value of such trials. I see instances of new therapies being developed for many diseases, with some patients exhausting all options before entering a clinical trial that could save their lives. Some are very fortunate, and others are not, but without doing these trials and supporting research, the scientists will not make any progress.

How have you used your experience to bring goodness to the world?

My experience and sense of urgency led me to found an event called Uncork for a Cure which started in 2016. The event was an idea over a glass of bubbly with my first cousin and master sommelier, Madeline Triffon of Plum Market, and Luciano DelSignore of Bacco Ristorante and Pernoi. They believed in me to take this idea and leap. I felt this need to highlight and bring together great culinary leaders with the booming food scene in Detroit while aiding and elevating the need to support breast cancer. There was no event like this in the metro Detroit area. Breast cancer is so pervasive. The statistics have not changed. One in eight will be diagnosed in their lifetime. Since its inception, the annual event has grown tenfold, incorporating the city of Detroit's award-winning chefs, sommeliers and artists all uniting for one cause: breast cancer research and awareness. The hospitality industry has come together to show their support and meet this challenge. From great need can come great generosity.

In just five years, Uncork for a Cure along with our nonprofit, the Dynami Foundation, has raised over one million dollars funding six research studies on Lobular Breast Cancer, an underfunded and underresearched common subtype of breast cancer which accounts to 40k women diagnosed a year. We are determined to change this statistic on Lobular Breast Cancer and funding research is the only way. By collaborating with our community and supporting the researchers, physicians and continued patient outreach, we will further foster our direct impact locally and nationally.

Fantastic. Here is the main question of our interview. Based on your experiences and knowledge, what advice would you give to others who have recently been diagnosed with cancer? What are your "5 Things" You Need To Beat Cancer? Please share a story or example for each.

- You need to be CEO of yourself, build your team of experts, research the best care and clinical trials and generate a strategic plan that best suits you. I feel the more engaged you are, the more control you have—mentally and physically—over your care.
- Advocate and Educate yourself
- Find an outlet whether yoga, running, group class, or walking. It helps your mind process any pain, and learning to let go, to accept things you can't change and learning to love yourself and be content.

- Don't let fear paralyze you
- Be Bold. Take Chances. Life is so short.

You are a person of great influence. If you could inspire a movement that would bring the most amount of good to the greatest amount of people, what would that be?

In the next year, 280,000 women and men in the U.S. will receive a breast cancer diagnosis. One in 8 women in this country will be diagnosed in their lifetime. To me, the fight is personal. I ask the community to make it personal as well—that my story and the stories of those you love inspire you to keep fighting with me, to broaden the reach we have together. I have the strength to speak out, to share with you my story, and to represent all those who need our help and support. The story of my diagnosis is one of thousands, but if it helps you to put a face to the work ahead, I am glad to have shared it with you.

How can our readers further follow your work online?

The Dynami Foundation works all year long to educate and raise funds for research.

This November the Dynami Foundation is so thrilled to have an event again and to bring people together to celebrate. Indoor and outdoor space will be used to make sure everyone feels safe. We are also raffling off a F355 Classic Ferrari! It will be a very exciting evening!

www.dynamifoundation.org

Grant Lottering: I Survived (Melanoma) Cancer and Here Is How I Did It

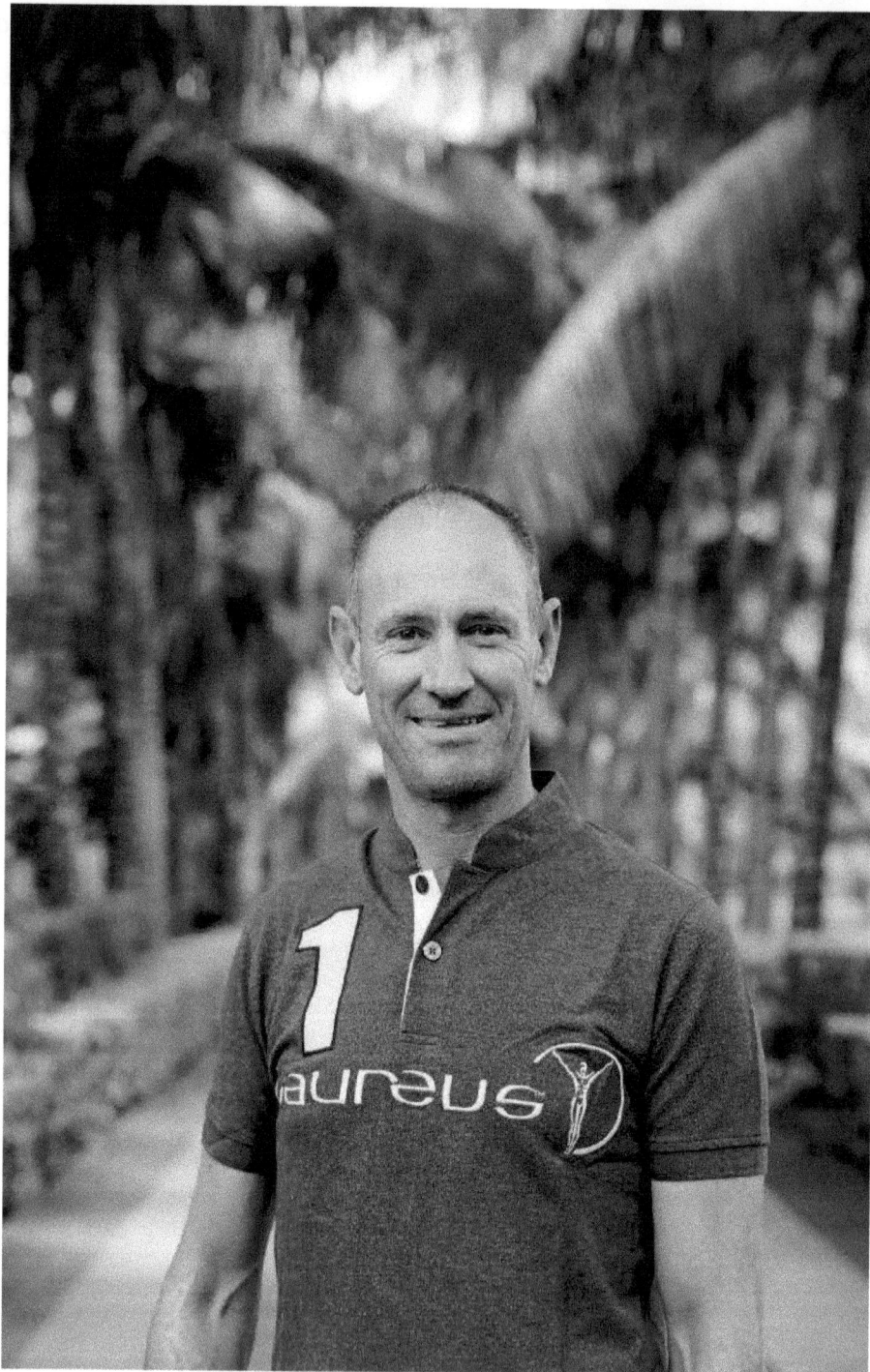

Make the decision to start looking after your body and to glorify God. So many people let go of their physical condition and don't live healthy until they get a medical scare. Do not wait until then. Your body and physical ability is a gift from God. Appreciate it, look after it and be grateful.

I had the pleasure of interviewing Grant Lottering, Springbok Cyclist and Laureus Sport for Good Ambassador. Grant's remarkable comeback from death on July 21, 2013 to conquering the French Alps, Pyrenees and now South Africa continues to astonish the medical profession and audiences alike. His remarkable story of survival and overcoming has attracted much media attention locally and world-wide, reaching over 33 million people through broadcast, print and online media. To date, he has raised millions for underprivileged children through his annual Im'possible Tours. What makes his accomplishments so remarkable is that he has undergone 12 surgeries between 2013–2018 due to his accident. In addition, he was diagnosed with cancer in December 2016 and had to deal with emergency cancer surgery.

Grant has shared his story 'From Death to the Top of the Alps' with audiences in over 11 countries to date at conferences and corporate events including the U.K., Singapore, Holland, Belgium, Germany, France, Mauritius, Zambia, Namibia and South Africa.

Thank you so much for joining us in this interview series! We really appreciate the courage it takes to publicly share your story. Before we start, our readers would love to "get to know you" a bit better. Can you tell us a bit about your background and your childhood backstory?

My passion for cycling developed when I was 12-years-old growing up in Johannesburg, South Africa. By the time I turned 18, I made junior Springbok colours (national colours) twice. By 20, I was a professional cyclist and raced in Europe in 1987–1989. Today, I am an Extreme Endurance Cyclist and Laureus Sport for Good Ambassador. My comeback from being declared dead on July 21, 2013, to conquering the French Alps, Pyrenees, South Africa, and now the USA continues to astonish the medical profession and audiences alike.

Described as a remarkable tale of survival and overcoming, my story has attracted much media attention worldwide, reaching over 60 million people through broadcast, print, and online media. To date, I am very proud and privileged to have raised millions of dollars for underprivileged children in disadvantaged communities in South Africa. Since my accident in 2013, I have undergone 12 surgeries. In addition, I had to overcome emergency cancer surgery.

Can you please give us your favorite "Life Lesson Quote?" Can you share how that was relevant to you in your life?

It is a bible verse in Proverbs: "Acknowledge God in your plans, and He will direct your paths." I realized that life is much more fulfilling when it's not just about you and your accomplishments. This principle keeps me grounded and humbled knowing that ultimately, we do not control tomorrow.

Let's now shift to the main part of our discussion about surviving cancer. Do you feel comfortable sharing with us the story surrounding how you found out that you had cancer?

Absolutely.

What was the scariest part of that event? What did you think was the worst thing that could happen to you?

When my surgeon called me two days after my biopsy and said the result was not good. He said, "You have a very aggressive, invasive melanoma and it has grown dangerously deep. You must come in as soon as possible for urgent surgery. Can we make arrangements for tomorrow?" At that moment I realized that I am now fighting an invisible disease, not just fractures, and rehabilitative surgeries as I have been doing since my accident in 2013 (11 surgeries). Being mentally strong and supremely determined, in hindsight, it was much easier to overcome those surgeries as they are visible; I feel it. I can do physical therapy and rehab because I see the improvements. It is measurable. Now, I had to deal with a killer which is not visible, and it had the potential to end my cycling career right there.

How did you react in the short term?

It was a frightening prospect at first. I went for surgery the next day and woke up in hospital with an 8 cm x 4 cm hole in my left hamstring. I have to admit I was concerned for the coming 12 months to see if I would be clear. I lost a lot of sleep those first few weeks!

After the dust settled, what coping mechanisms did you use? What did you do to cope physically, mentally, emotionally, and spiritually?

Having overcome so much since surviving that near-fatal accident on July 21st, 2013, I told myself, *God has got this, and this is just another setback that you will overcome. God's purpose for my life will be fulfilled, rest in Him and wait on Him.*

I have dedicated my life to cycling through some of the most challenging terrains, pushing myself to new extremes, and setting new records. I have been fortunate to complete extreme endurance rides across the world in aid of charities such as Laureus Sport for Good Foundation and the Reach for a Dream Foundation in South Africa. In addition, my partnership with UHSM Health Share has contributed to strengthening my relationship with God and helped share my inspirational story and testimony of the second chance at the life God has given me to audiences. Through this partnership, I have promoted healthy means of coping emotionally and spirituality with holistic well-being.

Is there a particular person you are grateful towards who helped you learn to cope and heal? Can you share a story about that?

My brother Glenn, who is 3 years older than me and lives in Holland. When he heard of my accident in Trento, Italy in 2013 he immediately traveled to be with me while I spent 9 days in ICU. Since then, he has been at every one of my Im'possible Tours and has been a pillar of encouragement and support. He himself had to deal with skin cancer and was a voice of reason and wisdom on many occasions. We have a very special bond of friendship and trust and when I need an ear of encouragement, he is the one I turn to.

In my own cancer struggle, I sometimes used the idea of embodiment to help me cope.

Let's take a minute to look at cancer from an embodiment perspective. If your cancer had a message for you, what do you think it would want or say?

For me, there was a very important lesson given my situation. Since 2013, I have proven medical professionals wrong by not only getting back on a bike but cycling further and longer than ever before. My mental strength and focus played a massive part in pushing my own physical and mental boundaries. As a result of the success I achieved, I grew in confidence and learned that very little is impossible when you are mentally strong and committed. When I suddenly had to deal with cancer, it was a humbling experience, and getting back on my knees made me realize that tomorrow is never guaranteed, that no matter how much we achieve and overcome, we need God in our lives. That is what cancer taught me.

How have you used your experience to bring goodness to the world?

God has given me a second chance at life. He made it possible for me to continue using my gift and talent to ride a bicycle.

How my accident did not leave me paralyzed remains a mystery, but it was clear very early on that God planned on using my talent and testimony to be relevant, to challenge, and to inspire people. Today, I live with intent and purpose. Whatever cycling project I plan to do with my sponsors, the core focus is always to raise money for underprivileged children. Secondly, to share my testimony and life story with businesses and at conferences that we all get second chances in life. If we live a life of gratitude, it becomes difficult to find things to complain about. I have been fortunate to share my story with corporations, conferences, and churches in over 12 countries across the world.

What are a few of the biggest misconceptions and myths out there about fighting cancer that you would like to dispel?

"I am healthy and fit, and the thought that I could have cancer doesn't exist."

Since I was given the all-clear at the end of 2017—after a year and multiple rounds of blood tests—I have been going for annual preventative check-ups and blood tests. People don't take preventative care seriously, which causes them to postpone or put off annual check-ups.

Fantastic. Here is the main question of our interview. Based on your experiences and knowledge, what advice would you give to others who have recently been diagnosed with cancer? What are your "5 Things" You Need To Beat Cancer? Please share a story or example for each.

1. You need to be mentally strong—become your own biggest fan and refuse to let the disease into your mind so to speak (I think my own story and details shared above speaks to this).
2. Now, more than ever have a vision of where you are going with your life, and clear goals to keep you focused on tomorrow, and not what you are dealing with daily. After my accident, after my diagnosis and the real threat that my cycling career could be seriously interrupted, I had to make sure my focus was not on where I was or the situation I was in,

but where I saw myself tomorrow. In other words, keeping my mental focus on tomorrow, and doing whatever I can today, to get there.

3. Surround yourself with positive people who will encourage and uplift your spirits, rather than share their worries and concerns about your condition and the 'what if's.

4. Make the decision to start looking after your body and to glorify God. So many people let go of their physical condition and don't live healthy until they get a medical scare. Do not wait until then. Your body and physical ability are a gift from God. Appreciate it, look after it and be grateful.

5. GIVE GOD 1ST PLACE IN YOUR LIFE. Both mentally and physically. If you apply step 4 in your life, you are allowing God to put His super, on your natural. That is when healing, overcoming and victory comes from. I've experienced that first-hand every year when I attempt my extreme endurance Im'possible Tours. Considering I ride 600+ miles over 20 - 30 mountains without stopping or sleeping, I never would have been able to do on my own, given my physical condition, since my accidents. Every time I start a tour, I feel God's supernatural strength carrying me, enabling me to complete what I start. To honour Him as a result.

You are a person of great influence. If you could inspire a movement that would bring the most amount of good to the greatest amount of people, what would that be?

To encourage people to become more outward-focused. Every one of us has the ability to make a positive difference in others' lives. There is always someone worse off than we are, no matter what situation we find ourselves in.

We are very blessed that some very prominent names in Business, VC funding, Sports, and Entertainment read this column. Is there a person in the world, or in the US with whom you would love to have a private breakfast or lunch, and why?

Without a doubt, Greg LeMond! He was the very first American to win the Tour de France in 1986. After Greg was accidentally shot in the back in 1987 by his father-in-law while hunting, he was written off as a professional cyclist in Europe. Yet, in 1989 he made the biggest comeback ever seen in professional cycling by winning the Tour de France by 8 seconds and the World Championships! The following year in 1990, he won his 3rd Tour de France with over 50 shotgun pellets still in his body. He was my cycling hero in the eighties, and it's special knowing we both overcame death and fought our way back from scratch.

How can our readers further follow your work online?

The best place is to visit my website www.grantlottering.com. Hyperlinks to all my social media handles are on my homepage as well as links to my YouTube videos of my testimony and my Im'possible Tours.

Howard Katz: I Survived (Pancreatic) Cancer and Here Is How I Did It

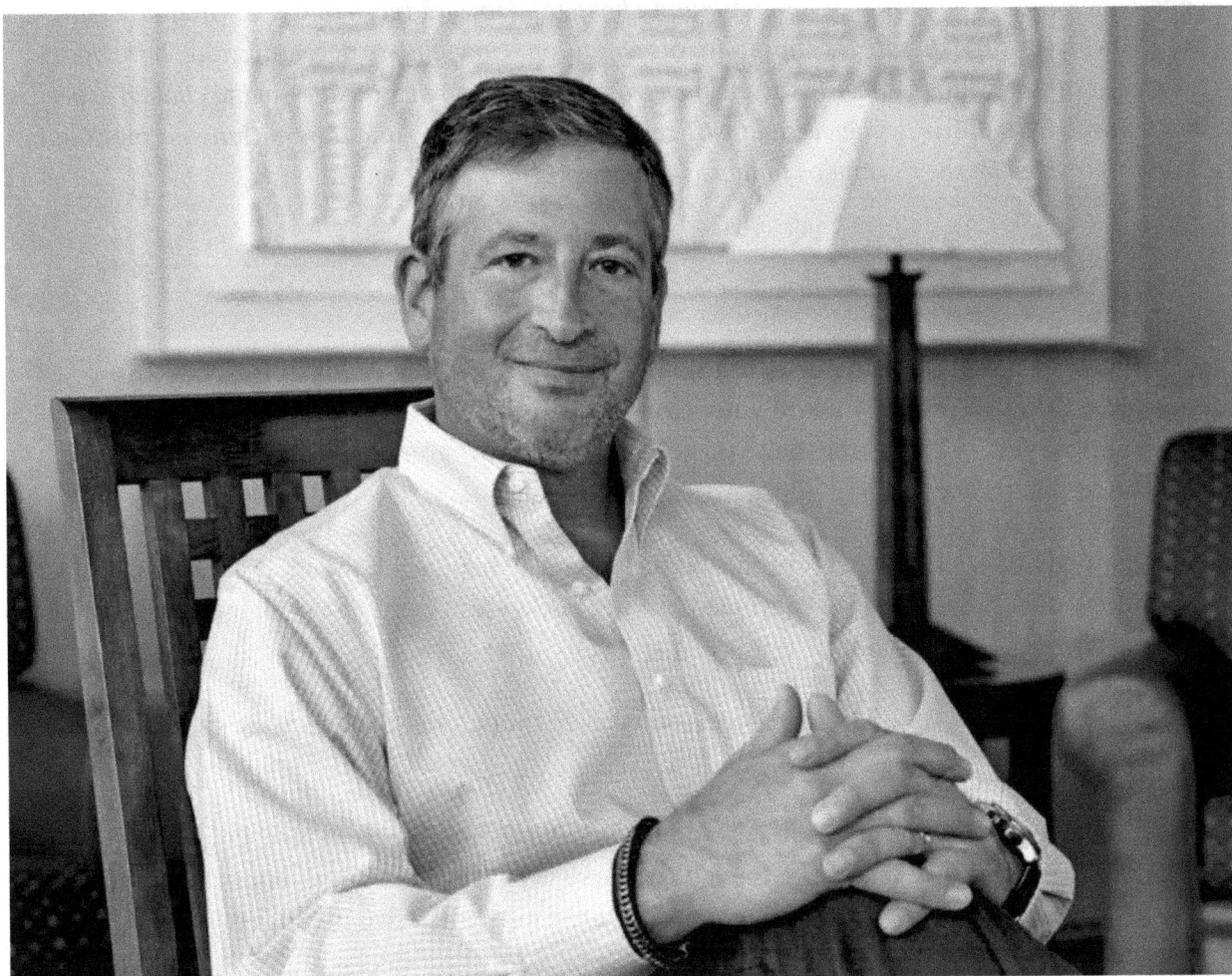

Find strength in winning small battles. When you're at a low point, focus not on your survival but on winning the little battles in your treatment and recovery. Finding the strength to get yourself through the next hour or day or week can be uplifting when you accomplish it. For a longer-term approach focus on how you're going to give back once you get through your battle. I motivated myself by looking forward to helping others. I remember thinking, 'once I beat this, I'm going to help other people figure out how to beat cancer.' I'll never give back as much as I've received, but I can try.

I had the pleasure of interviewing Howard Katz. Howard is a nine-year survivor of Stage 4 pancreatic cancer. Diagnosed at his community hospital, Howard received a poor prognosis, given the 3% five-year survival rate for those with his condition. Unwilling to accept his fate, he sought treatment at Karmanos Cancer Institute in Detroit, where he credits the life-saving clinical expertise and innovative treatments pioneered at NCI centers like Karmanos and the continuous emotional support provided by the Karmanos family as the reasons he's alive today.

Thank you so much for joining us in this interview series! We really appreciate the courage it takes to publicly share your story. Before we start, our readers would love to "get to know you" a bit better. Can you tell us a bit about your background and your childhood backstory?

I grew up in a nice suburb of Boston, and had a typical, happy childhood. I played sports all through childhood and even continued playing hockey and lacrosse through college at Bates College in Lewiston, Maine.

I've always been a big fan of Boston sports teams, even though I've lived in Michigan for almost 20 years.

I came to Michigan because I was relocated for work. I'd spent 17 years in New England working in regional sales for Chrysler, but as the industry joke says, "If you rise high enough in the auto industry, your reward is a transfer to Detroit." So, after more than two decades my family is still here and we love it.

I've been married to my best friend and love of my life for 36 years and we have two great daughters, ages 31 and 29. We moved here when they were 10 and 12 years old. It stings me a little bit that my kids consider themselves Michiganders, but we visit back home every summer. Travel is one of our passions and my career has provided the opportunity to travel extensively in the US and internationally.

I turned 60 in June.

Can you please give us your favorite "Life Lesson Quote?" Can you share how that was relevant to you in your life?

I have several, all attributed to my mother. We always joked in my family about "Nanna's words of wisdom." She had lots of little sayings, but one that I kept coming back to in my cancer fight was, "If you think you can't, you're right." In other words, your attitude about any challenge is everything.

I've tried to share that lesson with my kids and to live by it. Mom also used to say, "I'll tell you what you can't do. Otherwise you give it your best." Of course, I don't remember her ever telling me there was something I couldn't do.

In my life, as I've approached daunting or challenging situations, I always remember my mother's mantra, that you can do anything you put your mind to and if you do your best, no one can ask for more. Whether it's a career or personal challenge, attack it aggressively and do your best to succeed, keeping in mind that you define your own success. It's not defined by other people.

Let's now shift to the main part of our discussion about surviving cancer. Do you feel comfortable sharing with us the story surrounding how you found out that you had cancer?

My diagnosis was in July 2012. I was 51 years old. It was a pretty stressful time in my life. I had been recruited away from Chrysler to an executive position in Indiana, running sales and business development for a commercial truck manufacturer. My wife Cynthia and I were supposed to relocate there eventually. The girls were out of the house by then, so until we knew this job was a good long-term fit, and we could find a place we both wanted to live, I leased an apartment and drove the three hours down on Monday morning and back on Friday night.

I recall one Friday on my drive home from Indiana that I had a bad stomachache. I remember thinking I should go to the doctor. I thought I probably had an ulcer, which I didn't consider too serious. With all the stress of the weekly commutes, the new job, living on my own, not eating very well, entertaining customers and clients until late at night—a lifestyle I had lived most of my working life—I assumed an ulcer was likely, but very treatable. I went to my primary care physician about a week later and he said, "You're over 50 and you've never had a colonoscopy, let's start there."

So, the colonoscopy was ordered, and an endoscopy quickly followed.

When the endoscopy results came back, they said they had found some "cancerous tendencies," and referred me to a surgeon. This is where my denial began. Most people would have heard, *you have cancer,* but I never heard that. What I heard was, *we found something and now we need to go in and address it.*

I went to the surgeon, still not fully comprehending what was going on. My presurgical consult was with his physician assistant. She brought out a diagram of the digestive system and pointed out the pancreas and said, "The tumor is blocking the head of the pancreas and the bile ducts from your gallbladder."

My wife had already understood it was pancreatic cancer, but not me. They said the goal of the surgery was to remove the tumor at the head of my pancreas. Up to this point nobody had used the term "pancreatic cancer." What I heard was, *if we remove that tumor, you're home free.* Today I'm sure that's not what they said, but it's what I heard.

The next step was the operation, called a Whipple procedure—a six to seven hour surgery to remove the head of the pancreas, the first part of the small intestine, the gallbladder and bile duct. I never had major surgery, only relatively minor surgeries on my ankle and rotator cuff, but nothing invasive like this. When they put me in the full body warming suit, I realized the seriousness of this procedure and my condition. Less than an hour into the surgery, the surgeon came out and told my wife he couldn't continue the surgery because they found metastasis throughout my liver and spleen and there was no way surgically to remove all the tumors. He closed me up and referred me to an oncologist.

When I woke up, my wife was at my bedside by herself. I remember asking something like, "Are we all set?"

That's when she told me they couldn't finish the surgery. She told me, "You have cancer, it's in your pancreas, liver and spleen and they have to attack this medically."

That was shocking, but I was still somewhat in denial. I thought, *well, I'll have more treatment and then I'll be fine. It never occurred to me that I might die.* I didn't look at the internet, and I didn't do a lot of research on pancreatic cancer because I knew it was very serious and I didn't want to know the odds. Lots of famous people, like Steve Jobs and more recently, Alex Trebek had this disease, both of whom passed away. It's definitely not the cancer one would choose if they got to pick from a list.

What was the scariest part of that event? What did you think was the worst thing that could happen to you?

My recovery from surgery took a month, during which I started doing some research. The scariest part was finding out my cancer had a 5% survival rate. Dying was a very realistic possibility for people with my diagnosis.

We immediately started interviewing oncologists. I was unpleasantly shocked by my first experience. The oncologist came in with a resident and the resident did most of the talking while the oncologist sat back. He said, "You've got a very serious cancer. We can treat it with chemotherapy, but you're not a candidate for radiation because your tumors aren't isolated. They're spread out into multiple organs. But the outcome for this treatment is often uncertain."

We didn't like that answer. I had four weeks to recover from the surgery, and in that time, we decided to continue interviewing oncologists.

Although we'd lived in Michigan for 10 years, we have no family here, so we had no history of dealing with serious illness locally, and where to go for the best cancer treatment isn't something you think about until you have to.

Through a friend of a friend we learned about Karmanos Cancer Institute in Detroit. I didn't know at the time it was an NCI-Designated Cancer Center or even what that meant. We were able to get an appointment that week with an oncologist at the Institute. His comment to me was much more positive than my first experience. He said, "No question that with Stage 4 disease your case is very serious, but you're younger and stronger than most who get this diagnosis at a much later age. Therefore, we think you can handle a much more aggressive treatment regimen, which will give you the best possible chance for a successful outcome."

And, right away, he started me on a very aggressive chemotherapy regimen of Folfurinox, a combination treatment of several chemotherapy drugs used for pancreatic and bowel cancers. The side effects are significant: nausea, weight loss, lack of appetite and the development of peripheral neuropathy. It's supposed to be a twelve-course regimen over multiple months, but I had treatment every two to three weeks. Each chemo treatment was an eight hour infusion session. After about eight treatments, I had lost almost 70 pounds and, I'll be honest, I thought I was going to die of malnutrition before the cancer got me. I couldn't eat, and anything I tried to force down passed through me. I was also freezing cold the whole time. I was in my bed 24/7 bundled up in fleeces, socks, hats and gloves, shivering, sweating and crawling to the bathroom. It was a miserable time, but I kept telling myself this (whatever I was dealing with at the moment) is the worst part of a terrible journey. If I can get through this minute, this hour, and this day, there's light at the end of the tunnel, and it isn't necessarily a train.

After about half of the scheduled treatments I had an MRI, but it didn't show that anything was really changing with my cancer. But my Karmanos team was never negative. I remember asking my oncologist, "If this doesn't work, how long do I have?" He refused to answer that question because he said, "There are no absolutes during treatment. Every patient is an individual and every case is different so quoting averages and statistics is neither accurate nor helpful."

After eight treatments and months of hell, my oncologist was concerned about my declining health. He said it was time to consider my "quality of life," and he recommended I stop the treatments. I responded, "Quality of life and chemotherapy shouldn't go in the same sentence, they cannot coexist." I said I'd worry about "quality of life" after I finished the chemotherapy.

My impression at the time was the talk about "quality of life" was a euphemism for dying comfortably, and I wasn't there yet. I considered discontinuing the treatment equivalent to giving up, and I wasn't there yet either. However, after ten chemo treatments, I was physically and emotionally beaten up to the point where I came to agree with him and said, "No mas." I was exhausted and couldn't afford any more weight loss. Dr. Philip explained that even if we discontinued active treatment, the Folfurinox was by now entrenched in my system and would continue to have an impact on my disease. He prescribed Xeloda, an oral chemotherapy that could continue to address the disease, but with less dramatic side effects.

However, about this time we started to see signs of hope. The latest scans showed some shrinkage in the tumors; it appeared that the chemo had started to work. In the scan after that, the tumors had shrunk dramatically. Most of the liver tumors had cleared completely and the tumor on my pancreas had shrunk considerably. After one more check, probably six months after Folfurinox treatment had stopped, I was tumor-free. I had gained 30 pounds back and was slowly starting to feel stronger. I remained on Xeloda for 18 months.

My biggest fear during all this was if I was going to die from the treatment, not the cancer. I was losing weight and strength so quickly and had neuropathy. I couldn't walk well, and I couldn't pick things up, and even after treatment I was miserable. It was clear to me I was never going to be the same physically and mentally as I was before cancer, and that was daunting. Even today, after nine years, my recall isn't what it used to be, and the neuropathy keeps my hands and feet numb, making walking and things requiring manual dexterity difficult, but I often say this condition is far better than the alternative. Any day you see the green side of the grass has the potential to be a good day so rather than dwelling on the residual effects of cancer treatments I've chosen to be grateful.

How did you react in the short term?

I was always thinking positively but was worried about what life would be like after this experience, even if my cancer was cured. Would I be permanently disabled? Would I be able to do the things I always loved to do? Would I be able to care for my family, financially, emotionally and physically?

These thoughts were scary. I had disability and life insurance policies that would take care of my family financially whether I survived or not, which was reassuring, but the harsh reality that this is what I had to think about was upsetting. I decided to try the best I could to push those thoughts aside and focus on the moment, not looking too far into the future.

After the dust settled, what coping mechanisms did you use? What did you do to cope physically, mentally, emotionally and spiritually?

During my treatment my goal was to maintain a positive attitude. I would not allow myself to believe I would be among the 95% who don't survive pancreatic cancer. Admittedly, my rationale was convoluted, but there were several thoughts I tried to keep in my head in order to hold onto a positive outlook. They included:

- I'm not going to die. Dying is for other people. If 5% of patients with my disease do survive, why shouldn't I be in the 5% rather than the 95%?
- Statistics are not really numbers, they're people. Statistics include the whole universe of those affected, and while they call attention to the majority—those who lost their battle—they also include the survivors. I'll simply be a statistic who survived and not one who didn't.
- I did the math in my head. Though it's probably not very accurate, from statistics I had come across, I calculated that about 50,000 people are diagnosed with pancreatic cancer annually and 40,000 die from it annually. That leaves 10,000 survivors. How hard could it be to be one in 10,000? I'd spent my life competing to be number one, being number 9,999 didn't sound too hard to achieve.

This was mentally, emotionally and, I think, physically therapeutic.

Also, counseling helped considerably—not only for me, but for my wife and my entire family. I do have faith, and I don't discount its importance. Being Jewish, I talked to many people at my synagogue, and they provided much-needed emotional support. More importantly, they supported my family. I didn't have to worry about anything. Through "Caring Community," an active group at our temple, Temple Kol Ami in West Bloomfield, Michigan, individuals volunteered to prepare meals for the family, and brought them to our home daily for several months. They kept my wife engaged, relieving the constant weight of my situation.

I also want to credit Kathleen Hardy, an oncology social worker at Karmanos who worked with my family and me throughout my treatment and the months that followed. She shared perspectives that really helped put me on a path toward survival and recovery that would have been difficult without her help. She shared other survivor stories and constantly focused on the strength of my family and my amazing support system, and how I should draw inspiration from the sincere effort and caring of others. For so long I had been self-absorbed in my treatment and condition. Kathleen opened my eyes to all the wonderful things that were still around me, especially my family and all the people who were doing kind things to make our life easier.

Is there a particular person you are grateful towards who helped you learn to cope and heal? Can you share a story about that?

I'm lucky there were many people who helped me through this difficult experience. My wife Cynthia was my rock. She shows quiet strength and that's motivating to me. She doesn't dwell on any of the negatives. She just approaches everything on a day-to-day basis. Her attitude in dealing with adversity has always been, *this is what we have to face and we're going to take it on and deal with it. It doesn't help to get too dramatic or histrionic, just do what you have to do to deal with your problems and get through them.* As a software engineer, Cynthia is very calculating and direct. She looks at every challenge, big or small, and determines the best approach to address it successfully. In this way we complement each other very well. My wife is logical, organized and systematic, whereas I am emotional, dramatic, and creative.

Another key person was Kathleen, the social worker who helped me understand you get to choose how you approach challenges. You can make the choice to be positive versus negative, and you can choose to be around people who provide strength and empathy, versus the well-intentioned people who express sympathy. Sympathy from others is genuine, and you must appreciate the sincerity that accompanies it, but too much sympathy alone can validate feeling sorry for yourself. While everyone will have times they struggle with the "Why Me?" syndrome, ultimately it only leads you toward dwelling on your problems, and away from the positivity and inner strength you need to take them on.

I'm also incredibly grateful for my two daughters who gave me the inspiration to keep fighting. When I was diagnosed, my oldest daughter Sarah had just graduated college and started a new job in North Carolina. She made the incredibly unselfish choice to come home to support Cynthia and help focus on my care.

My younger daughter Emily was starting her junior year in college and was about to leave for six months in Thailand on a once in a lifetime study abroad program living with native peoples, in the city, in the rainforest and on the coast, studying environmental sustainability and how the lifestyles of these diverse cultures impact it. Initially, Emily wanted to cancel her travel and stay home to support me and help Cynthia. It took some time, but ultimately, we convinced her it was more therapeutic for me to know she was having such an enriching experience and allowing my disease to rob her of this opportunity would be more distressing to me. We pointed out that we could be in touch through Skype daily and that she could be home in a day if the need arose. Her decision to go halfway around the world at a time when the family was facing cancer was so courageous, it actually inspired me. Through her experience abroad, she was able to look at the world differently and she taught me there are lots of different ways to cope with personal struggles and that the easiest choices are not always the best ones. That resonated with me and became a source of needed encouragement.

In my own cancer struggle, I sometimes used the idea of embodiment to help me cope. Let's take a minute to look at cancer from an embodiment perspective. If your cancer had a message for you, what do you think it would want or say?

This is a tough one to answer, but I envision my cancer saying to me, "Hey you beat me. There aren't many who do. I'm successful at what I do. I kill 95% of the people I engage with, but you beat me."

It's a strange way to think about it, but it's one of my favorite takeaways. I won this battle.

What did you learn about yourself from this very difficult experience? How has cancer shaped your worldview? What has it taught you that you might never have considered before? Can you please explain with a story or example?

My journey has completely changed the way I look at the world. I'm a better person as a result of surviving cancer than I was before.

I think it's because when you're facing something you know will kill you if it "wins," you're able to see the things that are truly important. Those important things become obvious, as if they are in a spotlight, and the other things we all deal with—jobs, careers, finances—are relegated to the dark. While those "other things" can change your life, they don't change what's really important: family, friends and helping others the way others have helped you. My cancer caused me to turn the telescope around. Instead of looking through the end that magnifies your view, you look through the other end, which makes your field of vision much wider and objects you're traditionally focused on much smaller, further away and less significant. I became aware of all the support I had, which I was oblivious to when I was focused on my old daily routine. When my battle was ongoing, I was singularly focused, but now I can look back and see how much I depended on others to survive.

How have you used your experience to bring goodness to the world?

I don't take anything for granted. Today I appreciate the sun rising and the birds chirping. I always thought that kind of thing was too touchy-feely, but now I appreciate people with a mindset that values "the little things." Over time, careers and daily problems take over and it's easy to lose focus on what is truly important; not you, but others, and helping people who face struggles. I don't know if you could say I've brought goodness to the world, but personally, this journey has led me to truly living in the present and being attentive to the important things around us.

When I had cancer, I didn't like it when people told me, "Live in the now and focus on getting to tomorrow." I didn't want to live for tomorrow. I wanted to live for the future. That way I could look forward to my long, happy life without the struggles of cancer. I was only half right. In battling to survive, the strategy of short-term focus, going back to the idea of getting through this minute, this hour, this day, is very powerful because each day you can survive gets you closer to the "light at the end of the tunnel," which represented for me emerging from the darkness of cancer back into the light where you can enjoy "quality of life."

Today I sit on the Karmanos Cancer Institute's Patient and Family Advisory Council (PFAC), to help current cancer patients and their caregivers by providing the best possible environment for them to manage their personal battles. I also volunteered in the Karmanos Infusion Center. I'm not a formal counselor, but I have gotten strength from talking to people who are facing similar struggles to what I faced. Because I've been there and I understand what they're going through I think I can appreciate their fears, concerns and challenges, and I can provide a different type of empathy by recounting some of the strategies that helped me when I was facing what these people are dealing with right now. It is very gratifying.

What are a few of the biggest misconceptions and myths out there about fighting cancer that you would like to dispel?

Survivability for pancreatic cancer is improving. I'm living proof that the perception of pancreatic cancer as a definite death sentence needs to be dispelled. When I talk to current patients, I want to tell them to hold on to hope and never give up. Another misconception about fighting cancer is that good medicine is the exclusive path to survival. It's a necessary component of the "Survival Plan," but it's not the only component. Positive attitude, the sincere feeling that you can and will defeat cancer, is as necessary a component to survival as the medicine.

Another misconception is that you're in the battle with cancer by yourself, even though there may be many people caring and wanting to help. This is not true. If you can figure out how to take the genuine caring and help that other people want to give, you can turn that into a powerful tool to bolster your own strength and your ability to continue a long and exhausting fight. When I talk to patients and caregivers, I want to provide hope, but I'm straight with people. There's no guarantee that believing you will survive means you will, but I am convinced if you believe you're not going to make it, you're right, and if you believe you will make it, you give yourself a much better chance.

Fantastic. Here is the main question of our interview. Based on your experiences and knowledge, what advice would you give to others who have recently been diagnosed with cancer? What are your "5 Things" You Need To Beat Cancer? Please share a story or example for each.

1. Attitude: If you think you can't, you'll always be right. It goes for battling cancer, too. Adopting as positive an attitude as possible will increase your chances for a better outcome.
2. Accept help, and appreciate it, wherever it may come from: As badly as you're feeling, make the effort to see, appreciate and acknowledge the kindness and good intentions of all those who send good wishes or express the desire to help. Just being aware of all the

support you have can bolster your strength.

3. Specialized treatment: Find the best treatment you can from the best medical resources available. Go to a provider that specializes in cancer exclusively, ideally an NCI designated cancer hospital. Also, find an oncologist that specializes in your type of cancer. At NCI-designated cancer centers you will find the most specialists, the best research, the most clinical trials, and the greatest variety of alternative therapies as well as emotional support.

4. Take a holistic approach: Not just to cancer but to life: emotional, spiritual and physical. Try anything and everything to address your cancer and the side effects of your treatment. You have nothing to lose and everything to gain. I opened myself up to trying anything — acupuncture, massage and reiki treatments, music therapy, art therapy, mindfulness training, counseling, support groups — I was there. I've even become close friends with several of the men in my support group who are either survivors or still actively in treatment. My wife also goes to a Karmanos support group specifically for spouses and caregivers. At Karmanos, once you're a patient, you're always a patient. Nine years from my initial diagnosis and I'm still going to art therapy classes and support groups there.

5. Find strength in winning small battles: When you're at a low point, focus not on your survival but on winning the little battles in your treatment and recovery. Finding the strength to get yourself through the next hour or day or week can be uplifting when you accomplish it. For a longer-term approach focus on how you're going to give back once you get through your battle. I motivated myself by looking forward to helping others. I remember thinking, *once I beat this; I'm going to help other people figure out how to beat cancer.* I'll never give back as much as I've received, but I can try.

You are a person of great influence. If you could inspire a movement that would bring the most amount of good to the greatest amount of people, what would that be?

To give back. I had to stop working at 51, long before I was ready.

Once I recovered from cancer I was left with a huge hole in time and my self-worth suffered. I looked for things I could do to give back. I volunteer with Karmanos on the PFAC, and I talk with cancer patients and their families. I volunteer at my Temple because of all the support members of the congregation who provided for my family and me. I work on food insecurity by driving a truck to pick up food from retail locations like supermarkets and wholesale clubs where it's not going to be used, and redistributing it to food pantries, homeless shelters and neighborhood food banks where it's desperately needed and guaranteed to be used and not thrown away.

I'm not so concerned with starting a movement, but if I can help just a few people to believe they can overcome things that are overwhelming, be it cancer, hunger or anything needing people's time and attention, I am helping change the world.

We are very blessed that some very prominent names in Business, VC funding, Sports and Entertainment read this column. Is there a person in the world, or in the US with whom you would love to have a private breakfast or lunch, and why?

There is no one person. I'm interested in meeting anyone who can help make things better because I want to support and learn from them. I just want to be a part of positive change. I would love to meet and learn from anyone who espouses those things.

How can our readers further follow your work online?

I'm just a very lucky guy who survived cancer. I don't have a website and I'm not on Twitter, though I do have a Facebook page and an Instagram account, which I almost never check. And besides, with my chemo brain, I can never remember my usernames or passwords anyway.

Jaclyn Downs: I Survived (Lymphoma) Cancer and Here Is How I Did It

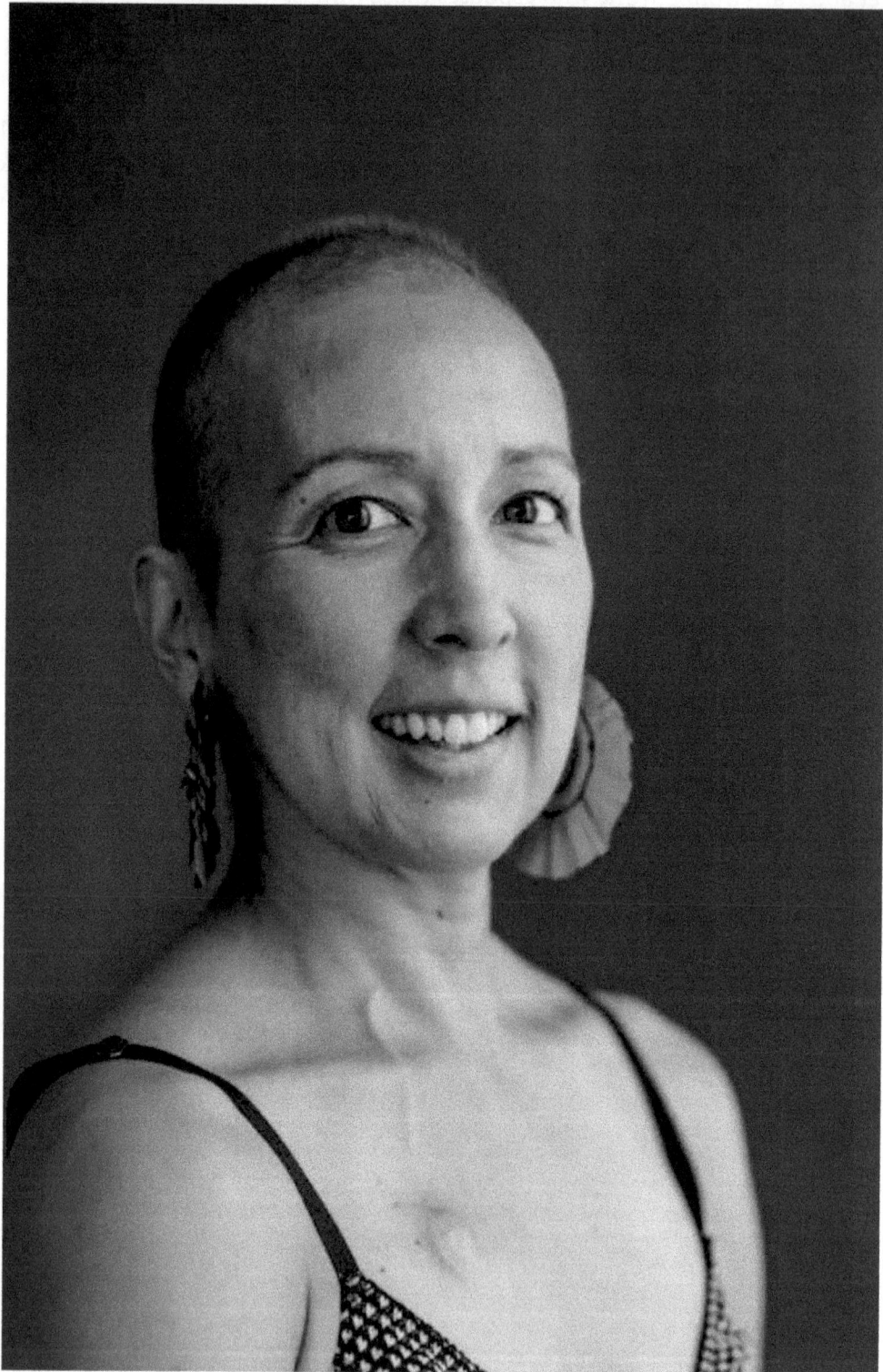

Photo Credits: Linette Kielinski

Get a second opinion, or even a third one. Although I was already going to an academic hospital, I still wanted to get a second opinion from another academic hospital in the area, so I contacted Johns Hopkins. With all my test results sent to them, they confirmed that they would do the same treatment protocol that Penn suggested for me, so I felt confident in my decision. I wanted to be sure that I wouldn't ever be left wondering, "what if?"

I had the pleasure of interviewing Jaclyn Downs. Jaclyn is a Functional Genomic Nutritionist that specializes in fertility and reproductive health. She is the author of "Solving 'Unexplained' Infertility: Your 12 Week Functional Fertility Plan."

Thank you so much for joining us in this interview series! We really appreciate the courage it takes to publicly share your story. Before we start, our readers would love to "get to know you" a bit better. Can you tell us a bit about your background and your childhood backstory?

I was born and raised around Central Pennsylvania. My parents had three children, of which I am the youngest. They divorced when I was a toddler. They both remarried within a few years, creating blended family trials and dramas that can often occur. My mom was a stay-at-home mom, and my father worked in the nutritional supplement industry. Growing up, even though I knew I was loved as a daughter and sister, I don't remember feeling much of a sense of adoration or being a priority in either household, although I still consider myself to have had a very typical suburban childhood. My two older brothers were best friends; combined with all other family dynamics, caused me to be a very independent person.

Because I had always felt that there was so much more for life to offer me outside of small town suburbia, I chose to attend college at Drexel University in Philadelphia. I had wanted to study nutrition or psychology, but the nutrition education that Drexel provided (which was based upon the USDA's subsidized nutrition) did not resonate with me, so I majored in psychology, learning about human nature. That's when I really began to grow into myself.

Along the course of my psychology education, I was introduced to a relatively new field of study (this was the late 1990s), called psychoneuroimmunology. This field explores how immune cells are regulated by neurotransmitters and hormones. Psychoneuroimmunology explains holistic health from a scientific perspective, far beyond nutrition. Learning about this field solidified my desire to work as a holistic health practitioner. After Drexel, I attended grad school for holistic nutrition and have since been furthering my nutrition education in the ever-evolving field.

Can you please give us your favorite "Life Lesson Quote?" Can you share how that was relevant to you in your life?

"It is impossible to feel grateful and depressed in the same breath." While everyone gets down on things from time to time, I have been blessed to not have experienced long-term depression, and it may be due to holding this quote very close. Whatever may be challenging or depressing in my life, I know that there are millions of people that would jump at the chance to trade "problems" with me. Although I have seen people struggle to come up with even one thing they are thankful for, most people stick with the big ones, like health, family, and home. I could go on and on about how grateful I am to be able to speak, see, hold a job, have functioning legs, ride a bike, have a bike to ride, sleep on a bed (and one with sheets!), read, have the social ability to have friends, hear the cicadas on a hot summer day, go to a grocery store whenever I want to, have water at the turn of a knob (and access to filters), and be able to make the hundreds of small choices I unconsciously and consciously make each and every day.

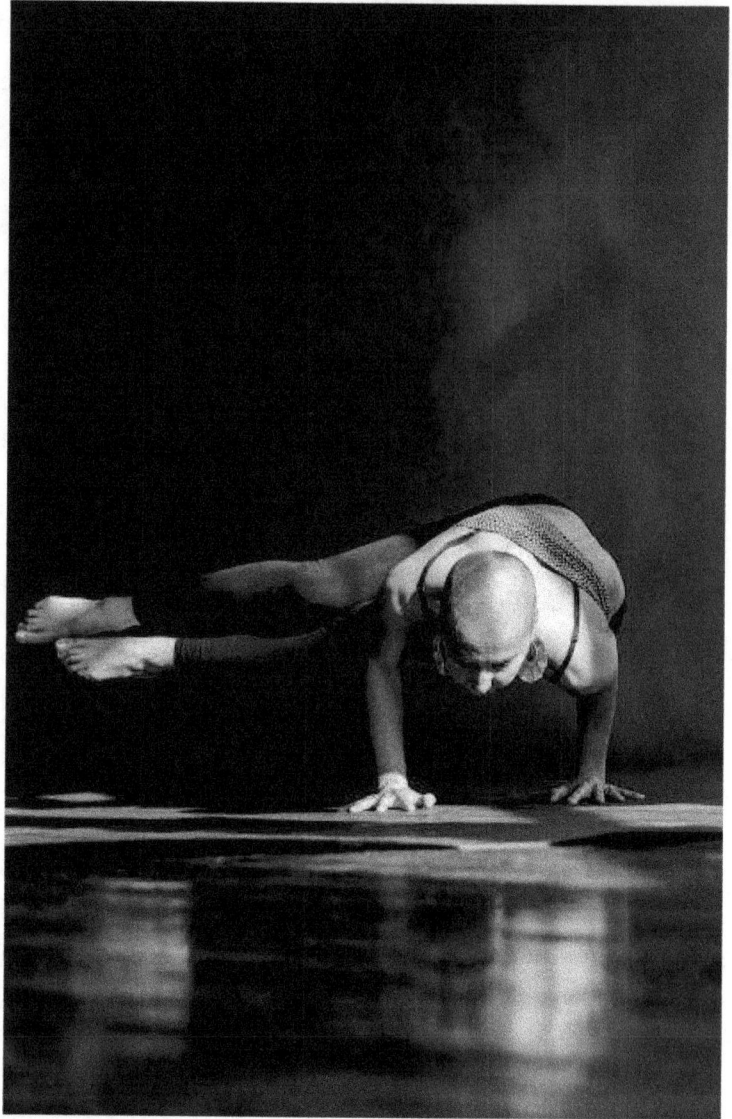

Let's now shift to the main part of our discussion about surviving cancer. Do you feel comfortable sharing with us the story surrounding how you found out that you had cancer?

Absolutely! In the Spring of 2020, shortly after COVID had shut everything down, it started with what felt like I had slightly overworked or tweaked a muscle on my ride side, below my armpit. I couldn't figure out what I had done to it. I would notice it doing small things like pushing down the hand soap pump or pulling my freezer door open. I was still able to do advanced yoga classes and ride my bike with no issues. As weeks went on, the discomfort became more evident. I remember doing hard bike rides on my bike trainer for about 20 minutes, working up a great sweat and then showering, and then, only after that period of about 15 minutes post-ride, I would be lying on my bed in pain for just a few minutes, until it passed. As time went on, the pain started to follow a line, from below my armpit to the center of my chest. I finally went to my family doctor. I described my experiences that brought me to him. I had told him there was about three days in April (it was now June) that I had the slightest crinkle in my lung at the top of my exhales, but that my breathing was now fine and clear ever since. He ordered some blood work and a chest x-ray. I told him my lungs felt fine, but he just wanted to double-check. He also ordered routine bloodwork. Because he was a very open minded and kind doctor, he ordered every other blood marker I requested, which were many; since us functional nutrition practitioners really like our lab work!

As a nutritionist, I'm proud to say that all my bloodwork came back normal! But the chest x-ray did not. A CAT scan was ordered immediately. A few days later I had CAT scan results that indicated a malignant tumor the size of a grapefruit that was eating away at my 4th rib. A biopsy was scheduled, along with a barrage of other tests and scans. I was diagnosed with Diffuse Large B-cell Non-Hodgkin's Lymphoma and scheduled to meet with an oncologist to discuss chemotherapy. I had always thought that I would never do chemo if I got cancer, but because the tumor was growing so quickly and my discomfort was constant (not the pain), I could hardly wait to start. By the week before I started chemo, I had to walk with a folded-up pillow under my arm for comfort and use multiple ice packs throughout the day.

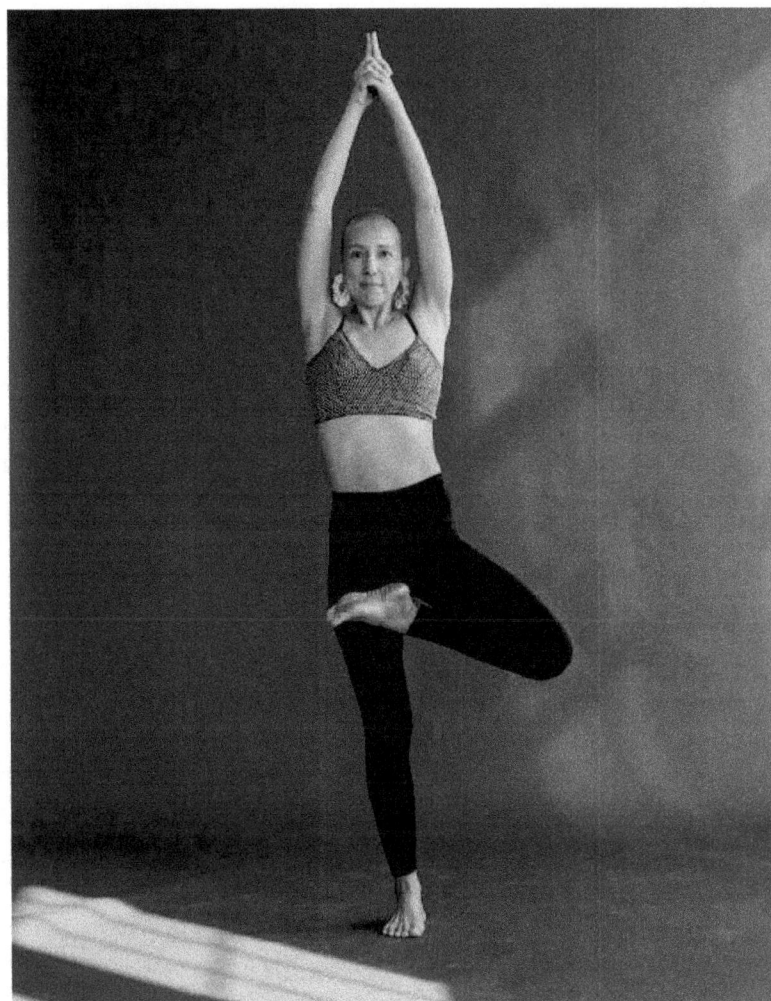

What was the scariest part of that event? What did you think was the worst thing that could happen to you?

The scariest part was the tumor was growing so quickly (my oncologist said it likely hadn't been very long at all since its inception), I began to wonder how much time I would have and what life would be like without me for my husband and two young daughters (four and eight at that time). Because it was a rarer form of NHL, they weren't sure how the tumor would respond to chemo.

How did you react in the short term?

I was undergoing so many tests that I was just moving from one appointment to the next, waiting for the next piece of information. I sought a second opinion with Johns Hopkins, where they concurred with the treatment that my local hospital proposed. I assembled my team. I was lucky to be referred to talk with an oncologist at University of Pennsylvania (which my local hospital was affiliated with) that specialized in Diffuse Large B-cell NHL, and that was open to me working with an integrative MD that was a friend and colleague.

After the dust settled, what coping mechanisms did you use? What did you do to cope physically, mentally, emotionally, and spiritually?

A TON! I did so many adjunct therapies. I did craniosacral therapy, positive affirmations, guided meditations, Qi Gong, and infrared sauna (always followed by a freezing cold shower). I learned that the chemo drugs stay in the body for about a week, so I did not use the sauna the first week following each chemo treatment, only the second and third weeks, as my six chemo treatments were each three weeks apart.

I did a few acupuncture treatments, one of which was mind blowing because my child-self appeared in my mind and I got to talk to her and hug her and acknowledge her feelings. Because I had a psychology degree, I was able to, years ago, mentally understand why certain people acted the way they did and treated me the way they did. I was able to mentally compartmentalize and make sense of it. But I never acknowledged how it affected me and my child-self. I felt a wondrous sense of release and closure after that session.

My journey also included reading *Love, Medicine, and Miracles* by Dr. Bernie Siegel, *Cancer and the New Biology of Water* by Dr. Thomas Cowan, *Falling Upward* by Richard Rohr, and I listened to a couple of Dr. Joe Dispenza's books, which reawakened my spiritual light (spirituality and religion can be two completely separate things in my opinion) that had gone dim over the past decade.

Physically, I still felt pretty good overall. The first couple days after each of the 6 chemo treatments, I would feel like I had a mild hangover, but I never vomited or had to take nausea medication. Actually, I was still doing yoga and roller skating my girls to school. I even learned to drop in on a half-pipe (skate ramp) during that time!

Since my oncologist was open to communication with my integrative doctor, I was able to take certain supplements that had clinical research behind them for being effective on cancer. Just like with the sauna, I would only take them after the first week post-chemo treatment.

Is there a particular person you are grateful towards who helped you learn to cope and heal? Can you share a story about that?

My integrative doctor, Dr. Lari Young. I felt very confident and so incredibly blessed to have her walking that journey beside me, guiding me, being a voice of reason. I met her when she lectured at my colleague's Functional Genomics Conference and immediately loved her energy. I have the utmost respect for her. She went through grad school at Dartmouth as a single mom with young children! She was one of the first people I called when I received my diagnosis. She gave me grounded perspective and listed my options. She took time out of her busy schedule to make time to talk to me, sometimes for over an hour. Doctors like her are rare gems.

I'm also grateful for my oncologist who was more than willing to communicate with her and be open-minded about my "alternative" treatments and options.

In my own cancer struggle, I sometimes used the idea of embodiment to help me cope. Let's take a minute to look at cancer from an embodiment perspective. If your cancer had a message for you, what do you think it would want or say?

This is a great question because I actually talked about this in one of the YouTube videos I made to keep family and friends apprised of my journey! Very early on, when I was lying in bed, mentally asking the cancerous tumor why it was there, it was as if I was hollering to it from across a large room. Then one night, further along in my journey and on a little bit of medical marijuana, I placed my hand on my side ribs, over the tumor area, and asked it again, as if I was sitting closely with it, able to speak softly and have a conversation with it. This made me ponder whether marijuana's successes with cancer are due to the phytocannabinoid (plant) compounds that it contains, or the way it changes our headspace and outlook. I surmised that it was much of both!

Either way, my takeaway was that my cancer was a way to get me to address and reawaken the energetic part of my body. Not like an energy level, but like, what sort of energetic imprint would I make if I was able to stamp it onto a canvas. As a functional nutritionist with a psychology degree, I had the body and mind covered, but as I said previously, had a spirit (energetic self) that dimmed down to almost nothing over the past decade or so.

What did you learn about yourself from this very difficult experience? How has cancer shaped your worldview? What has it taught you that you might never have considered before? Can you please explain with a story or example?

When you have young children, it is not uncommon to feel inundated by daily responsibilities. Your life seems no longer your own, your time is no longer your own, as you put yourself on hold to meet the needs of your family. I loosely kept in touch with a couple close friends, and I had a small pool of friends and acquaintances to schedule regular play dates with, but no longer felt a

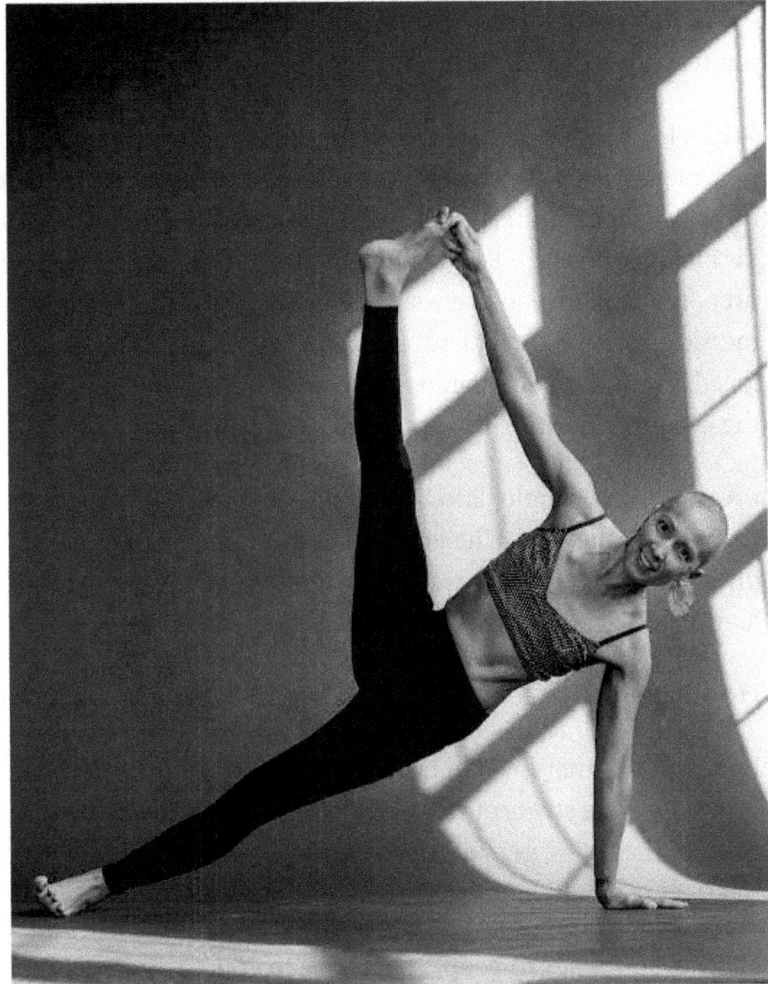

connection to my wider community. I felt limited amounts of love because I was not putting love out into the world or into myself. I was just tired to the core.

When I got cancer, a dear friend set up a meal train for the week following each of my six chemo treatments. She was an adamant voice for my new dietary restrictions so I didn't have to be (no meat, no sugar, low carb, and all organic, as NHL has been associated with pesticide and herbicide exposure). Friends I hadn't talked to in years rose to the occasion and brought meals prepared with love, or they sent gift cards for meals. People dropped off care packages and sent messages of love and encouragement. These acts of love and support made me know I was still loved, even despite not emitting love and fun vitality the way I used to years ago. I felt loved to the core and I know this supported my healing.

I realized that people didn't judge me for getting wrapped up in my own life, just as I didn't judge them when they did. The love and adoration and support are still there even in prolonged physical absence. I have wondered if my cancer was a way to let me know I am still loved and loveable. Even if it wasn't, that was a nice side effect of it.

How have you used your experience to bring goodness to the world?

I often doubt that I would have done so very well throughout my cancer journey if I didn't have insurance. The stress of cancer bills would have limited my ability to explore my stressors, do adjunct therapies, get additional testing, and buy therapeutic supplements. Each of my six chemo treatments would have been $60,000 a pop!

My heart goes out to people that have to endure not only the physical and emotional burden that cancer causes, but an even heavier financial burden that compounds the physical and emotional burden that not having insurance brings. My charities of choice are now contributing to crowdfunding that involves helping people pay for their cancer expenses so they and their families can focus on ensuring they feel the comfort and positivity that is needed to conquer cancer.

What are a few of the biggest misconceptions and myths out there about fighting cancer that you would like to dispel?

Buying something with a "pink ribbon" may be perpetuating the problem. The companies that don the pink ribbon are often making money off the very things that can cause cancer — like pink M&M's and pink candy bar wrappers. Bitch, please! Sugar feeds cancer.

And the pink fast food chicken buckets? Even The American Institute for Cancer Research states that to prevent cancer, one should focus on eating mostly plant-based foods and staying away from sugary foods and fast food.

They aren't looking to spread awareness about breast cancer as much as they are looking to profit from it. We don't need to spread awareness about breast cancer when almost everyone knows at least one person that has had breast cancer. How about we raise awareness about cancer prevention?

Fantastic. Here is the main question of our interview. Based on your experiences and knowledge, what advice would you give to others who have recently been diagnosed with cancer? What are your "5 Things" You Need To Beat Cancer? Please share a story or example for each.

- Get a second opinion, or even a third one. Although I was already going to an academic hospital, I still wanted to get a second opinion from another academic hospital in the area, so I contacted Johns Hopkins. With all my test results sent to them, they confirmed that they would do the same treatment protocol that Penn suggested for me, so I felt confident in my decision. I wanted to be sure that I wouldn't ever be left wondering, "what if?"
- Assemble a team—I was lucky to have options. My local hospital had me consult with an oncologist at University of Pennsylvania that specialized in my particular type of lymphoma. After speaking with him, I asked him if he could be my oncologist and then jumped ship from my local hospital. With my oncologist, integrative doctor, and craniosacral therapist (I explain why below) as my main practitioners, I was able to feel like I had all my bases covered for the best possible outcome.
- Explore the woo-woo—we are holistic beings. Just because some of us aren't aware of the energy we are emitting and how past negative experiences can shape our current state of health, it does not mean it isn't possible. If we explore, we may be able to identify a reason why our bodies allowed cancer to proliferate. Bernie Siegel, a surgical oncologist, wrote about this in his book *Love, Medicine, and Miracles.* My family doctor recommended this book to me, and I highly recommend it for anyone that has had a cancer diagnosis.
- Get proactive about your health and self-care—I write in my book that I define self-care as creating wellness for yourself physically, mentally, and emotionally. True self-care isn't wine and chocolates. It is putting in the work to ensure you create a life that doesn't require damage control by dieting, or "escape" with alcohol or addictions. Not doing so can feed cancer or let it thrive in your body. If you have cancer, I highly recommend starting by avoiding sugar and letting go of things that won't matter a month from now. I realized that I was focusing so much on how I wanted things to be for my family (like avoiding toxins and limiting screen time every day) that it was overriding my connection with them. Keeping this in mind is like strengthening a weak muscle; it doesn't just happen overnight. It needs to be worked.
- Consider dental health and history—I've mentioned my craniosacral therapist a few times in this interview. I don't have others to compare her to, but she has been such a (literally) amazing force in my cancer journey, and afterwards, helping to bring my body back to balance after what feels like the aftermath of a battle. My tumor and the rib it moved into were on my upper right torso, as was my port. After I beat cancer, she helped to clear out the trauma that area of my body experienced, both the emotional PTSD of that area, as well as the physical trauma to the muscle and tissue that the port and tumor created.

But that's not even the amazing part about her! Since my cancer occurred during COVID, I had a mask on during my appointments. At the end of one session, she asked me if I had ever had any root canals. I said that I hadn't. She then asked if I had any major dental work and I told her that I went to Mexico to get a mercury filling removed about 12 or 13 years ago. She asked, "On the top left?" and I was completely stunned. "How did you know?!" I asked her. She said that my immune system was reacting to it and that I should get it checked out. I told her that I had had dentists take x-rays in the past, and nothing noteworthy ever came back. She said that I needed a 3D cone beam scan to be able to pick up on any infections beyond the roots of the teeth. Long story short, my cone beam showed an infection above my (dead) tooth that had been there so long that it ate through the bone to my sinus cavity. You better believe I promptly made an appointment to get that pulled! Although I don't know for sure that infection caused or contributed to my cancer, studies have shown that oral health may affect the incidence of various types of cancer. I certainly didn't want to keep burdening my immune system for fear of the cancer returning.

You are a person of great influence. If you could inspire a movement that would bring the most amount of good to the greatest amount of people, what would that be?

To be able to inspire change in the corporations and companies that are creating cancer causing materials and toxic waste. To get them to truly feel that if their products are making people sick or causing death, they should re-evaluate their purpose. I'm thrilled that organic and "eco-friendly" products are becoming more popular (although, so is "greenwashing"), and that our consumer purchasing power has the ability to cause a company to change, but I would love to be able to inspire these companies to take more initiative instead of following purchasing trends. With their financial power and media influence, they could create change on a much faster and far larger scale.

Additionally, if we continue to "shit in our nest," our earth will not be habitable, and their profits are going to sharply drop as the population drops (or cancer bills increase) anyway.

We are very blessed that some very prominent names in Business, VC funding, Sports, and Entertainment read this column. Is there a person in the world, or in the US with whom you would love to have a private breakfast or lunch, and why?

Woody Harrelson. He is using his status to inspire people to create a better earth. If the earth is laden with toxins, all living beings will receive those toxins. Many of these toxins are known endocrine disrupting chemicals (intersex/hermaphrodite frogs are not uncommon these days) and cancer-causing agents that are in our food, water, and air. Woody's been doing eco-activism since before it was "cool." I liked him on *Cheers* as an actor and hunky celebrity, but once I learned about his radical activism with *Earth First!*, I was smitten. Then to find out that he was an avid yogi and cyclist like myself, how could he not be at the top of my list of people I'd like to have a meal with?

How can our readers further follow your work online?

My book, *Solving 'Unexplained' Infertility: Your 12 Week Functional Fertility Plan* is in editing/reviewing stage currently and will be available for purchase digitally and hard copy, as well as audio versions.

My website is www.JaclynDowns.com and my Facebook: FunctionalFertilitySolutions

Jaculin H. Jones: I Survived (Breast) Cancer and Here Is How I Did It

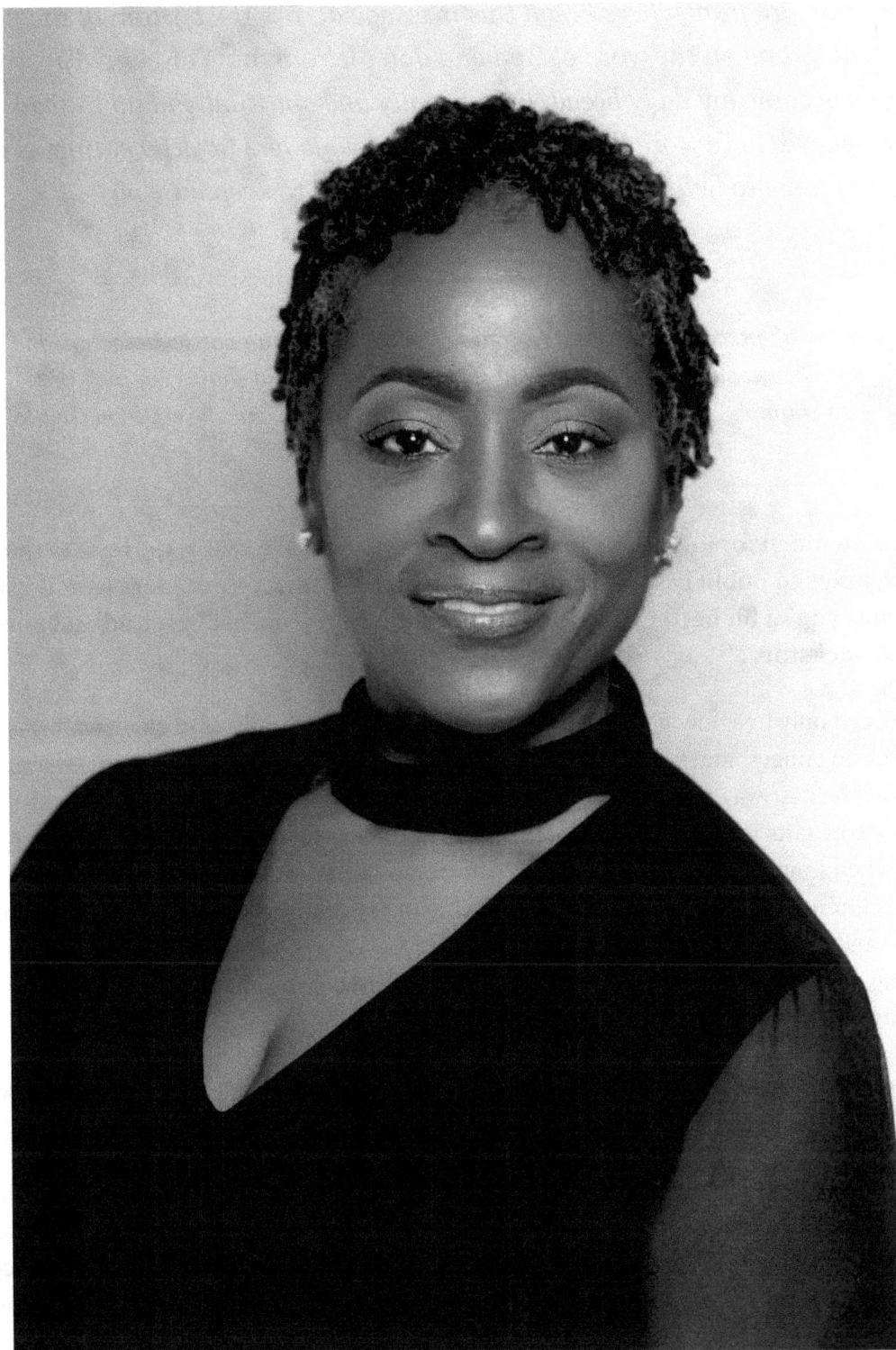

The dust from a cancer diagnosis never settles. That's the truth, but my resolve was to win. I had to level set my mind. I took the liberty to watch a television program while completing my warm-up before working out. This was right after meeting with my team of physicians who discussed

the course of treatment. As I surfed across the television, I stopped at a Christian program where I read this message across the bottom of the screen: "Stand on the word of God and don't let anything else in." Those words became my daily bread. Emotionally and spiritually I had to read and believe God's word. I also used exercise, yoga and healthy eating as a driving force to help me physically. My goal was to keep moving.

I had the pleasure of interviewing Jaculin H. Jones. The after-life of an aortic dissection and Triple Negative Breast Cancer survivor is nothing short of amazing. Jaculin shares her inspiring journey from tragedy to triumph. Surviving cancer was a matter of her will and she willed herself to live.

Thank you so much for joining us in this interview series! We really appreciate the courage it takes to publicly share your story. Before we start, our readers would love to "get to know you" a bit better. Can you tell us a bit about your background and your childhood backstory?

One can only imagine what life was like growing up in a family of 10 children. I was the ninth youngest and while we experienced our own family dysfunction, in retrospect it was the best way to be raised. There was never a dull moment. I was quite an athlete, but my true gifts were singing and acting. I carried these talents into college and continued the same when I moved from New Jersey to Maryland as a new bride. Together my husband and I had two children. Our lives became their lives, which kept us quite busy. My career was in healthcare and the experience I garnered was needed to help me navigate through the life-threatening conditions that plagued my body. I'm so blessed to be alive and present in the world to share my story.

Can you please give us your favorite "Life Lesson Quote?" Can you share how that was relevant to you in your life?

My life lesson quote is, "You can make it!" While this may sound cliché, I can now say without reservation one can make it. After the aortic dissection, I never thought that 15 months later I would be diagnosed with Triple Negative Breast Cancer. There I was wondering how this could have happened. I had a choice to make and I chose to believe. If I survived what should have killed me, then I was going to make it through this.

Let's now shift to the main part of our discussion about surviving cancer. Do you feel comfortable sharing with us the story surrounding how you found out that you had cancer?

I began experiencing unexpected ringing in my ears shortly after the aortic dissection repair. Recovering from such a traumatic experience, I could only attribute the change to my aorta. After following up with the vascular surgeon and to my relief it was not related, I was advised to see an ENT (ear, nose and throat) physician. Upon scheduling the appointment, I was informed that it was also time for my routine mammogram. I had no concerns and felt no lumps, so I didn't think twice about getting the exam. After getting the mammogram, I received a call requesting that I return for a follow-up mammogram. It wasn't the first time I had to repeat a mammogram, so I still had no worries. Two weeks later I had the mammogram, ultrasound and biopsy all on the same day. A few days later I received a call from the radiologist advising that cancer was found in my right breast. It was Ductal Carcinoma. At that moment, I felt a three second sting in the pit of my stomach. Then I asked, "What Next?"

What was the scariest part of that event? What did you think was the worst thing that could happen to you?

The threat of death is always scary when you're not ready. There were three things that were the scariest parts of this event. Upon learning that Triple Negative Breast Cancer was one the most aggressive forms of breast cancer and that chemotherapy and radiation would be the most effective form of treatment instantly caused a level of anxiety. Then I had to make the decision to have either a mastectomy or lumpectomy. I felt like a part of my femininity was being stripped away. After careful consideration, I elected to have the lumpectomy.

What became scary was the two lumps found in my breast following surgery, which were not there prior to having my routine mammogram. I later learned that they were called oil cyst which can occur as a result of the surgery. Every year when I get my mammogram, I have to settle my mind to win because I can still feel one remaining lump. But, it's also a reminder that I made it through such a dark time.

How did you react in the short term?

In the short-term, I had to remember that I had history with God. If He took me through the aortic dissection and the associated cutting edge surgery, I could depend on Him to take me through the cancer diagnosis.

After the dust settled, what coping mechanisms did you use? What did you do to cope physically, mentally, emotionally, and spiritually?

The dust from a cancer diagnosis never settles. That's the truth, but my resolve was to win. I had to level set my mind. I took the liberty to watch television program while completing my warm-up before working out. This was right after meeting with my team of physicians who discussed the course of treatment. As I surfed across the television, I stopped at a Christian program where I read this message across the bottom of the screen: "Stand on the word of God and don't let anything else in." Those words became my daily bread. Emotionally and spiritually I had to read and believe God's word. I used exercise, yoga and healthy eating as a driving force to help me physically. My goal was to keep moving.

Is there a particular person you are grateful towards who helped you learn to cope and heal? Can you share a story about that?

I'm so grateful for my husband who I honor and respect. Family, church family and friends were right by my side. My daughter was second to none. She spoke life into me while undergoing chemotherapy treatment as my hair began to fall out. When I looked into the faces of my family and knowing they were rooting for me, I had to make it through this event. Deborah, a co-worker who I met just two months prior to the diagnosis was very instrumental. It was as if God sent her just for me. She helped me understand and prepared me for what to expect because she was also a breast cancer survivor. She spared no expense in helping me get through this.

In my own cancer struggle, I sometimes used the idea of embodiment to help me cope. Let's take a minute to look at cancer from an embodiment perspective. If your cancer had a message for you, what do you think it would want or say?

I make it very clear that this is not "my" cancer. I acknowledge the reality that this happened to me, but it's not for me to own. But, if cancer had a message it would be, "I should have never tried it!"

What did you learn about yourself from this very difficult experience? How has cancer shaped your worldview? What has it taught you that you might never have considered before? Can you please explain with a story or example?

What I learned about myself is that I'm stronger than I think. My world was turned upside down and I could have given up, but cancer taught me how to better persevere. A cancer diagnosis gave me a greater heart of compassion. Cancer taught me to never give up and to extend the same hope for someone else. I can now speak what I have experienced. I had someone close to me die from breast cancer and it hurt me deeply, but because I'm still here, I can tell anyone that they can make it.

How have you used your experience to bring goodness to the world?

Since the cancer diagnosis, I've written an abbreviated memoir called, *And It Is So: The Power of His Promise.* Writing was the only way I could articulate this journey. My desire is to share how awesome this journey has been in hopes of encouraging others to believe. I also released two solo singles called, *Urgency* and *Thank You for the Good Life.* The cancer diagnosis gave me the courage to release songs I had written some time ago. Oh, the audacity of a cancer survivor!

In November 2020, I began a YouTube channel called, "Promise In Me Unleashed." By sharing stories from ordinary people doing extraordinary things, I believe others will be encouraged to live out their God-given purpose.

What are a few of the biggest misconceptions and myths out there about fighting cancer that you would like to dispel?

I think one of the biggest misconceptions is that cancer can only be in remission, but not cured.

Another myth is the use of other alternative and effective treatments outside of chemotherapy and radiation. Research is happening, but the implementation of other treatments has been slower in the mainstream medical community. I'm not insinuating that man-made medicines don't work, but there is less attention being paid to natural cures than to medicines that ravage the body while attempting to cure it.

Fantastic. Here is the main question of our interview. Based on your experiences and knowledge, what advice would you give to others who have recently been diagnosed with cancer? What are your "5 Things" You Need To Beat Cancer? Please share a story or example for each.

1. Declare yourself a winner.
2. Collaborate with a team of physicians to determine the best course of treatment. Also include your family on the decision making. Ultimately you make the final decisions.
3. Reach out to networks of support like Susan G. Komen, National Breast Cancer Foundation (NBCF), American Cancer Society, churches, other organizations, family and friend.
4. Eat well, rest well and exercise.
5. Stand on the word of God and don't let anything else in.

You are a person of great influence. If you could inspire a movement that would bring the most amount of good to the greatest amount of people, what would that be?

The "STAND" Movement. Stand Tall and Never Doubt.

We are very blessed that some very prominent names in Business, VC funding, Sports, and Entertainment read this column. Is there a person in the world, or in the US with whom you would love to have a private breakfast or lunch, and why?

Viola Davis is the one person I would love to have a private breakfast or lunch. As a lover of the arts, I'm always impressed and wonder what goes through her mind as she owns and brings to life every character she plays. I believe her off screen life impacts her on screen performances. She also has a spirit of compassion as observed through her philanthropic work.

How can our readers further follow your work online?

www.jaculinhjones.com. Facebook: Jaculin Jones. Instagram: @JaculinHJones

Scan the QR code to view my "5 Things" To Beat Cancer YouTube video:

Janelle Hail of National Breast Cancer Foundation (NBCF): A Story of Hope and Inspiration

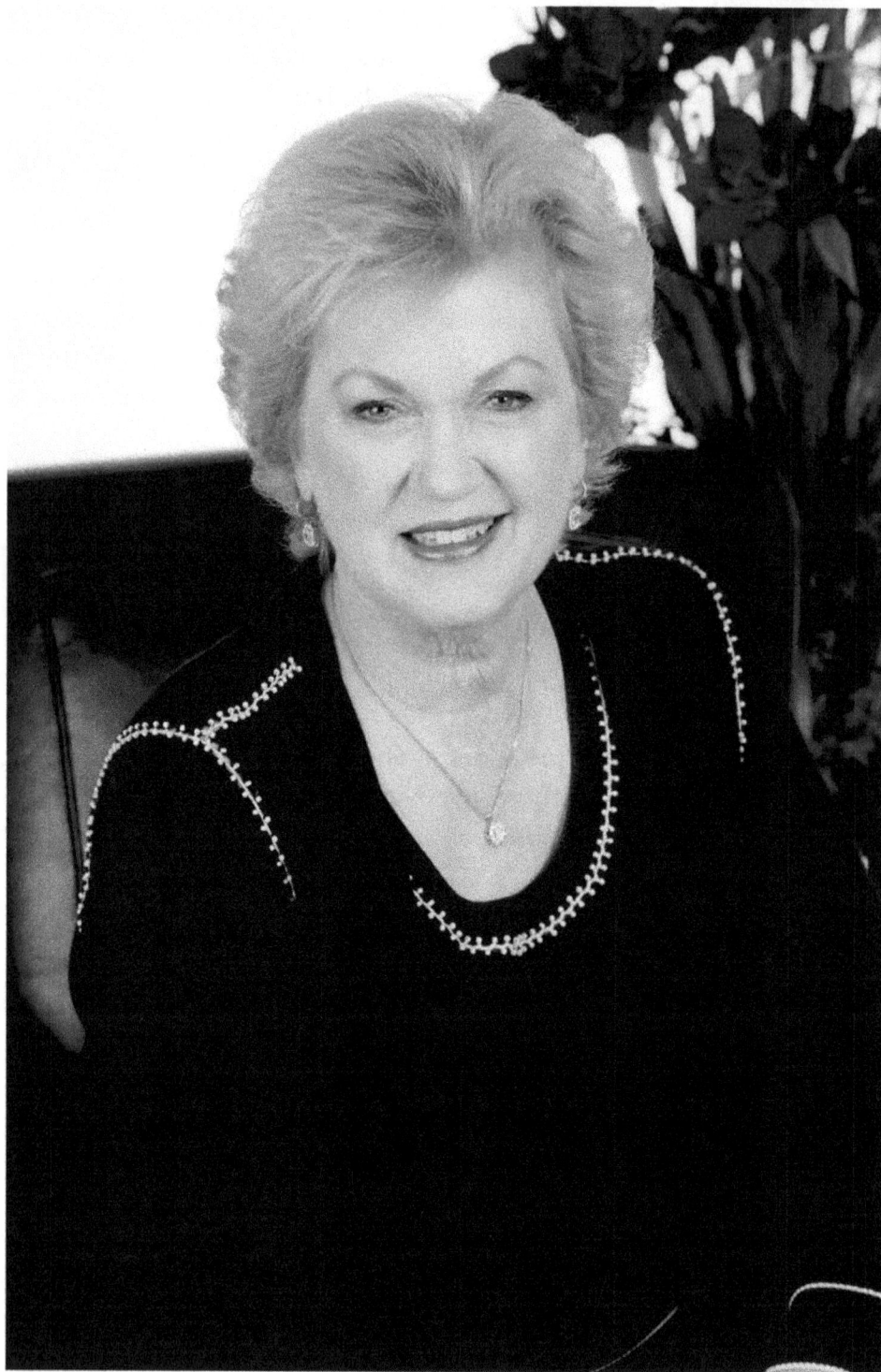

Run away from bad attitudes and unhealthy thoughts that fuel the fire of fear. Fear can be the most destructive force to deal with. It can keep a person frozen in procrastination and indecision. I have met many women who waited a long time to get medical help and jeopardized their health

doing so. I have heard women say they didn't go to the doctor for fear of what they might find. Early detection can help eliminate later stages of breast cancer.

I had the pleasure of interviewing Janelle Hail. Janelle is a forty-one-year breast cancer survivor, CEO and Chairman of the Board of National Breast Cancer Foundation (NBCF). Janelle and her late husband Neal founded NBCF in 1991 with a mission to help women now and inspire hope to those affected by breast cancer through early detection, education, and support services. The NBCF worldwide headquarters is in Frisco, Texas, where they offer medical services to needy women through their hospital network across the United States and support services for breast cancer patients throughout the United States and worldwide.

Thank you so much for joining us in this interview series! We really appreciate the courage it takes to publicly share your story. Before we start, our readers would love to "get to know you" a bit better. Can you tell us a bit about your background and your childhood backstory?

I grew up in Lubbock, Texas, with my parents and a brother who is five years older. Neal and I met while I was attending Texas Tech University as a freshman. After four years in the Navy, Neal had transferred in his senior year of college from Texas Christian University to Texas Tech University. We fell in love and married within the year when he was 26 and I was 19. We had 52 years of marriage until Neal passed away in 2018.

Can you please give us your favorite "Life Lesson Quote?" Can you share how that was relevant to you in your life?

One of my favorite life lesson quotes is, "Our pathways often twist through stormy landscapes; but when we look back, we'll see a thousand miles of miracles and answered prayers." –David Jeremiah

Many times, when you are in the middle of the storms of life, all you can see are the billowing clouds and rugged landscape you must climb over. As I have learned to trust God with my life, I can see that He was there all the time helping me move forward and bringing about beauty in my life.

Let's now shift to the main part of our discussion about surviving cancer. Do you feel comfortable sharing with us the story surrounding how you found out that you had cancer?

I encountered breast cancer when I was 34 years old and married with three sons, ages 3, 10, and 13. One night as I was getting ready for bed, I remembered learning about breast healthcare from my health class in junior high school. I was surprised to discover a lump in my breast that night, as I had always taken care of my health, ate well, and exercised.

At that point in my life things were wonderful. We were building our dream home in another city with my husband, Neal, traveling back and forth to oversee the progress. Suddenly our lives were rudely interrupted with a health issue that led me along a dark, unknown pathway.

I called my doctor the next day for an appointment to find out what was going on with my body. With some mounting female health issues, my doctor recommended a hysterectomy and a biopsy of the breast lump at the same time. It's still hard to believe that there was no internet in 1980. Every answer had to come from one's doctor. For some reason, I wasn't concerned about the biopsy. I figured if there was a problem, the lump could be removed, and my hysterectomy would take care of the other issues. How naïve could I have been? That was the way of thinking back then. Get a good doctor to fix you up, and you'll be on your way to life again.

When I rolled out of recovery from hysterectomy surgery and settled into my room at the hospital, I awakened at 6:01 a.m. to see my husband, mother, and mother-in-law standing at my bedside. My first thought was how nice it was for them to come see me this early.

That wasn't why they were there. Neal leaned over my bed and tenderly whispered, "Janelle, they found cancer." I will always remember the kindness in his eyes as he kissed me on the cheek.

"What? Tell me what I have to do to get rid of it," I said. There were few options. One was to have a mastectomy. The other, a lumpectomy, which had only been around a few years without enough data to prove its long-term effectiveness.

I said a quick prayer, *God, please help me know what to do.* A clear answer came to me to have the mastectomy.

Two days later I returned to surgery, this time to have a mastectomy. With no complications, I planned to resume life. But my life would never be the same again. The changing course of my life started the day I went home from the hospital. Too many things had happened at one time!

What was the scariest part of that event? What did you think was the worst thing that could happen to you?

When Neal told me I had breast cancer, fear of death gripped me. I had no knowledge of the disease, and there were no resources available except what my doctor told me. Eleven years later when Neal and I founded National Breast Cancer Foundation, we wanted to give those resources to women so they could make informed decisions about their own healthcare. We wanted to replace fear of the disease with hope through early detection, which saved my life.

How did you react in the short term?

I had no choice when I left the hospital but to take care of my family. My husband needed his wife; my children needed their mother.

After dinner one night at dusk, I stood at my kitchen sink washing dishes. There were few trees in West Texas, but one small tree outside my kitchen window caught my eye. There was only one red leaf remaining on the tree, and it seemed to dance in the fall breeze. My emotions were as scattered as the pile of leaves on the ground beneath the tree. I said, "I want my life to be like that leaf, brilliant until the end."

The memory of that red leaf drifted through the years with me until we founded NBCF and incorporated it into our logo, representing life, growth, and hope for the future. I never imagined that an ordinary event like washing dishes would give me an epiphany before NBCF was ever conceived.

After the dust settled, what coping mechanisms did you use? What did you do to cope physically, mentally, emotionally, and spiritually?

As my life began to move forward from the first day I went home from the hospital, I followed the natural pathway in front of me. I volunteered at a local hospital to fill the empty void of life with the enjoyment of giving to others while learning the ways of the hospital and how to communicate with doctors. Little did I know that I would work with medical facilities and doctors across the world in four continents in future years.

I spent eleven years involved with the National Speakers Association, learning everything possible to advance my skills. During that time, I also attended numerous writer conferences and continue today to study the art of writing.

There are no books, no manuals, and no advice that solves the emotional, mental, physical, and spiritual aloneness following such a loss. I felt sadness over losing my breast, a once lovely part of my young body. I had fearful thoughts that my husband would leave me, and people would have nothing to do with me. Doctors could only treat the body, not the spirit. I did what I have done since I became a Christian at the age of nine. I prayed and trusted the Lord to guide my life.

One morning as I dressed for the day, I caught a glimpse of my broken body in the mirror. I stopped, took a deep breath, and looked down at my feet as I said aloud, "I have two feet to go places, two hands to work, a mind to think, and a mouth to speak. I will use all of those to do the will of God in my life." That was a turning point for me. No longer did I look at my brokenness, but rather saw myself from the heart of my Heavenly Father who loved me as I was. That was my "move forward moment."

Is there a particular person you are grateful towards who helped you learn to cope and heal? Can you share a story about that?

My husband, Neal, loved me and encouraged me every step of the way. I was concerned about how losing a breast affected him. A few years previously, he nearly died during gallbladder surgery, leaving him with an 18" scar across his stomach.

He said to me one day, "Tell me, Janelle. Does my scar bother you?"

"No, it doesn't. I don't even notice it," I said.

"That's the way I feel about your scar, too. I only see my beautiful wife. You are the same woman I have always loved," he said.

When we founded NBCF years later, we realized there were many women with no support, so caring for those affected by breast cancer all the way through their journey became the heartbeat of NBCF.

In my own cancer struggle, I sometimes used the idea of embodiment to help me cope. Let's take a minute to look at cancer from an embodiment perspective. If your cancer had a message for you, what do you think it would want or say?

I looked at cancer as my enemy, one that wanted to destroy me. I imagined cancer saying to me, "I will kill you. You don't stand a chance against my powers."

Here's what I said to cancer, "You are not going to kill me. I am going after you and will hunt you down in the darkest parts of the earth, shining a bright light of education on you so women will not live with fear of the unknown and can make healthy decisions. I will be your Number One enemy!"

Today that is exactly what we have done at NBCF. We educate women and their families about early detection, offering support services, and help on their journey through breast cancer.

What did you learn about yourself from this very difficult experience? How has cancer shaped your worldview? What has it taught you that you might never have considered before? Can you please explain with a story or example?

Dealing with breast cancer revamped my worldview. I was always on the outside of the disease looking at others who had breast cancer, feeling sorry for them, but helpless to do anything about it. Now I was on the inside of the disease looking out at the pain and desperation that I experienced, along with others.

Helping others has become my life work.

How have you used your experience to bring goodness to the world?

My patience and understanding have greatly increased since breast cancer. I am freer to let go of petty issues that many times are unnecessary burdens and have a clear focus on my purpose of life. I found that looking only at my own losses can easily breed bitterness, hatred, and other negative attitudes. Helping others brings the joy out of my heart and a smile on my face. I know that through National Breast Cancer Foundation I am enriching the lives of women worldwide.

What are a few of the biggest misconceptions and myths out there about fighting cancer that you would like to dispel?

Here are a couple of misconceptions about breast cancer:

Before education on breast cancer emerged for the public to research on the internet, people thought they could catch cancer from another person, which is not the case.

People think breast cancer is an automatic death sentence. There are 3.8 million breast cancer survivors today. NBCF has developed local and national support groups for survivors to empower women with help and hope on their journey.

The internet is an amazing tool where we give correct information on our website, nbcf.org. We dispel the helplessness people feel when they don't know where to go for help. We provide support services at every stage of their disease and give them hope. No woman should have to face breast cancer alone, and we are here to be the emotional and physical support they need with options to make wise choices.

Fantastic. Here is the main question of our interview. Based on your experiences and knowledge, what advice would you give to others who have recently been diagnosed with cancer? What are your "5 Things" You Need To Beat Cancer? Please share a story or example for each.

Things You Need to Beat Cancer:

1. Seek medical help as soon as you discover something different about your breasts, such as a nipple discharge, a dimpling of the tissue, a redness, or other unusual symptoms. I have thought often about what would have happened if I had not followed through with medical help when I first found my lump. There would be no National Breast Cancer Foundation. As we celebrate NBCF's 30th anniversary, we have given funding for 305,000 breast cancer screenings and diagnostic services and 1.7 million patient navigation services.

2. Reach out to people who will surround you with care and help. When women come to us for help, we find a way to connect them with resources. People frequently tell us that NBCF makes them feel loved and accepted. When you have once experienced that kind of care, you can't help but give it away to others. Our volunteers tirelessly pack Hope Kits filled with thoughtful and comforting gifts and encouraging notes for thousands of breast cancer patients throughout the United States.

3. End bad habits such as overeating, excessive alcohol, smoking, and other things that deteriorate your health. Bad habits are distracting and can easily derail good health practices. Happiness comes from inside a person and flows outward, creating a better lifestyle and draws good people your way.

4. The best gift you can give those you love is to take care of yourself. It is time to turn your attention to preventative healthcare. We knew of a mother who died while saving up money she stored in an old coffee can so she could buy her son tennis shoes instead of using it to get a mammogram. Neglecting one's own health can lead to tragedy for those you love.

5. Run away from bad attitudes and unhealthy thoughts that fuel the fire of fear. Fear can be the most destructive force to deal with. It can keep a person frozen in procrastination and indecision. I have met many women who waited a long time to get medical help and jeopardized their health doing so. I have heard women say they didn't go to the doctor for

fear of what they might find. Early detection can help eliminate later stages of breast cancer.

You are a person of great influence. If you could inspire a movement that would bring the most amount of good to the greatest amount of people, what would that be?

Early stages of breast cancer offer more options for a healthy outcome.

Take care of your body and educate others around. Early detection saves lives!

We are very blessed that some very prominent names in Business, VC funding, Sports, and Entertainment read this column. Is there a person in the world, or in the US with whom you would love to have a private breakfast or lunch, and why?

I would be honored to have breakfast or lunch with Jerry Jenkins, 21-time New York Times bestselling author who has written nearly 200 books with over 72 million copies sold. He is one of the most successful writers of our time and generously shares his knowledge and skills through The Jerry Jenkins Writers Guild.

How can our readers further follow your work online?

Readers can follow my work on www.nbcf.org

Javacia Harris Bowser of See Jane Write: I Survived (Breast) Cancer and Here Is How I Did It

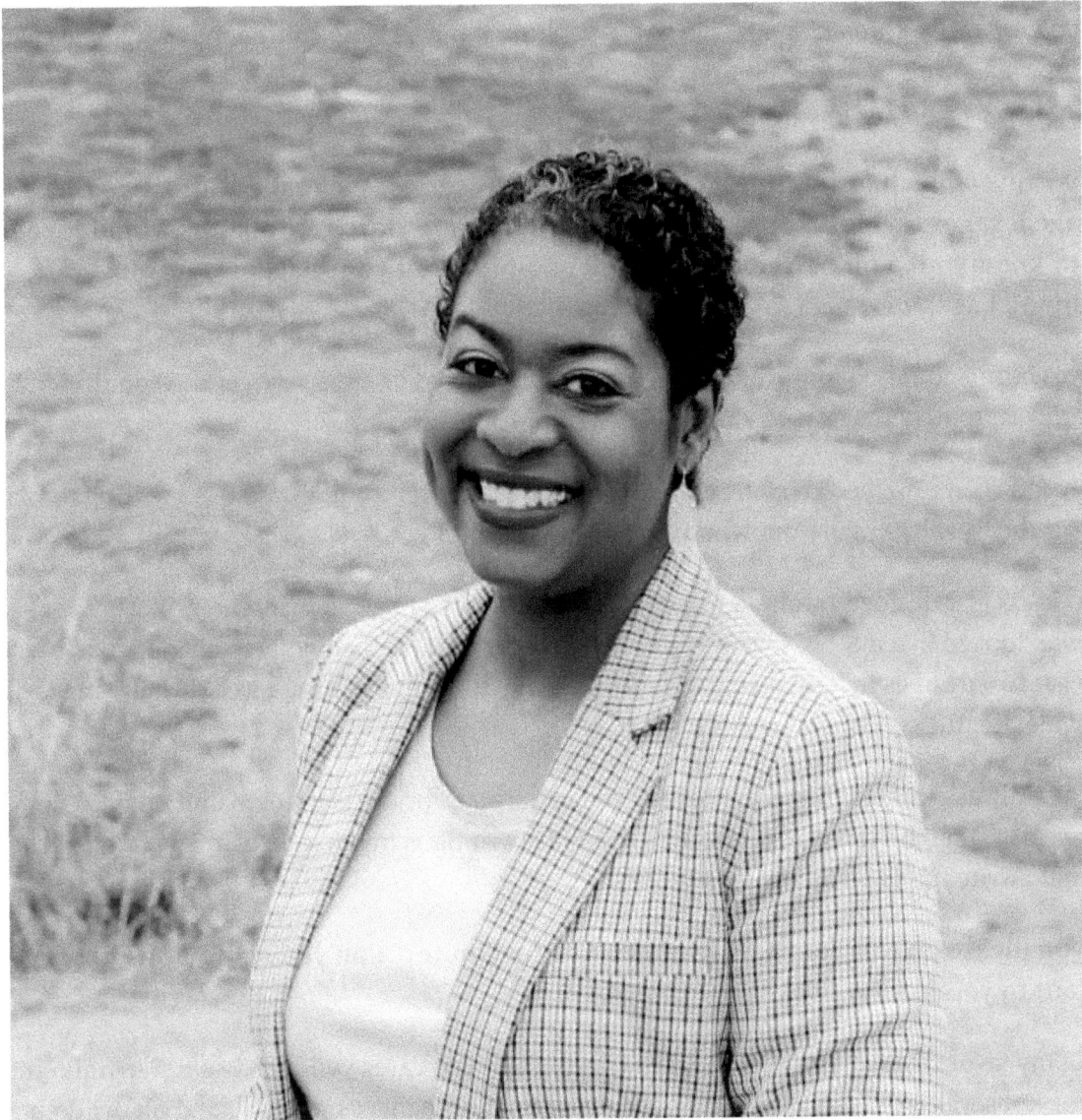

Persistence— "Nevertheless, she persisted" is my cancer-fighting mantra. To me "beating cancer" isn't about not dying. Beating cancer means living your life as well as you can with whatever time you have left. Even while I was going through treatment I continued writing and walking for exercise because I refused to let cancer take those things away from me. Find a way to continue doing at least one of the things you love in spite of cancer.

I had the pleasure of interviewing Javacia Harris Bowser. Javacia is an award-winning freelance journalist and the founder of See Jane Write, a website, coaching service, and community for women who write. Her forthcoming essay collection 'Find Your Way Back: How to Write Your Way Through Anything' chronicles how she has used writing to cope with cancer and everything else life has thrown her way.

Thank you so much for joining us in this interview series! We really appreciate the courage it takes to publicly share your story. Before we start, our readers would love to "get to know you" a bit better. Can you tell us a bit about your background and your childhood backstory?

I was born and raised in Birmingham, Alabama. I've lived in cities all over the country, but I returned to my hometown in 2009. I am a proud Southern girl.

My mom says I've been writing since I could sit up straight. I've always used writing to make sense of the world, to figure out who I am and what I think.

When I was 15, I decided I wanted to be a journalist. I loved reading magazines, but I never saw girls who looked like me. So, I wanted to work for the media so I could help change that. I went on to get two degrees in journalism and I worked as a staff reporter for a weekly news magazine in Louisville, Kentucky.

But I also always wanted to teach. So, I left the newsroom for the classroom and taught English for 10 years. Though I loved working with students, writing is my first love. In 2019, I quit teaching so I could write full-time on my own terms.

Can you please give us your favorite "Life Lesson Quote?" Can you share how that was relevant to you in your life?

One of my favorite quotes is, "Do one thing every day that scares you." It's usually attributed to Eleanor Roosevelt. And this quote has pushed me to take chances on myself and on my dreams. In 2019, for example, when I left my job as an English teacher to be a full-time freelance writer and to work on expanding See Jane Write I was taking a huge risk. But it was worth it.

Let's now shift to the main part of our discussion about surviving cancer. Do you feel comfortable sharing with us the story surrounding how you found out that you had cancer?

I was diagnosed with breast cancer on January 24, 2020. I hadn't found a lump in my breast because I wasn't looking for one. I was only 38 and, in my mind, breast cancer wasn't something I needed to worry about until I turned 40. The mammogram I got earlier that month was meant to just be a baseline, something I did because my doctor thought I should. But that mammogram led to another one, which led to an ultrasound, which led to a biopsy, which led to a doctor telling me that I had cancer.

What was the scariest part of that event? What did you think was the worst thing that could happen to you?

Honestly, when I was first diagnosed, I wasn't scared. I was just angry. I was mad that cancer was interrupting my life. During active treatment, I wasn't afraid because I was so focused on just getting through chemo and radiation. The fear didn't come until many months later. Once treatment was done, I became consumed with the fear that the cancer would return. Honestly, this is something I continue to struggle with.

The fear isn't a fear of death itself. My fear is that cancer will make life not worth living. But a friend of mine helped me realize that cancer will only do that if I let it.

How did you react in the short term?

When I was first diagnosed, I tried to just throw myself into my work and not think about what was happening to me, but that didn't last long.

After the dust settled, what coping mechanisms did you use? What did you do to cope physically, mentally, emotionally, and spiritually?

Once I started chemotherapy, I had to truly face my diagnosis. Being a workaholic was no longer an option because my energy levels were so low. I knew I had to find a way to cope physically, mentally, emotionally, and spiritually. I prayed and read scripture often. I journaled a lot. Specifically, I did a lot of scripting—that's a type of journaling where you write about your desired future as if it already exists. Doing that gave me a sense of hope. I also wrote blog posts and essays for my own website and some digital publications. Sharing my story was empowering. I felt as if I was taking my power back from cancer. I also walked for exercise for at least 30 minutes every single day. This was like moving meditation for me and helped me feel more like myself.

Is there a particular person you are grateful towards who helped you learn to cope and heal? Can you share a story about that?

My husband was absolutely amazing. He was the best caregiver I could have asked for.

My cousin Tasha (who's more like a sister) was also great. She sent me funny videos every single day to help keep my spirits up and we would often text each other while I was sitting in the chemo chair. Most of all, she never treated me like a sick person.

In my own cancer struggle, I sometimes used the idea of embodiment to help me cope. Let's take a minute to look at cancer from an embodiment perspective. If your cancer had a message for you, what do you think it would want or say?

My answer to that depends on my mood, honestly. Some days I feel like cancer is there laughing at me and taunting me. But other days I feel that cancer is reminding me to give myself a break and to not tether my worth to productivity. The year I was going through treatment I was forced to rest and to work less and yet I made more money than I had in previous years. Cancer forced me to find ways to work smarter, not harder.

What did you learn about yourself from this very difficult experience? How has cancer shaped your worldview? What has it taught you that you might never have considered before? Can you please explain with a story or example?

Cancer taught me that I'm stronger than I thought I was. Before my diagnosis, I would say, "At least it's not cancer" ALL THE TIME. And not in a flippant way. I truly thought that cancer was the one thing I could never handle. So, when something bad did happen to me—even when I was diagnosed with lupus in 2008—I would tell myself to not freak out because it wasn't cancer. Then on January 24, 2020, it was cancer. But I handled that, too!

How have you used your experience to bring goodness to the world?

I've been doing all I can to help other breast cancer survivors and thrivers—whether that's sharing my story, answering questions about surgery and treatment, or doing advocacy work with organizations like Tigerlily Foundation.

What are a few of the biggest misconceptions and myths out there about fighting cancer that you would like to dispel?

The biggest misconception is that after you complete active treatment, you're "done with cancer." Even if your doctor declares that there's no evidence of disease you still don't feel "cancer-free." Cancer still sits on your shoulder whispering in your ear that it could return at any moment and interrupt your life and turn your world upside down again. But instead of letting this get me down, I use it as motivation to live life to the fullest while I still can.

Fantastic. Here is the main question of our interview. Based on your experiences and knowledge, what advice would you give to others who have recently been diagnosed with cancer? What are your "5 Things" You Need To Beat Cancer? Please share a story or example for each.

Five things you need to beat cancer include a playlist, your people, a sense of purpose, prayer, and persistence.

1. Playlist

Shortly after my diagnosis, I made a playlist because every battle needs a fight song. Destiny Child's "Survivor" was at the top of my list. I would listen to these songs as I went on my daily walks.

2. People

You need your people. As I mentioned, my husband and cousin Tasha were incredible. Because of the pandemic, I couldn't hang out with friends or family while I was going through treatment, but the women of the See Jane Write community made sure I never felt alone by sending me gifts, inspirational messages and more.

3. Purpose

Cancer is stupid (that's even the title of my cancer playlist). In most cases it's nearly impossible to figure out why cancer decided to attack your body. So it's important to try to find some sense of purpose in it all. For me, that meant sharing my story to encourage other women.

4. Prayer

When going through cancer treatment it's important to prioritize your own well-being while also finding a way to focus on something bigger than yourself. For me it was my faith. I wrote in my prayer journal daily. I read scripture daily and scribbled my favorite bible verses on pink index cards and carried them with me to every treatment.

5. Persistence

"Nevertheless, she persisted" is my cancer-fighting mantra. To me "beating cancer" isn't about not dying. Beating cancer means living your life as well as you can with whatever time you have left. Even while I was going through treatment I continued writing and walking for exercise because I refused to let cancer take those things away from me. Find a way to continue doing at least one of the things you love in spite of cancer.

You are a person of great influence. If you could inspire a movement that would bring the most amount of good to the greatest amount of people, what would that be?

I believe that focusing on helping women—economically, politically, and socially—brings the most amount of good to the greatest amount of people. Research shows that when women move forward, their communities move forward with them.

We are very blessed that some very prominent names in Business, VC funding, Sports, and Entertainment read this column. Is there a person in the world, or in the US with whom you would love to have a private breakfast or lunch, and why?

I would love to have a private brunch with Elaine Welteroth. Even though she's much younger than I am, I look up to her for so many reasons. Her career shows how you can start in magazine journalism and then go anywhere you want by building your brand, believing in yourself, and staying true to yourself.

How can our readers further follow your work online?

You can find me online at www.seejanewrite.net and www.javacia.com and on Instagram: @seejavaciawrite

Jennifer Brown of PinnacleCare: I Survived (Ovarian) Cancer and Here Is How I Did It

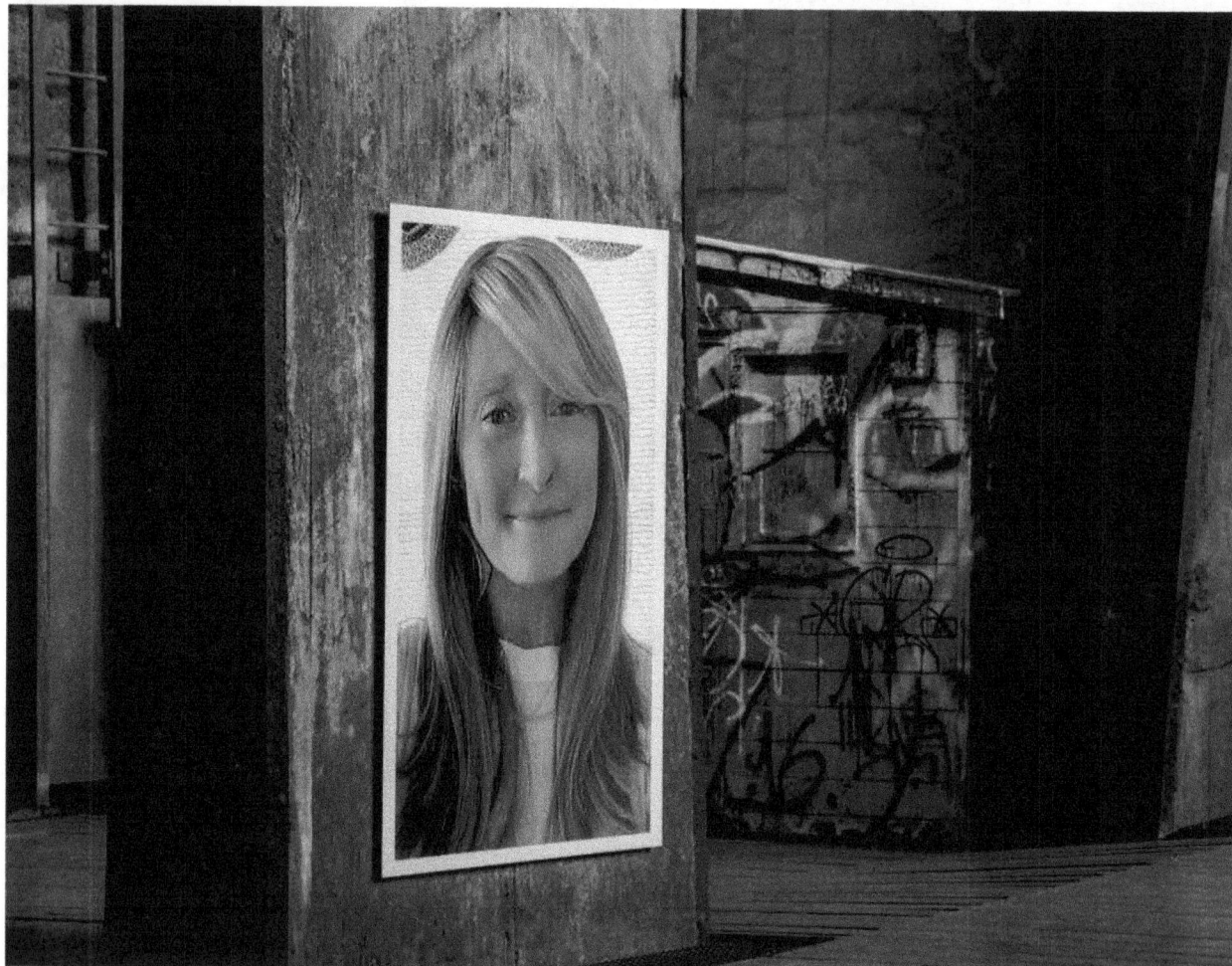

Learn how to graciously receive care—especially during chemo. You need to let the people you love and who love you the most take care of you—don't fight it. Accept their love and care because they want to share in your journey. Your friends, parents, husband, and children all feel the pain of a serious cancer diagnosis along with you, and you need to let them in so they can grieve and recover, as well.

I had the pleasure of interviewing Jennifer Brown. Jennifer experienced a life-threatening challenge after being diagnosed with ovarian cancer late last February 2020. She is Vice President of Marketing at PinnacleCare, a company that provides compassionate health advisory support to people facing serious medical challenges, and was able to tap into their expertise for assurance throughout her cancer journey. She has never let her cancer diagnosis define her or hold her back from her next great adventure... just stay tuned!

Thank you so much for joining us in this interview series! We really appreciate the courage it takes to publicly share your story. Before we start, our readers would love to "get to know you" a bit better. Can you tell us a bit about your background and your childhood backstory?

I grew up in the Baltimore suburbs with a typical childhood tale: lovely family that valued education and encouraged adventure. Post college, I moved to Aspen, CO, to meet a boy from NYC who is my husband of 30 years. After living in Europe and several cities in the US, I found my way back to "Charm City" to raise my family and further my career and life adventures. I'm a mother, wife, sister, daughter, athlete, and executive who intimately understands survival — both as a mother who lost a child and more recently as a cancer survivor.

Can you please give us your favorite "Life Lesson Quote?" Can you share how that was relevant to you in your life?

"There are no passengers on spaceship earth. We are all crew." This is by Marshall McLuhan. I've never been one to be passive; I'm proactive and engaged in every aspect of my life, and I'm comfortable as my own advocate. I also understand that I'm in the driver's seat when it comes to getting beyond cancer...it's up to me to get through and put it behind me.

Let's now shift to the main part of our discussion about surviving cancer. Do you feel comfortable sharing with us the story surrounding how you found out that you had cancer?

Sure...I've always been a super-fit, healthy person. I'm a marathon runner and cyclist and work out every day — but towards the end of January, I developed a constant cough. I didn't feel sick, but the cough just wouldn't go away.

I saw my primary care physician who, suspecting pneumonia, prescribed an antibiotic. I asked for a chest X-ray, but he didn't feel it was needed. Five days later, I was no better and was seen by another doctor in the practice, who prescribed an inhaler and steroids — but again, no chest X-ray. After a week, my condition hadn't improved, so I went to urgent care, and this doctor in fact saved my life. She was concerned that there was fluid in my chest, and it could be an issue with my heart, so I went to the local ER where I finally got that chest X-ray plus CT scans. The scans literally showed two liters of fluid in my chest, which after pathology, revealed malignant cells. A full CT scan that followed found a 15 cm mass in my ovaries. I was in shock — I had advanced stage 4 ovarian cancer. I went into the ER with a cough and came out with cancer! I was lucky, though.

I had a team of experts behind me and contacted the CEO/Chief medical Officer at PinnacleCare, who confirmed I was seeing the best physician for my cancer diagnosis and on the right treatment path.

What was the scariest part of that event? What did you think was the worst thing that could happen to you?

Honestly, the most frightening part was knowing in my heart that something was happening and that I needed to advocate for myself until finally someone recognized that it was serious and recommended the right next steps. Until then, I was not being heard and cancer was not even on my radar. The worst I could imagine was that I had some kind of metabolic deficiency or disorder.

How did you react in the short term?

Practically and strategically, I'm good at "compartmentalizing," so I was in the moment with each test, procedure, and specialist appointment—they came fast, one after another (amazing how quickly/easily you get answers and access when they know you have the big C and it's really, really, bad). Within two weeks of the confirmed diagnosis on February 14th, I had had major surgery and was readying myself for the next treatment after recovering: chemo. I was basically on autopilot, and little did I suspect when discharged from the hospital on March 1st that literally two weeks later, the entire world would shut down with COVID-19!

After the dust settled, what coping mechanisms did you use? What did you do to cope physically, mentally, emotionally, and spiritually?

Coping came easy for me:

- Physically, I'm a "go-hard"—once I was cleared from surgery, I got back on the bike every day for 15–20 miles. No rest for the weary!
- Mentally, I'm a marketing professional in the healthcare industry and working full time and being incredibly busy (because we were helping others during COVID) was the fuel for getting me through. Plus, everybody around the world had to work from home to with me. No FOMO here...I was essentially going through treatment and recovery under the camouflage of COVID-19!
- Emotionally, I'm so lucky to have an incredible family and great friends who surrounded me with 24/7 love and took care of me. It was the first time ever both my husband and son were home working as well, so it was pretty much a lot of togetherness during quarantine... like everyone else.
- Spiritually, I practiced mindfulness, which was a wonderful way to stay balanced and calm. But you see, I have a unique perspective because I lost my 22-year-old daughter Olivia five years ago. Olivia survived for 19 years after a traumatic brain injury, and watching and caring for her when she was so broken and living through so much pain for almost two decades changed how I synthesized my own discomfort and fear. I was never afraid because I knew she was watching over me. I managed chemo treatment well because I knew she had gone through so much more. And I was not afraid of dying because I knew she was on the other side if my cancer won the war.

Is there a particular person you are grateful towards who helped you learn to cope and heal? Can you share a story about that?

Most of us live for our children, and although there is no specific story to share, I do know that when going through cancer treatment (especially chemo), it became even clearer how important it was for me to get through this "mess" so that I could watch my son grow, mature, and become the wonderful husband and father I know he will be—especially after losing my sweet daughter, I wanted another chance to someday be a grandmother. That was my steadfast goal and that was the motivation for me to cope and heal because my son is truly my hero and champion.

In my own cancer struggle, I sometimes used the idea of embodiment to help me cope. Let's take a minute to look at cancer from an embodiment perspective. If your cancer had a message for you, what do you think it would want or say?

That no matter what you do (I'm very healthy, active, and fit), and even though you've chosen to live a "good" life doing decent and kind things, you can't control an "out of control" circumstance. Sometimes bad things happen to good people—sh&t happens. I believe cancer was telling me, "Here we go again—but remember, you have much to be thankful for." You need to remember gratitude even when facing cancer.

What did you learn about yourself from this very difficult experience? How has cancer shaped your worldview? What has it taught you that you might never have considered before? Can you please explain with a story or example?

What I can pull away from the experience is that I now consciously "choose" to be more present. Since you're not guaranteed a long life, you need to make the most of the time you have—especially when it comes to family and being there for the older loved ones in your life who need you. Being that I'm in the club that nobody wants to join—the club of parents who have lost a child—I want to ensure that I'm present and there to help my parents as they age in place, so they don't have to face losing a child, as well.

How have you used your experience to bring goodness to the world?

By being completely open and transparent in sharing my story... at least for anyone interested in listening! Sharing my story is hopefully going to push others to advocate for themselves when they know something is just not right.

What are a few of the biggest misconceptions and myths out there about fighting cancer that you would like to dispel?

First and foremost, cancer is not a death sentence. Fifteen years ago my stage 4 ovarian cancer most likely would have been a death sentence; yet with innovative genetic testing, treatment, and therapies (I'm BRCA 1 and being treated with PARP Inhibitors), I'm moving beyond the diagnosis, and cancer is now a footnote, no longer a headline in my life story.

Fantastic. Here is the main question of our interview. Based on your experiences and

knowledge, what advice would you give to others who have recently been diagnosed with cancer? What are your "5 Things" You Need to Beat Cancer? Please share a story or example for each.

1. It's never too late to be healthy and in good shape. Being that I'm somewhat of a beast as far as fitness goes, I began my cancer journey physically in good shape, and then picked up my workout routine as soon as I was cleared post-surgery. I'm convinced that my fitness is part of my success in beating cancer.

2. It was easier to focus on getting through the current treatment du jour, rather than the bigger picture of getting through the entire illness. For me, I set a goal of getting through each chemo session only, so I had a little victory each time. I won by focusing on each battle rather than the whole war.

3. Losing my hair was nothing short of catastrophic for me. When I looked in a mirror, I felt as if the person I knew had disappeared—this was a stranger. I had a great wig, but hats helped the most—especially because it was during COVID, and I was basically home for 14 months. Wearing hats from my son's college lacrosse teams somehow seemed more normal. That said, since completing chemo last August, my hair is growing and the wig I have has been awesome as I re-enter the outside world.

4. Learn how to graciously receive care—especially during chemo. You need to let the people you love and who love you the most take care of you—don't fight it. Accept their love and care because they want to share in your journey. Your friends, parents, husband, and children all feel the pain of a serious cancer diagnosis along with you, and you need to let them in so they can grieve and recover, as well.

5. Work was the one great distraction and the great equalizer for me during COVID. If you're able to dig in deep at work to get your mind off the severity of your illness, it is an enormous help in your day-to-day emotional well-being. For me, it served as the great equalizer, too, because going through cancer during COVID meant that everyone else was working from home and collaborating over ZOOM, not just me. I shared my diagnosis with several people in my company, but the workday looked the same for us all and it gave me a huge sense of normalcy in an otherwise chaotic situation. Work is good, and it's also okay to say no and rest whenever you need it.

You are a person of great influence. If you could inspire a movement that would bring the most amount of good to the greatest amount of people, what would that be?

I've been a longtime caregiver and caretaker, and when it was time for me to be taken care of, I knew enough about it to let my loved ones in. It made everything easier, more graceful. I think people need to prepare for their caregiving roles more thoughtfully and thoroughly because becoming a caregiver sneaks up on you, yet it's one of the most important and potentially fulfilling jobs you'll ever have.

We are very blessed that some very prominent names in Business, VC funding, Sports, and Entertainment read this column. Is there a person in the world, or in the US with whom you would love to have a private breakfast or lunch, and why?

I would love the opportunity to meet and enjoy a conversation with George Noory, who helped me through countless sleepless nights by listening to his syndicated radio program Coast to Coast AM. He's opened my mind to many "considerations," as well as expanded my spiritual universe. On his show, I was introduced to James Doty, MD, whose teachings on mindfulness helped me through both the loss of my child, as well as through cancer. I'm eternally grateful.

How can our readers further follow your work online?

My LinkedIn profile is www.linkedin.com/in/jennifer-brown-4864346 and I would love to connect with your readers!

Joanna Chanis: I Survived (Breast) Cancer and Here Is How I Did It

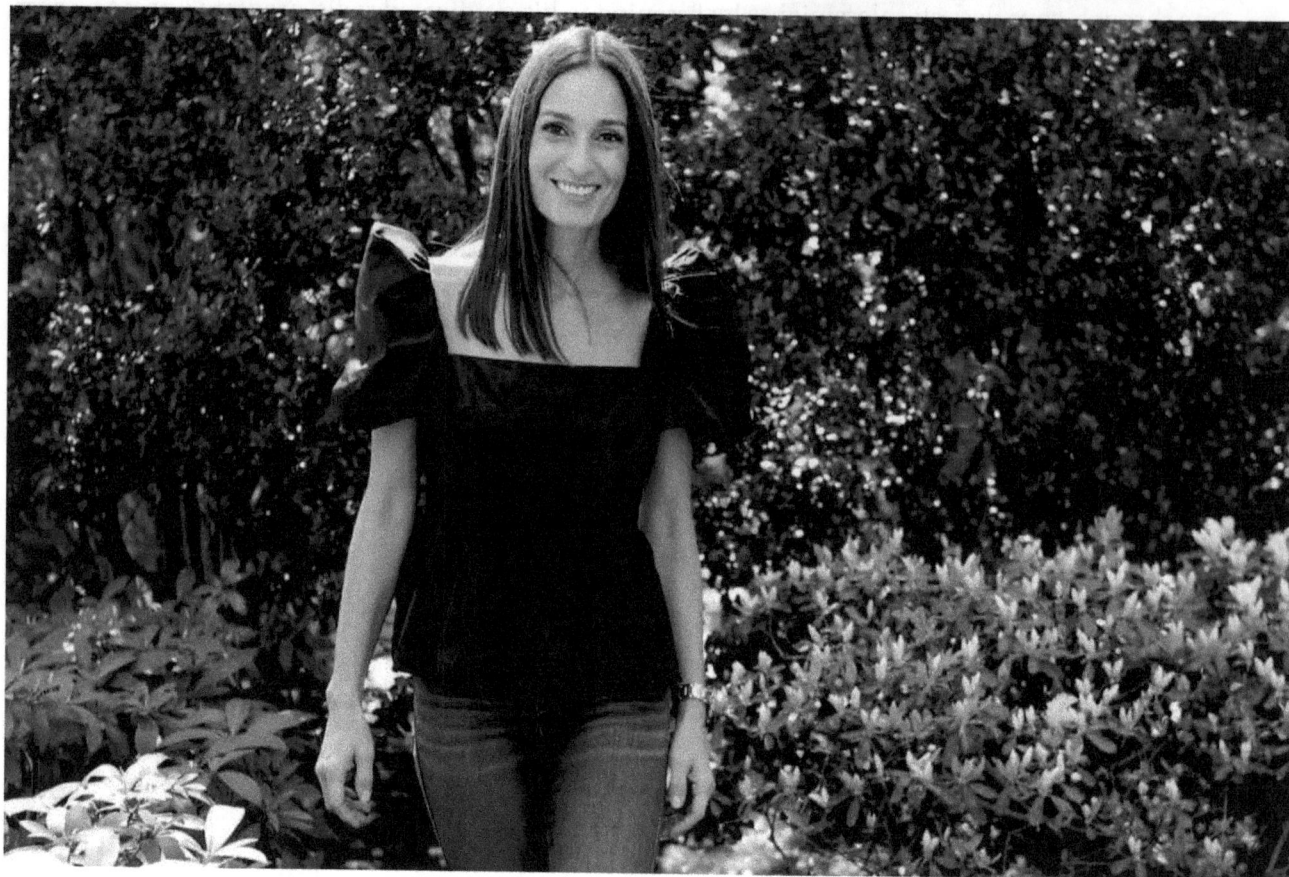

Learn and practice "The Mindset Mentor Method." I developed this method so that I could heal from cancer and come out better on the other side. My book was inspired by a woman who was going through a similar diagnosis as me just a few weeks behind. I would share this methodology with her and watch her have similar results healing and navigating her cancer. She encouraged me to share it with others and said, "You helped me pick me up from my knees and stand tall." I am so happy to report that she is now healthy, happy, and a dear friend.

I had the pleasure of interviewing Joanna Chanis. Joanna, professional mentor and resilience expert, helps young adults and entrepreneurs through hard things—anything from career changes to cancer. Author of The Waiting Room Book, Joanna has healed from cancer, carrying the lessons learned from her journey into every aspect of life. As a professional speaker, corporate teams and young adults have found Joanna's story powerful, utilizing the realistic problem-solving tools and values to teach their teams how to have healthy resilience, overcome challenges, and increase productivity.

Thank you so much for joining us in this interview series! We really appreciate the courage it takes to publicly share your story. Before we start, our readers would love to "get to know you" a bit better. Can you tell us a bit about your background and your childhood backstory?

Thank you so much for having me and allowing me to share my story in order to help others. I was born and raised in Worcester, Massachusetts in a large Greek-American community. My mother, who is an immigrant, raised my younger sister and me while taking care of my father who had progressive MS and was wheelchair-bound and eventually bedridden for the majority of my childhood. He died when I was 16 years old. She worked very hard to provide for us, but it was an extremely stressful childhood. When my father died, I immediately grew up in that instant, as I believe all teenagers do when they lose a parent.

I moved to Boston in 1990 when I was 17 to go to college and have lived there ever since. It was a whole new world for me, so different than how I grew up. I immediately fell in love with the city and knew that was where I belonged. I got married at the age of 25 and have two daughters that I raised in Boston. My career has been super interesting and diverse. I started in corporate sales and sales management and transitioned to being an entrepreneur when my girls were little so I could have more flexibility to be with them. I owned and operated a high-volume restaurant then invented, developed, and launched an app. When I was diagnosed with breast cancer in 2019, my entire life changed, and I knew my purpose was clear. I needed to heal and learn what cancer was trying to teach me so I could live the life I was intended to live, and then help others do the same. I became an author, and now I am a corporate speaker and a professional mentor who helps women get through hard things from career changes to cancer. I teach the method that I developed and give them a clear framework and tools to get through any challenge and come out better on the other side, no matter what. It is the most rewarding and incredible feeling to see someone thriving after going through hardship, and the fact that I can be part of helping them is so fulfilling.

Can you please give us your favorite "Life Lesson Quote?" Can you share how that was relevant to you in your life?

"The Truth Shall Set You Free"

My life from the outside looking in looked "perfect." I worked 24/7 to make it look that way. In fact, I had done that since I was a little girl. No matter how bad things got at home when I was a kid, I could always clean myself up and "pull it together" and show up like everything was great. You can imagine that in 47 years of doing that, I became an expert. There is a fine line between looking at the bright side and flat out lying to yourself.

I am a practical optimist by nature. Combine that with wanting to make something work that was just never meant to, and you have a woman that lied to herself and to everyone around her. The image I put forth became my driving force. Well, there is nothing to shake that up more than cancer. It makes you see things differently. Through it, I finally gave myself permission to say the truth and from there my whole life changed.

Let's now shift to the main part of our discussion about surviving cancer. Do you feel comfortable sharing with us the story surrounding how you found out that you had cancer?

Yes, I am very comfortable sharing. I wrote a book about the time between the initial diagnosis and my double mastectomy surgery called *The Waiting Room Book* so that other women would never have to "wait" alone. Finding the cancer and then all the testing and waiting that leads to more testing and waiting after the cancer diagnosis for me was the hardest part. In the opening of the book, I describe the moment that my doctor called me with the news that a routine biopsy for what they thought was a fibroadenoma was indeed cancer. My primary care doctor had felt it in my annual checkup so that's what got the wheels going. I have had regular mammograms since I was 32 years old because of a swollen milk duct after the birth of my youngest daughter. My breasts were lumpy and dense so there were other times in the past that I had to have biopsies and ultrasounds in addition to mammograms. I was always so stressed and worried that one day this call would come, and in September of 2019, it did.

What was the scariest part of that event? What did you think was the worst thing that could happen to you?

There were so many scary parts, but I think the scariest was having to tell my daughters. Having grown up with a parent that was sick and who had died while I was around their age was beyond scary. I knew how they were feeling firsthand, and that made everything so much harder. I thought the worst thing that could have happened to me was that I would become very sick and die.

How did you react in the short term?

My initial instinct was to make sure I could process all this before I told my daughters. You see, the phone call from my doctor was in the early evening, right around the time that they were expected home from the first day of their sophomore and junior years of high school. So, I knew I needed to get out of the house before they got home. I called my husband and my best friend, and the three of us created a plan to give me some initial space for a few hours. I describe the whole evening in my book; it was a night that I will never forget because it revealed a lot about what was to come. My marriage was not in a good place and hadn't been for many years. I had been able to overlook things that somehow now I just couldn't anymore. Cancer is the greatest truth-teller.

After the dust settled, what coping mechanisms did you use? What did you do to cope physically, mentally, emotionally, and spiritually?

This is exactly what I wrote about in my book! I made so many changes in all of these avenues that completely transformed my life.

Physically, I was in great shape. I practiced Pilates, yoga, and took Soul Cycle classes three times each week. Once I was diagnosed, I didn't crave any of those things. Instead, I ordered a rebounder and started to bounce each day. I have kept this as part of my routine today. I took long walks which I still do without any technology. I walk for about an hour four days per week.

Mentally, I had a secret weapon that literally saved me. I am a Transcendental Meditator and relied heavily on this practice. I remember thinking how incredibly lucky I was to have this as part of my life. I still feel that way today, and it has deepened my commitment to meditate daily. This is a game-changer.

Emotionally, I relied heavily on my friends and my little sister. I am incredibly blessed to have these humans in my lifeboat. I always knew how incredible they were, but they went above and beyond to support and love me. It was a silver lining for sure.

Spiritually, I prayed...and prayed...and prayed! I have a very deep connection to my faith and to God, so this part was natural for me. I was able to form a prayer circle based on the book *The Power of Eight* by Lynne McTaggart. This circle came together so easily and includes women from every part of my life and every religious background. After I was healed, the circle stayed together, and now we pray for others. It is one of the best parts of my life.

Is there a particular person you are grateful towards who helped you learn to cope and heal? Can you share a story about that?

There are many people that I am grateful for throughout my healing journey, and I would never be able to find the words to describe how much love and support I received from my friends, family, and community. However, there was one very special connection that I made during this time that helped me to heal from the inside out. Her name is Apollonia and I saw her once a week during the 10 weeks between my diagnosis and surgery. She was so important in my healing that I dedicated an entire chapter in my book to the first session we had. Her ability to help me energetically was so vital that I would make the trip each week from Boston to New York.

Apollonia and I met a few days after my diagnosis. A dear friend who had healed from cancer had insisted I work with her. I still remember my trembling legs in the Uber on the way to her apartment in Harlem. I didn't even ask my friend what it was that Apollonia actually did so I had no idea what to expect. I just knew that I had to see her. After we met, I immediately knew I was in the best hands possible. That first session she "worked" on me using different energetic healing methods, and I was hooked.

When I came out of the room, my friends that were waiting for me said, "You look like a completely different person." I felt that was the moment that I knew I was going to be able to heal and grow through my cancer journey.

In my own cancer struggle, I sometimes used the idea of embodiment to help me cope. Let's take a minute to look at cancer from an embodiment perspective. If your cancer had a message for you, what do you think it would want or say?

I am so sorry that you had to go through cancer, and I wish you good health today and every day. I agree with you 100%! In fact, I always refer to my cancer as my greatest teacher. I knew that if I had handled cancer the way I had handled every other crisis in my life that I wouldn't fully heal, and I would have missed "the point."

Cancer's message to me was to teach me how to be authentically grateful. You see, I always considered myself a grateful person, but I realized that although I would say I was grateful, I didn't really feel grateful. I believe that by surrendering to and accepting cancer, it taught me how to find authentic gratitude, no matter what the circumstance. I didn't realize it at the time, but once I had applied this methodology to cancer, I was able to use it in every other aspect of my life.

I have had tremendous results in my health and personal and professional life by using this "mindset mentor method." People around me noticed, and I started to teach it to them, as well. The results are phenomenal. I have helped many people since teaching them this three-step method. It has allowed me to get through cancer, the pandemic lockdown, divorce, and come out better on the other side. Plus, I use it for the little things, too, like being stuck in traffic. It works on any challenge. I believe that if I had this method when I was younger, I would have had a much happier and easier life...and who knows, maybe I could have avoided cancer altogether. I was always stressed out before, and I believe there is nothing worse for your health than stress.

What did you learn about yourself from this very difficult experience? How has cancer shaped your worldview? What has it taught you that you might never have considered before? Can you please explain with a story or example?

I learned how to relax. Cancer has changed my worldview because it is the great equalizer. It doesn't care what you look like, how much money you have, what kind of car you drive, how many followers you have on social media, or what your dreams are. I remember one of the first times I walked into the "cancer floor" at Massachusetts General Hospital; I looked around at all the different people. It was pre-pandemic, so I could see everyone's faces. I thought, *what is the common link here?* I was in a room filled with adults of all ages, races, sizes, and backgrounds, and the one thing we all had in common...cancer. I spent most of my life worrying about how things "looked," pretending everything was okay when it wasn't. At that moment when I looked around the room at my new "tribe," I realized it was something inside that connected us that was far deeper than anything we could see on the outside. We were all doing the same thing, trying to heal ourselves. I have carried this with me ever since that day.

How have you used your experience to bring goodness to the world?

It is now my purpose and mission to do exactly that. I am a mentor to women who have/had breast cancer and require a mastectomy and hormone suppression therapy. I teach them everything I learned and give them the support and tools to come out better on the other side. I have written *The Waiting Room Book* which is meant to feel like a friend is holding your hand throughout your diagnosis. It also gives you tools and practical advice on how to navigate everything from logistics to how to tell your kids. As a resilience expert, I speak to top performing corporate teams and help them reduce stress during the COVID crisis based on my method, "The Mindset Mentor Method," so they can relax and increase productivity. And I am SUPER excited to be launching The Women's Wellness Club. This is my passion project, and it was inspired by the group of young women that I mentor and fans of my podcast and YouTube channel *About Life with JO*. The mission is to teach women how to put themselves first while juggling all the demands of life, so they can stay healthy. It includes two live talks per month and one live cooking demonstration, with a custom monthly "toolkit" summarizing everything we covered so that they can be present in each session and don't have to worry about taking notes. This incredible community will have access to a private FB group where I will answer questions and come up with specific relevant content based on what the group needs.

What are a few of the biggest misconceptions and myths out there about fighting cancer that you would like to dispel?

The biggest myth and misconception is that you must "fight" it! It is what we are told to do by the media and all of the cancer propaganda out there, and it's so sad. Here you are getting this life-threatening diagnosis and they are sending you to war? How does that make sense? I think fighting of any kind only increases stress which helps cancer grow. I see it differently. In my experience cancer needs to be acknowledged and accepted without reservations, and from there you can work through it. I am no stranger to fighting, I had been fighting my entire life and, yet, I knew that if I approached cancer that way, I wouldn't fully heal. So, I set forth to find a better way, and I am so grateful that I did because it not only healed me but now is helping to heal so many others.

Fantastic. Here is the main question of our interview. Based on your experiences and knowledge, what advice would you give to others who have recently been diagnosed with cancer? What are your "5 Things" You Need To Beat Cancer? Please share a story or example for each.

1. Learn and practice "The Mindset Mentor Method." I developed this method so that I could heal from cancer and come out better on the other side. My book was inspired by a woman who was going through a similar diagnosis as me just a few weeks behind me. I would share this methodology with her and watch her have similar results healing and navigating her cancer. She encouraged me to share it with others and said, "You helped me pick me up from my knees and stand tall." I am so happy to report that she is now healthy, happy, and a dear friend.
2. Cut refined sugar out of your diet in all forms. I was always a "healthy eater," but after my diagnosis I made sure to focus on eating things that would help me heal. Nothing new here, as we hear this all the time. My two biggest influences and teachers on this subject were Dr. Mark Hyman and Anthony Williams. I developed a hybrid of both of their philosophies that has helped me tremendously, and I still stick to it 80% of the time.
3. Ask for help. I always thought I could do everything by myself. Well, I don't think that way now. Leaning on my incredible friends and family was one of the biggest gifts I received through this journey.

4. Forgive yourself and others. I chose to completely wipe the slate clean with every single hang up I had about myself. I forgave myself for all the mistakes I had been holding onto for decades. I also chose to forgive people that had hurt me. I did this for me without even engaging them. I think this is vital to all healing.
5. Believe in something bigger than yourself. You can call this anything you want, Higher Power, The Universe, Inner Guide; I call it God. Having a spiritual practice has been the foundation of my life, and in my hardest moments it is what got me up each time.

You are a person of great influence. If you could inspire a movement that would bring the most amount of good to the greatest amount of people, what would that be?

My dream is to inspire "The Mindset Mentor" movement, a community where people apply the method in every aspect of their lives so they can live a healthy, authentic, and satisfying life.

We are very blessed that some very prominent names in Business, VC funding, Sports, and Entertainment read this column. Is there a person in the world, or in the US with whom you would love to have a private breakfast or lunch, and why?

Arianna Huffington! She is my mentor, and I am so inspired by her work. We have so much in common. We are both Greek mothers of two daughters, gone through divorce, entrepreneurs, and turned our biggest health challenge into something that helps and inspires others. I have this vision of Arianna and me making spanakopita together while she gives me advice! A girl can dream, right?

How can our readers further follow your work online?

Please connect with me at www.Joannachanis.com. From there, you can see all my work, access The Women's Wellness Club, my book, podcast, YouTube, and Instagram.

Josh Mailman of WARMTH: I Survived (Pancreatic Neuroendocrine) Cancer and Here Is How I Did It

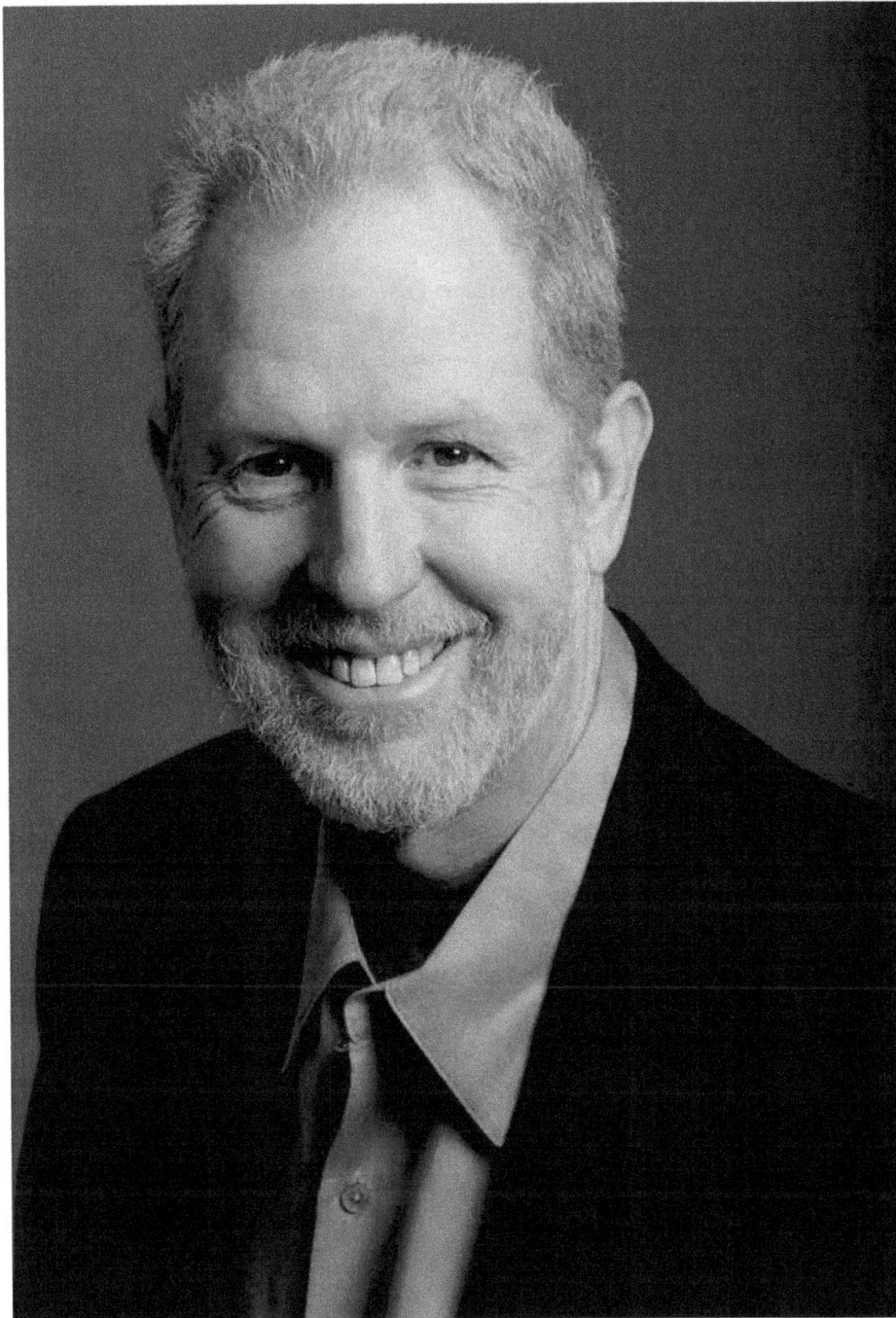

Never stop learning. Research your disease—research treatments. Don't be afraid to ask for a second opinion. Your journey might take you on unfamiliar roads. Many people are afraid of "Watch and Wait." I was told this at the start of my journey. I turned this into "Watch and Learn" so when the time came for action, I was prepared to make a decision.

I had the pleasure of interviewing Josh Mailman. Josh is an internationally recognized advocate for neuroendocrine tumor patients as well as an advocate for nuclear medicine and molecular imaging and integrative oncology. He is the inaugural chair of the Society of Nuclear Medicine and Molecular Imaging's (SNMMI) Patient Advocacy Advisory Board, a board member of the Neuroendocrine Tumor Research Foundation, President of NorCal CarciNET Community and COO of WARMTH. He has an MBA from the Anderson School of Management at UCLA and has been a technology entrepreneur for more than 20 years.

Thank you so much for joining us in this interview series! We really appreciate the courage it takes to publicly share your story. Before we start, our readers would love to "get to know you" a bit better. Can you tell us a bit about your background and your childhood backstory?

I am the youngest of four children and the only son in the family. My dad was a physician and my mom a registered nurse. I was always comfortable around medicine, as I went on patient "rounds" with my father in the hospital on the weekend. I played volleyball in high school and then kept playing at the beach during my college years. I was always healthy, and had only experienced medical issues due to injuries sustained from volleyball. I had knee surgery in my teens and shoulder surgery as an adult. Otherwise, I was just your average, 6'6" volleyball player from southern California.

Can you please give us your favorite "Life Lesson Quote?" Can you share how that was relevant to you in your life?

"Enjoy Every Sandwich" —Warren Zevon

Warren Zevon (lung cancer patient) made this comment on his last appearance on the David Letterman Show, when David had asked him for a "life lesson quote." It sums up what I tell other cancer patients—we need to do what we can to prolong the quantity and quality of our life, but in the end, we must enjoy what is around us, as that is really all that really matters.

Let's now shift to the main part of our discussion about surviving cancer. Do you feel comfortable sharing with us the story surrounding how you found out that you had cancer?

Happy to—as I hope my path through cancer can help others.

So the challenge of my cancer discovery was that I was feeling well. I was 46 years old and going in for my annual checkup. My physician felt something unusual under my rib cage, but she didn't think much of it. She recommended at some point to have an ultrasound, but it wasn't a rush. Six weeks later, I went to Urgent Care for a flu test. Since I needed an ultrasound too, it was suggested I get the ultrasound while I wait for my test results. I'm not worried at all at this point. Things turned scary when the technician wouldn't look me in the eye during the ultrasound. The Urgent Care physician would no longer look me in the eye either. I knew something was amiss.

The Urgent Care doctor put me in touch with my internist. He ordered a bunch of extra blood tests and told me that they needed to do more imaging scans and that everything was going to be alright.

The CT scan was scheduled for the following week. The waiting between the ultrasound and the CT scan was incredibly scary. Once the scan was complete, we knew it was a tumor on my pancreas that had spread into my liver.

What was the scariest part of that event? What did you think was the worst thing that could happen to you?

Waiting for the diagnosis was incredibly scary. I was pretty scared after they realized it was a tumor on my pancreas. Doctors weren't sure what it was for certain or if it was cancerous, but they did not seem to think it was going to be good. This waiting and uncertainty were very frightening. I waited another 10 days for a biopsy and another week until we found out what type of cancer I had. I have a very rare neuroendocrine tumor of the pancreas with metastatic disease to my liver. At the time of diagnosis, I had a larger-than softball size tumor on my pancreas and several hundred tumors on my liver. At that time, our son was only 10-months-old and I was fearful that I wouldn't be at his first birthday party.

Given the extent of my disease, I was not sure there were any surgical options available to me. I thought the worst thing that could happen to me is that I would not be alive to see my son reach his first birthday.

How did you react in the short term?

My background is in technology management. The way I manage most things is I try to get the most information that I can and make the best decisions based on that information. The fact that I had such a rare diagnosis was the scariest and most consequential issue I had ever faced in my life. I spent many hours researching and investigating answers and immersed myself in information to understand the disease.

After the dust settled, what coping mechanisms did you use? What did you do to cope physically, mentally, emotionally, and spiritually?

The dust never settles when you have a cancer diagnosis. In the early days, I would drive my road bike around the bay on the Bay Area Trail in California and just look at the beautiful water. I tried to calm myself on those rides. I have tremendous support from my wife, and from my family and friends. I also have an incredibly supportive medical team.

When I did find a support group that dealt with this rare type of cancer—I learned to lean on my support group friends as well. I was also really fortunate to be able to take advantage of the University of California San Francisco (USCF) Integrative Oncology Program where I learned about taking care of myself during this part of my life journey.

It was my support group that changed the arc of my journey with cancer. The group provided me with emotional support, encouraged me to learn more about my disease and explore educational conferences, and to meet with more patients and doctors. It was at an educational conference on my disease where I had heard a lecture from a leading nuclear medicine physician from Germany that changed my life and learned how I was to be medically treated going forward.

Is there a particular person you are grateful towards who helped you learn to cope and heal? Can you share a story about that?

There are so many people who help you and join the journey with you. Donald Abrams, M.D. at UCSF taught me how to take care of myself. My wife stood by me at every appointment and at every turn of my diagnosis and subsequent treatments. My friends and family were always there for me, as were members of my support group.

In my own cancer struggle, I sometimes used the idea of embodiment to help me cope. Let's take a minute to look at cancer from an embodiment perspective. If your cancer had a message for you, what do you think it would want or say?

Figure out what is important to you—what brings you joy and go do it. Don't put off something in the future or don't waste time on work that has little meaning for you—life is too short. In a sense, I have adapted this attitude—my planning horizon is no more than four times my imaging scan intervals.

What did you learn about yourself from this very difficult experience? How has cancer shaped your worldview? What has it taught you that you might never have considered before? Can you please explain with a story or example?

I learned to trust the tools that I had used in my life in this stressful situation. There are no easy answers or shortcuts: do your research, learn who to trust and who you want on your team.

I am, as are most that live in the United States and other developed countries, extremely fortunate to have quality health care and availability of treatment options. These options don't exist for most in the developing world and even for some in underserved communities. We must work with the medical community to make durable, affordable health care solutions that can be implemented worldwide.

Until I started working with healthcare nonprofits and speaking at international events, I had never fully considered the challenges in providing healthcare worldwide. The typical Western model of seeing a doctor annually for check-ups or when sick, and taking a treatment followed by another checkup is not viable in many other parts of the world. Most will see a doctor only when sick, but will barely be able to afford it, and many don't have the luxury of multiple treatment visits. Treatments need to be available and financially viable to these types of communities.

How have you used your experience to bring goodness to the world?

I'm leading a life of advocacy for others in my situation. I advocate for neuroendocrine tumor patients as well as advocate for nuclear medicine and molecular imaging and integrative oncology. I chair the Society of Nuclear Medicine and Molecular Imaging's (SNMMI) Patient Advocacy Advisory Board and am a board member of the Neuroendocrine Tumor Research Foundation, as well as the President of NorCal CarciNET Community and COO of WARMTH (World Association of Radiopharmaceuticals and Molecular Therapy).

I also work with the American Society of Clinical Oncology (ASCO) and the American Association of Clinical Researchers (AACR) to help train young clinical oncology researchers across all cancer types because it is vital that we train the next generation of researchers to keep making progress against all types of cancers.

What are a few of the biggest misconceptions and myths out there about fighting cancer that you would like to dispel?

First, it's a myth that you can't live with cancer. You can. I am. I've had cancer for 15 years. With the right treatment plan, you can still participate and thrive in life.

Second, it's a myth that there are miracle cures that can cure everything, including cancer, that are being kept from patients. There really aren't and the vast majority of all who work in the medical field would like people to live longer and have a better quality of life.

Third, go where your journey takes you. You want to ask questions and be open to learning something new. I was fortunate to meet with some of the leading experts in nuclear medicine at a patient conference. I asked questions and was open to learning more even though I knew very little at the time. The path that opened up for me changed the path of my cancer journey with new diagnostics that could image my disease and new treatment possibilities that could extend and improve the quality of my life.

Fourth, remember that the statistics that you see online or that your doctor may quote to you are for what came before. There are new treatments and methods going forward and your job is to live your best life and continue to seek advancement in care.

Fantastic. Here is the main question of our interview. Based on your experiences and knowledge, what advice would you give to others who have recently been diagnosed with cancer? What are your "5 Things" You Need To Beat Cancer? Please share a story or example for each.

1. Talk about it—to your medical team, to your family, to others who share your journey. Find a support group; find a way to reach out and help others who are walking a similar path as you. Learn how to talk to your medical team so that they can be more responsive to what you need. Learning to "Speak Up!" is something I am passionate about—I have even gone around the country giving talks on this topic (www.norcalcarcinet.org/speakingup). Many patients don't want to share their journey with family and friends, for me it was a great source of support. Yes, you might lose a few friends in the process but the ones who step up will be your true friends for life. Support groups can be extremely helpful as it gives you an opportunity to listen to and share experiences with others. The support group I went to encouraged me to educate myself in

addition to the information I was receiving from my medical team which led me to the treatment path that extended the quantity and quality of my life. In 2008, with the encouragement of my support group, I attended a patient education conference in Toronto, Canada 3,000+ miles from my home. There, I learned about new innovations in nuclear medicine occurring in Europe. Within six weeks, I was in Europe having a new type of imaging tracer for my disease. That one decision changed the course of my disease. Six months later, I was back in Europe having a type of nuclear medical therapy that was still investigational. I didn't know at the time but this was early in the development of theranostics (diagnostics/therapy) of my disease—which used the same nuclear medicine targeting agent for imaging and treatment of cancer. This not only changed the path of my disease, but it also changed it for tens of thousands of those that have come after me since the approval of theranostics in Europe and the United States in 2017–2018. Now this nuclear medicine technique is in clinical trials and heading towards approval in prostate cancer.

2. Never stop learning. Research your disease—research treatments. Don't be afraid to ask for a second opinion. Your journey might take you on unfamiliar roads. Many people are afraid of "Watch and Wait." I was told this at the start of my journey. I turned this into "Watch and Learn" so when the time came for action, I was prepared to make a decision.

3. Enjoy Every Sandwich. I am inspired by the words of the late singer-songwriter Warren Zevon who when asked by David Letterman if he had any wisdom that he wanted to share now that he was diagnosed with terminal cancer replied, "Enjoy Every Sandwich." I think Warren's message is simple—don't dwell on the past and enjoy where you are and every moment that you experience. While I have lived with cancer for more than 14 years I know that I will not live forever, so I try to enjoy every moment I have.

4. Remember, the majority of your body is well. While it is natural to focus on your cancer and what you need to manage your care, make sure to take care of yourself. When I was first diagnosed and had my first meeting with an integrative oncologist his philosophy was that my body was a garden and that cancer was a weed growing in my garden. My oncology team's job was to manage and remove the weeds as best as they could. His job (and mine too) was to tend the garden—making it a place of joy and beauty and not an easy place for weeds to grow. Cancer patients often tell me that their oncologists only see their cancer and not them. I let them know that that's okay, as their job is to weed out the cancer. Work with an integrative oncologist or a palliative care team to make sure all of YOU is taken care of so you can have the best "garden on the block."

5. Give back—If you survived cancer, it is because others before you gave their time, energy, or funding to make the advancements that have enabled you to survive and thrive. I have continually given back by participating in clinical trials and volunteering with medical societies to give patient's perspectives. I have also raised funds for and donated to cancer research. One of the nuclear medicine diagnostic clinical trials I raised funds for was approved in 2020.

You are a person of great influence. If you could inspire a movement that would bring the most amount of good to the greatest amount of people, what would that be?

I would make cancer diagnostics and care more affordable and available worldwide. I would educate more physicians and patients on the benefits of nuclear medicine and the emerging field of Theranostics which uses the targeting molecule to image and treat cancer.

We are very blessed that some very prominent names in Business, VC funding, Sports, and Entertainment read this column. Is there a person in the world, or in the US with whom you would love to have a private breakfast or lunch, and why?

I'd go with breakfast, as I am up early collaborating with friends in the nuclear medicine field around the globe. I'd love to have breakfast with Bill Gates to discuss his efforts on worldwide health initiatives. He has spent a great deal of energy and resources on tackling some of the world's largest health issues, like COVID and malaria—which combined has taken the lives of 4,000,000. How can I learn from what has and has not worked on controlling those infectious diseases and apply this to cancer which takes 10,000,000 lives annually? Is there a strategy for low-cost and durable cancer treatments so less lives can be lost to this deadly disease?

How can our readers further follow your work online?

You can follow me on Twitter: @globeseek or contact me at josh@norcalcarcinet.org

Scan the QR code to view my "5 Tips" I've Learned On My Journey With Cancer Vimeo video:

Judy Pearson: I Survived (Breast) Cancer and Here Is How I Did It

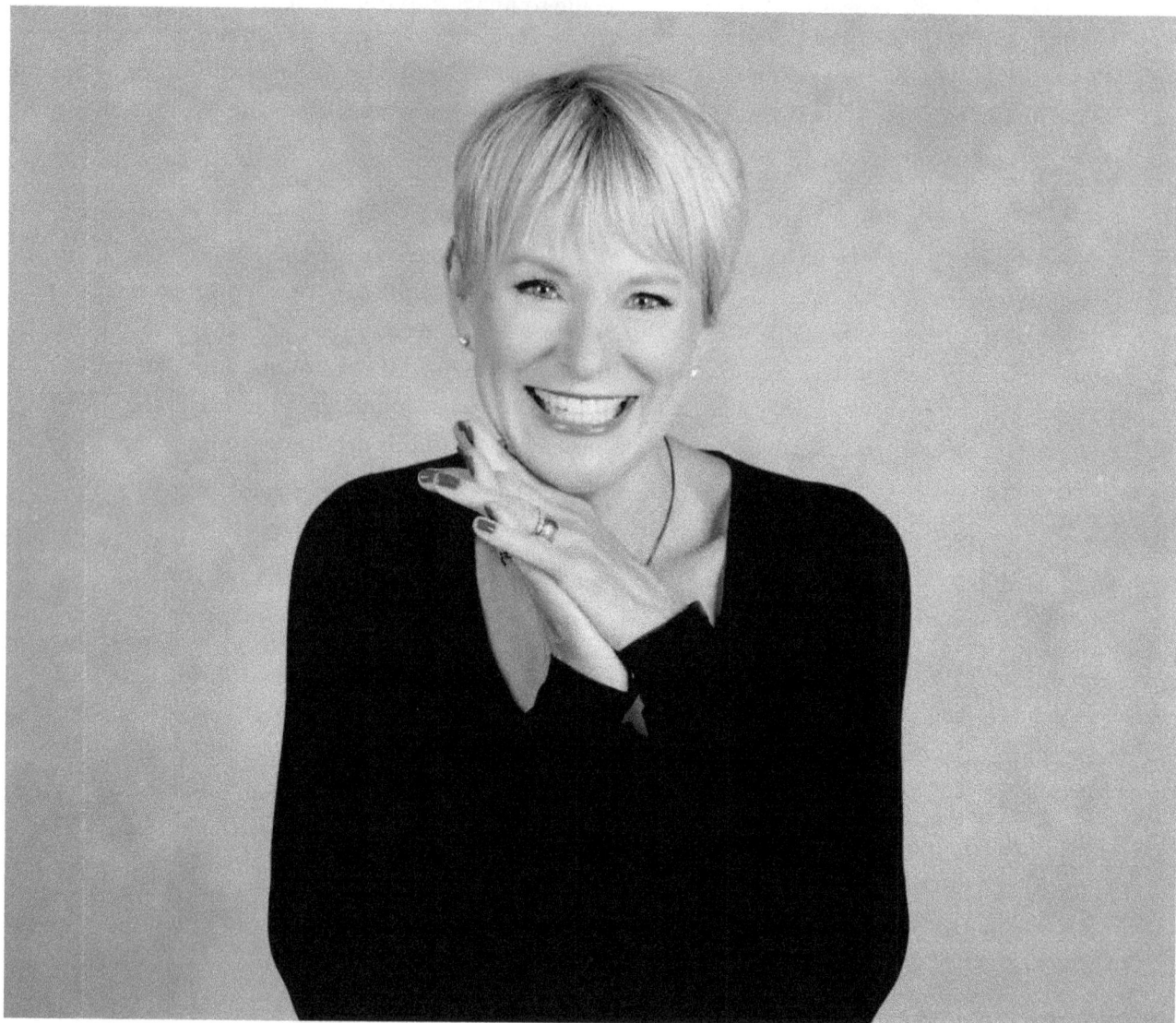

It's the darkest nights that produce the brightest stars. Focusing on the good things in a bad situation can make it easier. You may be bald from chemo, but now you can try a shorter hair do. Hospitals and treatment rooms can be a drag, but you're meeting new people, some of whom might just become great friends. Treatment is difficult, but how fortunate are we that it exists! In addition, what doctors learn from you could save lives in the future.

I had the pleasure of interviewing Judy Pearson. Judy is a storyteller and a cancer survivor. She learned that helping is healing and has spent her survivorship sharing that lesson. And in a remarkable twist of fate, that lesson is now reaching thousands.

Thank you so much for joining us in this interview series! We really appreciate the courage it takes to publicly share your story. Before we start, our readers would love to "get to know you" a bit better. Can you tell us a bit about your background and your childhood backstory?

As a Michigan girl, I'm a Spartan for life, having graduated from Michigan State University. I've always loved a good story. And while it took me a few career choices (as a high school French teacher, a basketball coach, an advertising executive and a voice-over talent), that love led me to become a published author. I write biographies about little known people who have done extraordinary things in their lives. One of my books has even been purchased for a movie.

Can you please give us your favorite "Life Lesson Quote?" Can you share how that was relevant to you in your life?

"It's only in the darkest night that you can best see the stars." The quote is attributed to many authors, but it's the meaning that's the most important. When we feel we're at the bottom, when everything seems as though it's slipping away, *that* is the moment you'll most clearly see the way forward.

Let's now shift to the main part of our discussion about surviving cancer. Do you feel comfortable sharing with us the story surrounding how you found out that you had cancer?

I had just married the man of my dreams (after a couple of divorces). I was living on the shores of Lake Michigan and had two grown sons of whom I was (and still am) extremely proud. Two months after a clean mammogram, I found a lump in my cleavage. A biopsy confirmed it was Triple Negative Breast Cancer, rare and extremely aggressive.

What was the scariest part of that event? What did you think was the worst thing that could happen to you?

(Laughing out loud) Scariest part? All of it was scary! I thought about my own mortality. Death was not in my immediate plan. I had so much more to do, so many more stories to tell. I wanted to love my husband into old age, enjoy my sons' successes, and watch my grandchildren grow.

How did you react in the short term?

And then I realized that if I hadn't found that lump myself, if it had been buried more deeply in my breast tissue and not noticeable till my next mammogram, death would have been a certainty.

Clearly, this wasn't my end. It was an experience that had meaning. And I was going to make it mean something for others, too.

Ironically during surgery, there was indeed more cancer found that the mammogram had completely missed. I have dense breast tissue (as do about 40% of all women). Mammography has difficulty detecting anomalies through dense tissue.

After the dust settled, what coping mechanisms did you use? What did you do to cope physically, mentally, emotionally, and spiritually?

Research! As I mentioned, I'm a biographer and do a lot of research for my books. I'm also someone who likes to be well-prepared for any contingency. Therefore, I had thoroughly researched my disease, reconstruction and treatment. But at no time did it occur to me to research survivorship. I just assumed at the end of it all, the old Judy would jump out of the chemo cake!

But the old Judy was nowhere to be found. Replacing her was a woman with night sweats, joint pain, brain fog, chronic fatigue AND insomnia. My oncologist offered more drugs to offset those, but I declined. It was the chemo drugs—which, I'm grateful to say, saved my life—that had gotten me there in the first place. I wanted to know what else was coming. So I began researching survivorship, and discovered other women survivors who were using their gifts of life and experience for the greater good. By helping others, they were healing themselves.

There is real, scientific research that has been done on the health benefits of volunteering. And it just makes sense. When you take the focus off yourself and your problems, and shine your energy out to others, your challenges seem to take a back seat.

Is there a particular person you are grateful towards who helped you learn to cope and heal? Can you share a story about that?

Without a doubt, it is my amazing husband. I actually told him he should probably get out of our new marriage as fast as he could. I might die and my personal landscape would be completely altered. I insisted this new world was NOT what he had signed up for. But he took my hands, looked me in the eyes, and said this was EXACTLY what he had signed up for. And we have slogged through the ups and downs together ever since.

What did you learn about yourself from this very difficult experience? How has cancer shaped your worldview? What has it taught you that you might never have considered before? Can you please explain with a story or example?

I've now met thousands of cancer survivors. And almost all of them have said what I've often said over the last decade: cancer was the best worst thing that ever happened to me. Two years before the disease came to call; I had gone through a difficult divorce (after 15 difficult years of marriage). I recovered to have a wonderful new life with my new husband.

Cancer has been the same, difficult but life-changing for the good. I thank God and the universe every day for all my blessings. I've learned there's not a minute to waste in life. I have jettisoned toxic situations and relationships. I focus on what matters to me (and those I love).

Psychologists often refer to it as post traumatic growth, the reverse experience of post-traumatic stress. And boy, have I grown!

How have you used your experience to bring goodness to the world?

I like to think so. When I discovered the "helping is healing" theory, I began volunteering, too. My volunteering experiences led me to create A 2nd Act, an organization whose sole mission is to celebrate and support women survivors of all cancers as they give back to the world around them. Our annual fundraising is a live, professionally produced storytelling event, with an ever-evolving cast of eight women survivors sharing their 2nd Acts (how they're giving back after cancer).

And A 2nd Act led me to a woman who became the inspiration for my latest biography, *From Shadows to Life: A Biography of the Cancer Survivorship Movement*. It begins with President Richard Nixon signing the National Cancer Act on December 23, 1971 (this year will be the 50th anniversary). The act infused unprecedented amounts of money into cancer research. But survivors faced horrible discrimination and isolation. A group came together to launch and lead a survivorship movement, much like the women's movement and the AIDS movement. This is their story.

What are a few of the biggest misconceptions and myths out there about fighting cancer that you would like to dispel?

First, that survivorship begins at diagnosis, as that's the moment we begin surviving cancer. There's no magic three or five year goal line to receive that title. The founders of the survivorship movement created that definition 35 years ago and it is accepted by the medical community today.

Secondly, as both my organization and my new biography clearly illustrate, cancer doesn't end when treatment does. Whether you have no evidence of disease, or you're told you must live with your cancer, the changes you've undergone are now a part of the fabric of your life. However, as I mentioned above, some of those changes can—and should—be used for good.

Fantastic. Here is the main question of our interview. Based on your experiences and knowledge, what advice would you give to others who have recently been diagnosed with cancer? What are your "5 Things" You Need To Beat Cancer? Please share a story or example for each.

1. As I said at the outset, it's the darkest nights that produce the brightest stars. Focusing on the good things in a bad situation can make it easier. You may be bald from chemo, but now you can try a shorter hair do. Hospitals and treatment rooms can be a drag, but you're meeting new people, some of whom might just become great friends. Treatment is difficult, but how fortunate are we that it exists! In addition, what doctors learn from you could save lives in the future.

2. Did you know you can even eat an elephant a bite at a time? In this case, the elephant is cancer, and at the outset, it can seem like a daunting, never-ending journey. But breaking it down to one day at a time makes it feel more manageable. I posted a sticky note in our bedroom with the number of chemo treatments I had left. Watching the number go down was greatly stress reducing.

3. One of the founders of the survivorship movement talked about the importance of "Veterans guiding the rookies." In other words, there are always survivors who can benefit from your knowledge and experience. Even if you're newly diagnosed, you're already a veteran. There will be others diagnosed tomorrow who could avail themselves from what you learned in the early stages. And for long-term survivors, you have lots of experience to share!

4. And if you jump on the "Veterans guiding the rookies" bandwagon, you're also on the "helping is healing" bandwagon. It's a win/win for everyone. And as we stress in A 2nd Act, your 2nd Act doesn't have to be big or cancer-related. Whatever makes your heart sing will have the healing benefits.

5. Finally, never forget to live life fully every day: smile more; take time to smell the roses; help a neighbor in need; give yourself the gift of joy.

You are a person of great influence. If you could inspire a movement that would bring the most amount of good to the greatest amount of people, what would that be?

Since the cancer survivorship movement has already been launched, I'll claim the 2nd Act movement. It doesn't matter what life challenge someone has faced, creating a 2nd Act by using the knowledge learned will help others with their challenges

We are very blessed that some very prominent names in Business, VC funding, Sports, and Entertainment read this column. Is there a person in the world, or in the US with whom you would love to have a private breakfast or lunch, and why?

There are MANY people I'd like to have time with. But at this moment, I'd love to have a one-on-one with the documentary producer Ken Burns. As a history buff, I've been impressed with all of his series. I'd like to know where his ideas come from, what makes his creativity thrive, and why he chose his profession.

How can our readers further follow your work online?

Prologues to all of my books can be found at www.JudithLPearson.com. To learn more, and to see the stories of our amazing storytellers, visit www.A2ndAct.org

Kelley Skoloda of KS Consulting & Capital: I Survived (Colon) Cancer and Here Is How I Did It

Do Your Research—Many people, including doctors, have suggested, "Don't Google your sickness." But how else can you best advocate for yourself if you haven't done your research, your homework? How will you know what questions to ask? How will you know what to expect? How will you know how to best prepare yourself? To me, forewarned is to be forearmed. Others may subscribe to the idea that ignorance is bliss, but I believe that knowledge is power, and it has always served me better than ignorance. Many cancer patients seem to see their doctors as the font of all knowledge. Doctors are certainly knowledgeable, though your doctor is one expert in a world and field of many.

I had the pleasure of interviewing Kelley Murray Skoloda. Kelley is a wife, mom, daughter, sister, aunt, author, angel investor, entrepreneur, CEO of KS Consulting & Capital and now, a cancer survivor. A consumer brand marketing expert, Kelley is passionate about her work and her family is the center of her life—she loves to golf, cook, travel, and enjoys cat humor. She is grateful every day for the love and support she received throughout her health challenges and hopes her story can be helpful to others navigating cancer.

Thank you so much for joining us in this interview series! We really appreciate the courage it takes to publicly share your story. Before we start, our readers would love to "get to know you" a bit better. Can you tell us a bit about your background and your childhood backstory?

My background is in public relations and brand marketing. Now I'm an entrepreneur and run my own consultancy, KS Consulting & Capital, which I absolutely love. For many years, I worked at a top, global PR agency. An avid angel investor, I am passionate about investing in women-led start-ups. I serve on several boards of directors and have been named one of the "most influential women in business" by the *Pittsburgh Post-Gazette*. I love to write and speak. My first book, *Too Busy to Shop: Marketing to Multi-Minding Women*, is a business book and I've spoken at global venues. I never imagined that my second book would be about surviving cancer, *A Way Back to Health: 12 Lessons from a Cancer Survivor*, which debuts on November 9 and is the true story of and lessons learned from my recent journey with cancer.

The oldest of four kids, I grew up mostly in Western Pennsylvania. We had a close-knit, Italian family with lots of family gatherings and great food. My dad was a drill instructor in the Marine Corps, so I learned discipline from an early age. I've been married for 31 years to a great husband and we are blessed with two amazing kids, and wonderful friends and family (and three cats).

Can you please give us your favorite "Life Lesson Quote?" Can you share how that was relevant to you in your life?

"This, too, shall pass, honey." One of my Nonnie's (grandmother) favorite sayings. Even though a cancer diagnosis and treatment took over my life in the worst way, it did pass and I'm here to share my story about it to make it a little easier for others who face similar challenges.

Let's now shift to the main part of our discussion about surviving cancer. Do you feel comfortable sharing with us the story surrounding how you found out that you had cancer?

I was the healthiest person I knew until I became a cancer patient. When I went in for my first routine colonoscopy, I was anxious, but not expecting anything out of the ordinary. No symptoms, no sickness, a lifelong healthy lifestyle. What could possibly go wrong? I had no idea colorectal cancer was incredibly common. I was diagnosed with colon cancer and, within just a few weeks had colectomy surgery, where a large section of my colon was removed, and then underwent chemo, which was worse than the cancer itself.

I still wrestle with sharing my story because I don't want the pain of reliving even a second of the ugliness. But what I have found is that there is pain in *not* sharing a part of my life that has forever changed who I am. After undergoing the full process, from diagnosis to surgery to chemo and back to health, I learned a great deal along the way. I witnessed other patients and their families struggling with challenges like I had experienced. They are lessons I never wanted or expected to learn, but they helped me, and based on the power of personal stories, could help others who are coping with a similar situation.

What was the scariest part of that event? What did you think was the worst thing that could happen to you?

Despite how often we hear or read the word "cancer," hearing the word associated with yourself is devastating and inconceivable. And fear. I had so much fear. The fear was so real and scary that it took my breath away and made me sick to my stomach. The fear took me to a place I'd never known before. Thinking that you might not be around to see your kids grow up is one of the worst and most sickening things that could happen.

How did you react in the short term?

When I first found out about the cancer, I felt like I was in a haze. It was too much to comprehend. When you are thrust into the world of cancer, it's absolutely overwhelming. I cried a lot. But, things happen fast after a cancer diagnosis, so I began to take action, without even knowing it.

After the dust settled, what coping mechanisms did you use? What did you do to cope physically, mentally, emotionally, and spiritually?

I researched, meditated, exercised, changed my diet, worked, sought second opinions, kept records and looked for miracles. In short, I took action. In fact, this exact question was the impetus for taking my cancer journey and turning it into a book, which details how surprising lessons paved the way for my recovery, shares helpful action steps and illuminates how personal stories can powerfully motivate and heal. Often overlooked actions, such as trusting your instincts, speaking up, getting a second opinion, and watching for miracles, can have a profound impact on recovery, help patients advocate for themselves, and help friends, family, and caregivers as they wrestle with cancer and its treatment.

Is there a particular person you are grateful towards who helped you learn to cope and heal? Can you share a story about that?

There are so many people for whom I am grateful. My husband, kids and mom who were with me every step of the way. My nephew, who patiently sat through my chemo treatments with me. The dear friends who made meals for us. The oncology nurse who treated me with such great care.

In my own cancer struggle, I sometimes used the idea of embodiment to help me cope. Let's take a minute to look at cancer from an embodiment perspective. If your cancer had a message for you, what do you think it would want or say?

I'm sorry you've had to deal with cancer, too. While I do not consider cancer a blessing, it has enabled me to practice gratitude on a whole new level and appreciate even small miracles and everyday life. My grandmother would say, "If you have your health, you have everything." That message truly resonates with me now.

What did you learn about yourself from this very difficult experience? How has cancer shaped your worldview? What has it taught you that you might never have considered before? Can you please explain with a story or example?

My story is about capturing and sharing my story.

Being a professional marketer and storyteller by trade and having previously published a book, the idea of writing a book about my cancer experience was almost second nature, though the idea of reliving the stories was scary. When I shared parts of my story on social media, I received dozens of responses, many about people who took action because of what they read. "I scheduled my colonoscopy," or "I encouraged my sister to get a colonoscopy," were common refrains. Those responses told me that my story could get people to take action.

Sometimes writing the story was too painful and I had to walk away.

Other times, the feeling of survival and a drive to share what could be helpful to others would win. In the end, what I learned was too compelling for me to keep to myself because I didn't know then what I do now and too many people are in the same situation.

How have you used your experience to bring goodness to the world?

I've seen the quote, "Stories help others. Share yours." While talking recently to a friend who had been diagnosed with breast cancer, she said she had read about my story on social media. She went on to say that she and her family had taken several of the actions that I recommended and that they helped her. It is my hope that by sharing my story, someone will find the help they need on their cancer journey.

What are a few of the biggest misconceptions and myths out there about fighting cancer that you would like to dispel?

1. Doctors know medicine, but only you know you best. You are your own best advocate.

2. Food and nutrition are rarely addressed by medical professionals. You'll need to seek ways to use the healing power of food and exercise.

3. So many people don't seek second opinions. I did and was so glad I did.

4. Cancer doesn't mean not looking good. When I looked good and got moving, I felt better. I did my best to get dressed, put on make-up, do my hair and go to work.

Fantastic. Here is the main question of our interview. Based on your experiences and knowledge, what advice would you give to others who have recently been diagnosed with cancer? What are your "5 Things" You Need To Beat Cancer? Please share a story or example for each.

1. Do Your Research

Many people, including doctors, have suggested, "Don't Google your sickness." But how else can you best advocate for yourself if you haven't done your research, your homework? How will you know what questions to ask? How will you know what to expect? How will you know how to best prepare yourself? To me, forewarned is to be forearmed. Others may subscribe to the idea that ignorance is bliss, but I believe that knowledge is power, and it has always served me better than ignorance. Many cancer patients seem to see their doctors as the font of all knowledge. Doctors are certainly knowledgeable, though your doctor is one expert in a world and field of many.

2. Get A Second Opinion

There are many objections and hurdles to seeking a second opinion—time, money, effort, lack of knowledge—and to many it still just feels uncomfortable. Cancer patients are already uncomfortable in so many ways that adding to the discomfort is not something they want to do. But it's worth the time and discomfort to push for a second opinion. I believe that second opinions made a big difference for me.

3. Watch for Miracles

I've tried to reground myself by recognizing that each and every facet of life is a miracle. You woke up this morning? Miracle. You are breathing? Miracle. Your family has enough food to eat? Miracle. A butterfly landed on a flower in my yard, enabling me to take a look at its beautiful and fragile wings? Miracle. Especially when you are facing cancer, every part of your life can produce miracles, if you look for and recognize them.

4. Prepare to Speak Up

One month into my chemo regimen, I was in dire straits due to side effects, and I found it hard to speak up. Self-doubt about my condition, a significant loss of energy, not getting much of a reaction from the medical team, and not wanting to be a pain in someone's ass all contributed to my reticence. But when I got to the point when my physical and mental ability to withstand treatment was fading, I had to find the strength to save myself. It's crazy that I had to get to such a breaking point before pressing harder to help.

Don't let yourself get to this point. If things don't seem right to you, then they aren't. Speak up for yourself, even if you feel like you are being a pain. Find the strength to speak up for yourself before you lose your strength altogether.

5. Trust Your Instincts and Take Action

In a serious medical situation, it may sound heretical to trust your instincts more than you trust your doctors. After all, medical professionals are highly educated and know more than we do. Decisions are made based on facts and data that we, as regular people, know little about. We have been trained to believe doctors know best. These commonly accepted principles are followed by many patients. Well, medical professionals may know more about medicine, and this is half the game, but they don't know the most about you.

You are a person of great influence. If you could inspire a movement that would bring the most amount of good to the greatest amount of people, what would that be?

Helping cancer patients, and patients of all kinds, advocate for themselves and helping in any way to enable sick children to get better.

We are very blessed that some very prominent names in Business, VC funding, Sports, and Entertainment read this column. Is there a person in the world, or in the US with whom you would love to have a private breakfast or lunch, and why?

While having a meal with my family is always my top choice, I'd welcome an opportunity to meet with a strong, successful female founder, mom, investor and philanthropist, like Sara Blakely.

How can our readers further follow your work online?

Thank you for asking. My new book about cancer, *A Way Back to Health*, is available beginning November 9 on Amazon. I often post on related topics on LinkedIn. Helpful videos can be found on my Kelley Skoloda YouTube channel. My business can be found at www.ksconsultingandcapital.com. Twitter: @kelleyskoloda, Instagram: @kelleyskoloda

Scan the QR code to view my "5 Things" To Beat Cancer YouTube video:

Kim Hunter Heard: I Survived (Breast) Cancer and Here Is How I Did It

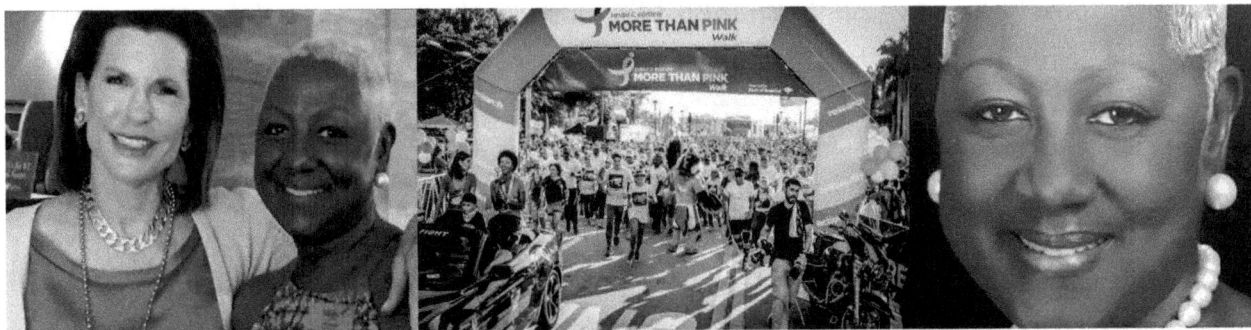

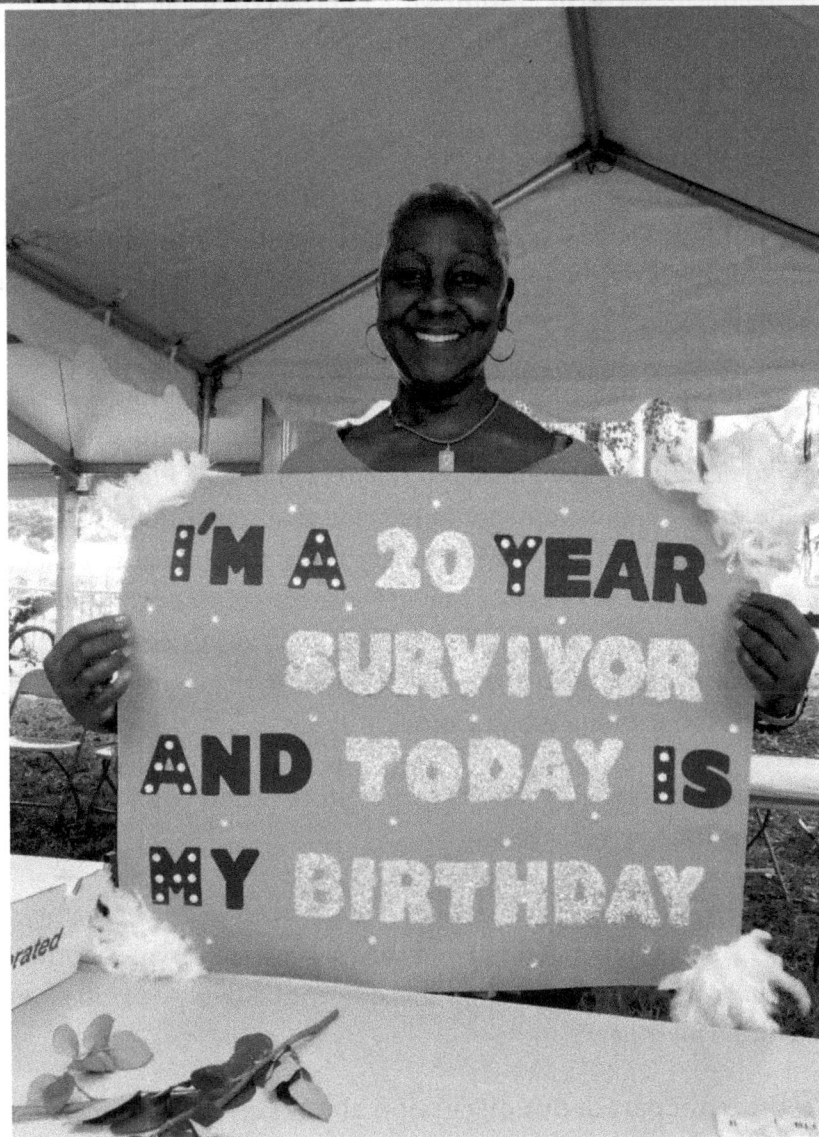

Surround yourself with positive people. Your village makes a huge difference. Allow loved ones to help you. Ask for what you need or want. Don't sweat the small stuff literally. Love yourself through the changes...the changes are not the sum total of you. You are so much

more. I still joke about mine and I am healthy and whole and grateful. Also, don't waste your moments fretting about what you cannot change. Embrace the new you, be thankful for the breath of life and celebrate your life. You are worth it and so much more!

I had the pleasure of interviewing Kim Hunter Heard. Kim is a 26 year breast cancer survivor. She was first diagnosed with Stage 2 DCIS at age 38, and despite growing up in a Bahamian culture that protested intensive treatment, she went forward with it and survived. She joined the Susan G. Komen organization in Miami 25 years ago and has been an active advocate for early detection ever since. All she asks from those that she has helped is to pay it forward.

Thank you so much for joining us in this interview series! We really appreciate the courage it takes to publicly share your story. Before we start, our readers would love to "get to know you" a bit better. Can you tell us a bit about your background and your childhood back story?

I am a military brat of Bahamian decent and when I grew up everything was cloaked in secrecy. I knew absolutely nothing about breast cancer when I was diagnosed and neither did my family. Wanting to make a positive impact on the lives of others, I had long been searching for my purpose in life, and I've since come to understand that often times we are already walking in our purpose and just haven't fully embraced it. Because of the disparities I encountered after my diagnosis, I was on a mission to remove some of those barriers for others. I jumped at the chance to join the Susan G. Komen family as we call it as soon as I discovered that they were already addressing disparities as it relates to people of color in the continuum of healthcare and so many other vital issues concerning breast cancer.

Can you please give us your favorite "Life Lesson Quote?" Can you share how that was relevant to you in your life?

My favorite quote is by Lailah Gifty Akita, "I devote my life in service to humanity." My mother always encouraged my sister, brother and I to dedicate our lives to service of others as she had. It's all I've ever known. When I happened upon this quote it perfectly described me and my passion to be an advocate for others.

Let's now shift to the main part of our discussion about surviving cancer. Do you feel comfortable sharing with us the story surrounding how you found out that you had cancer?

Absolutely, hopefully my story will lend inspiration, courage and hope to someone who's having a bend in their road. I'm borrowing from Helen Steiner Rice's Poem, *A Bend In The Road*. It has helped me through some difficult times. I found my lump doing a BSE or breast self-examination. It was quite painful. I was turned down by three doctor's offices because as I was told...1. I was too young (I wasn't 40 yet) to receive a baseline, 2. I didn't have a family history (my family didn't share medical history), and 3. pain is not an indicator of breast cancer, as I was told with quote fingers in the air. Finally at my fourth doctor's office, after saying no and seeing me start to cry, they agreed to humor me and give me a mammogram after telling me the lump was probably from shaving or deodorant. I was sure it wasn't as it was way too painful. Long story short, it was clear as day on the ultrasound and the biopsy confirmed that it was cancer. This was my first lesson in the importance of being my own best advocate! Had I not been steadfast by insisting I get the full diagnostic screening I would not be here today. I am elated to share that I have seen so many barriers removed since then. Specifically, these were the three I had to deal with: 1. I am happy to share that because of a piece of legislation called the Early Act passed in 2019, no woman regardless of age can be denied a mammogram. 2. Because of cultural research, which I personally participated in, it is accepted that many women do not have a known family history. 3. Globally, pain that won't go away is now recognized as a possible indicator of breast cancer (I personally know many survivors who said that pain was their indicator).

What was the scariest part of that event? What did you think was the worst thing that could happen to you?

By far the worst part of my journey was the chemo. I had Adriamycin, which is better known as the "Red Devil." I never thought cancer would kill me but I was certain that the chemo would. It was grueling but I kept praying and reminding myself that it was just a means to an end. Also, the look of hurt and fear in my family's faces especially my one and only child, my daughter, who was 19 at the time. She asked me why this had to happen to me and I told her I didn't have the answer but that I believed we were going to look back and laugh. We actually laughed our way through. She and my sister would rub my bald head and wait for the genie to pop out of the imaginary bottle. I know it sounds kinda silly but we took baby steps and it helped. It's true that laughter soothes the soul.

How did you react in the short term?

I was super debilitated, nauseous, weak, and wasn't eating, but whatever was in the chemo made me gain so much weight I looked like the Pillsbury dough girl. I played a game in my head by counting out the next treatment as soon as I had the current treatment. I know it sounds absolutely crazy but in the words of Malcolm X, "by any means necessary."

After the dust settled, what coping mechanisms did you use? What did you do to cope physically, mentally, emotionally, and spiritually?

The dust doesn't always settle completely! I still have residual side effects from treatment after 26 years. I have used and continue to use the same mechanisms to cope which are Faith, Hope & Love. I embrace these three things with all my heart. While I hope to inspire with my story let me be absolutely transparent, my journey has been very tough at times...BUT I'M STILL HERE!!!

Is there a particular person you are grateful towards who helped you learn to cope and heal? Can you share a story about that?

There are several…God, my Wing Girls/Angels who include my mother, my sister and my daughter.

In my own cancer struggle, I sometimes used the idea of embodiment to help me cope. Let's take a minute to look at cancer from an embodiment perspective. If your cancer had a message for you, what do you think it would want or say?

I never considered the idea of embodiment for my cancer. I was the one and only boss of my body and my message to cancer was to get the heck out and stay out. I prayed for a complete and total healing from cancer and I received it. I don't use the term remission because I have intentionally chosen to embrace my healing. I unequivocally believe Proverbs 23:7; "As a man thinketh in his heart, so is he."

What did you learn about yourself from this very difficult experience? How has cancer shaped your worldview? What has it taught you that you might never have considered before? Can you please explain with a story or example?

This difficult experience has taught me that regardless of what your diagnosis is, everybody is going through something; you can and I can get through this! Cancer has enhanced my world view by affording me the opportunity to meet/support survivors all over the world while being supported by them as well. We may speak different languages and live far apart but there is power in unity.

It has taught me that I can make a difference one woman or man at a time. I used to think that if I were to help people, I would need it to happen in mass. I have spoken in front of hundreds of people and to this day I am so very grateful when I speak with that one individual (usually there are many) who needs a gentle nudge to get that mammogram or follow up on one. I often personally drive women, who are a little frightened, to their appointment. I realized early in my journey that there's nothing more comforting during that time of uncertainty than the heartfelt pearls of wisdom from someone who has been down that road.

How have you used your experience to bring goodness to the world?

For 25 years I've been on a passionate mission to empower, engage, educate and support any woman or man (as you know men get breast cancer too) in need, to help save lives.

What are a few of the biggest misconceptions and myths out there about fighting cancer that you would like to dispel?

There are so many myths and misconceptions. I don't want to repeat them here it would almost feel like I'm reinforcing them. What I will say is Get Screened, Know Your History, Eat Healthy, and Exercise. These are all a part of a healthy lifestyle. It doesn't mean that you will never get cancer, but it sure increases your chances of not getting it. Another thing, yes a mammogram is uncomfortable, but I promise you it's not as uncomfortable as being on the other end of a chemo line or even getting fried by radiation.

Fantastic. Here is the main question of our interview. Based on your experiences and knowledge, what advice would you give to others who have recently been diagnosed with cancer? What are your "5 Things" You Need To Beat Cancer? Please share a story or example for each.

Surround yourself with positive people. Your village makes a huge difference. Allow loved ones to help you. Ask for what you need or want. Don't sweat the small stuff literally. Love yourself through the changes...the changes are not the sum total of you. You are so much more. I still joke about mine and I am healthy and whole and grateful. Also, don't waste your moments fretting about what you cannot change. Embrace the new you, be thankful for the breath of life and celebrate your life. You are worth it and so much more!

1. Be consistent with your care and treatment. Don't skip appointments.
2. Eat a healthy diet and maintain healthy weight as best you can.
3. Protect yourself from the sun.
4. Don't smoke or quit immediately if you already do.
5. REMEMBER THAT ATTITUDE IS EVERYTING.

When I was in treatment I never missed an appointment even though there were days I needed assistance with dressing for my appointment. At one point, I had chemo and radiation simultaneously. It was daunting. It took many conversations with myself, and I know you can do it too.

I had chemo every three weeks and I only had an appetite the last three days before the new treatment. What I refused to do was to put junk into my already challenged body. As I mentioned before, I think steroids were added to my chemo to keep me from wasting away and it had a super reverse result.

Instructions for chemo and radiation both warn you to avoid extensive sun exposure. I developed a hypersensitivity to the sun during my treatment. It's okay. I do my best to avoid the sun and I'm still here!

I wasn't a smoker but I remember having a blood clot (one of those bumps in the road) in my lungs and while on the oncology floor at the hospital, I would see other patients disconnect their IV to go outside to smoke. That's the part where you have to do your work. No one can do it for you!

You are a person of great influence. If you could inspire a movement that would bring the most amount of good to the greatest amount of people, what would that be?

I'm already dug in the movement to end breast cancer. In 2020 there were 2.3 million women diagnosed with breast cancer and roughly 700,000 deaths. When I embarked on this journey, my goal was and is to live in a world without breast cancer! We have saying that goes..."Until Every Story Is A Survivor Story" and I am committed to that.

We are very blessed that some very prominent names in Business, VC funding, Sports, and Entertainment read this column. Is there a person in the world, or in the US with whom you would love to have a private breakfast or lunch, and why?

Oprah Winfrey! She has exemplified generosity and I don't mean money. I heard a quote once that said, "Generosity is love in action." Ms. Winfrey leads by example, always pouring into others, empowering others, inspiring others, and creating new ideas and ways to reach more people. I often find myself reflecting on her pearls of wisdom or those of others she has invited to share.

How can we follow you online?

On Twitter: @KimHunterHeard1

Lisa Lurie: I Survived (Breast) Cancer and Here Is How I Did It

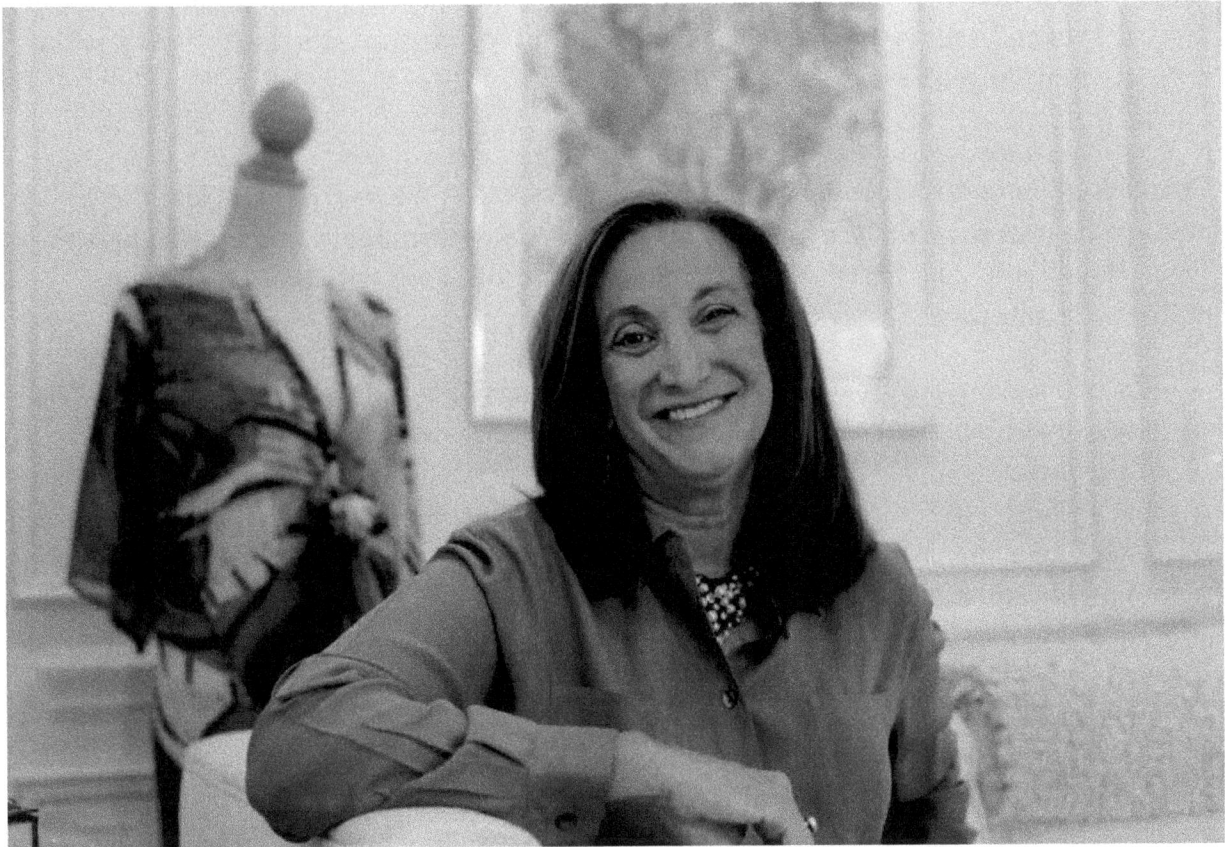

Be Kind & Good to Yourself—Cancer surgery, treatment and recovery can be all consuming. Please don't compare yourself to how other survivors have handled it. Focus on being kind and good to yourself instead. When I felt too fatigued to attend a school function or didn't want to join everyone for a holiday dinner, it was tempting to feel like I was letting my family down. The truth is that I was listening to my body and it was telling me to rest. In the end, recognizing what you need to do to get better and making it a priority benefits not only your recovery but everyone in your life.

I had the pleasure of interviewing Lisa Lurie. Lisa is a breast cancer survivor, patient advocate, author and Co-founder of Cancer Be Glammed. Cancer Be Glammed is the premier lifestyle company that educates and empowers women coping with all forms of cancer to recover with dignity, positive self-esteem and personal style.

Thank you so much for joining us in this interview series! We really appreciate the courage it takes to publicly share your story. Before we start, our readers would love to "get to know you" a bit better. Can you tell us a bit about your background and your childhood backstory?

I was very fortunate to grow up in a home surrounded by love and laughter. The middle child of two sisters, Janet and Ann, we argued and enjoyed each other in equal measure. They are still my best friends. My parents instilled in us a love of family. Family life and close personal relationships (I have been BFF's with my childhood friends for over 50 years) is at the core of who I am. Our house then and my house now pre-COVID had a revolving door. Everyone was welcome and popped in often. I thrive on that spontaneous, overly hectic and loud, warm closeness.

I was always interested in people's lives and their stories. I loved doing projects that involved creative writing and photography. In college, I realized that working in television would allow me to combine all three. I became a broadcast television writer, producer and director and then eventually worked as a corporate writer/producer until I became a freelancer. Television and video production taught me to "think on my feet," be better organized and to appreciate the struggles and achievements of life. These skills turned out to be valuable when I was diagnosed with cancer and even more so when I co-founded Cancer Be Glammed and became immersed in the cancer community.

Can you please give us your favorite "Life Lesson Quote?" Can you share how that was relevant to you in your life?

A life lesson quote that really resonates with me is "Life is not measured by the breaths you take but by the moments that take your breath away." Prior to having cancer and even more so since then, I have cherished the heart-stopping, life-changing moments in my life that helped shape who I am. These include holding my precious daughters Michelle and Gillian for the first time, celebrating their milestones as they went from preschoolers to caring, capable adults and crying with Brian my husband at my first post treatment scan that showed NED, No Evidence of Disease.

Let's now shift to the main part of our discussion about surviving cancer. Do you feel comfortable sharing with us the story surrounding how you found out that you had cancer?

During a breast self-exam, I felt a hard lump near the nipple in my right breast. Even though I had gone for a mammogram seven months prior, I spoke to my primary care doctor who decided to order a breast ultrasound. During the ultrasound, the radiologist performed a core biopsy to remove small amounts of tissue from various areas in the lump.

My husband Brian and I were very nervous about receiving the test results. I was out of the house the morning that my doctor called. When I got home, Brian told me that the doctor's office wanted me to call them. He wanted me to do it right away, and I just couldn't. I knew in my heart that the news would not be good and I desperately wanted to preserve a few more moments of calm before cancer turned our lives inside-out.

I had brought home lunch for us. I insisted that we sit down and eat together. When we were done choking down our sandwiches—I made the call. It turned out that I had Stage 2-Invasive Ductal Breast cancer. The Imaging Center recommended that I meet with a breast surgeon right away. Two weeks later I underwent a double mastectomy without reconstruction and started to prepare for chemotherapy.

What was the scariest part of that event? What did you think was the worst thing that could happen to you?

The scariest part of any cancer diagnosis is the fear of the unknown. At the heart of that is the fear that you won't survive. I felt like I could personally endure anything as long as I stayed alive for my family. The thought of leaving my husband and my daughters who were 13 and 9 years old at the time, almost broke me. It made me want to be strong and thrive for them.

How did you react in the short term?

A cancer diagnosis is like having your own personal tornado touch down and upend your life. From the moment that my doctor said, "You have cancer." I was thrown into a whirlwind of oncology appointments, medical tests, insurance phone calls, family planning, and decision-making. On the outside, I appeared focused and determined but inside I was screaming, "Oh my God. I have cancer!!!"

After the dust settled, what coping mechanisms did you use? What did you do to cope physically, mentally, emotionally, and spiritually?

I was able to draw strength from my close family. I tried very hard each day to keep my, "eye on the prize." For me that meant doing whatever it took to get through my surgery and treatment and to keep mentally moving forward. It was important for me to conserve my energy and rest while my daughters were at school so that I would be in better shape to spend time with Brian and them when they returned. I would see them off in the morning, rest during the day and then be refreshed to welcome them home after school.

For many people faith, spiritual practices, family bonds, sheer determination or even anger keeps them from getting sucked into the rabbit hole of despair. I have felt all of those things at different times. For me though, it almost always came down to this: I wanted to live (obviously) but I didn't want to die and leave behind a shattered family. Loving them (and their love) gave me purpose and strength. My immediate and extended family, my sisters, friends and relatives who are so precious to me kept me determined to do whatever I could to survive.

Is there a particular person you are grateful towards who helped you learn to cope and

heal? Can you share a story about that?

My go-to person then and always is my husband Brian. To the casual observer we may seem like opposites. He has a practical, thoughtful approach to life while I am more spontaneous and emotional, but in reality we make a good team. Coping with cancer forces you to juggle many balls in the air at one time while emotionally you have one hand tied behind your back. You need to be well informed and organized to stay on top of appointments, treatment, medication, side effects and family life while at the same time you are living under this cloud of pain, anxiety and at times, crippling fear.

Brian held not just me but our whole family together. He worked, took care of everyone, came to every appointment and chemo treatment and comforted me in the dark of night when I finally could shed the tears that I didn't want anyone to see.

"Brian and The Wig" is a story that is legendary among my family and friends. I knew that I was going to lose my hair from chemo. I was advised to cut it short and to get a wig prior to it falling out. Without a doubt, hair loss is one of the most devastating appearance related side effects of cancer. It makes your very private cancer public.

I knew that losing my hair would be particularly upsetting to my daughters Michelle and Gilly. I took them with me to the hair salon after I purchased a wig to see it styled and cut. The drive home was devastating. No one said one word. Radio silence. We were all too undone.

The next morning, the girls woke up and came to cuddle in my room. Brian had gone downstairs to bring up some breakfast. He came into the bedroom with a tray and...he was wearing the wig!!! We lost it. We couldn't stop laughing. For the rest of the day friends and family came over and they wore the wig. There is no way to overstate how important humor is when undergoing such a dramatic event. By Brian wearing the wig, it demystified it as a symbol of illness. I never got completely used to wearing it nor did my family but it never held the dread and sorrow that it initially did.

In my own cancer struggle, I sometimes used the idea of embodiment to help me cope. Let's take a minute to look at cancer from an embodiment perspective. If your cancer had a message for you, what do you think it would want or say?

I think that the message or worldview that cancer instilled in me is to fully appreciate the incredible kindness and humanity of people. From the dedicated doctors and nurses to the stranger at Trader Joes who bought me a bouquet of flowers because she felt "I deserved one." I was and I still am, awed and humbled by how people reached out to me and my family just to make each day a little brighter or easier.

If I had to sum it up, here is how cancer touched and transformed me. It is my own personal belief that "cancer is a not a gift, but the people that it brings into your life are." This discovery inspired me to pay it forward to lift up other patients, survivors and their families. It is the spark behind my co-founding of Cancer Be Glammed. I have no medical experience but I felt perhaps I could use my "life experience" to address the unmet lifestyle issues women and their families face from cancer and to empower them to have a well informed and better prepared recovery.

What did you learn about yourself from this very difficult experience? How has cancer shaped your worldview? What has it taught you that you might never have considered before? Can you please explain with a story or example?

A message that cancer patients and survivors often hear is, "Cancer does not define you." And yes, while I agree that I am so much more than my cancer I feel that this quote is too glib and somewhat dismissive. I learned that cancer impacts every aspect of a survivor's physical and mental health. It is a complicated disease that requires undergoing physical traumas like disfiguring surgeries, grueling treatments including chemotherapy and radiation and for many people years of follow-up medication. For patients coping with metastatic cancers—this is an ongoing reality.

For me and many other people, the emotional fallout of trying to cope with the ongoing fear of recurrence, regaining a positive body image and self-esteem following life-changing surgery and treatment, and finding a way to integrate your cancer experience into your life are some of the ongoing mental health challenges survivor's face. I lost my breasts, my ovaries, my physical strength, and temporarily my hair. I gained weight from treatment, was thrown into early menopause with its unpleasant symptoms, and continue to deal with medication-induced joint and muscle pain. In addition, I went from good bone health to having osteopenia and a high fracture risk. These are challenges that I will have to deal with the rest of my life. I am clearly not alone.

I learned that there is a great underserved need for the oncology community and mental health professionals to understand and support the lifestyle and/or psychosocial challenges of people coping with cancer. It sounds cliché but cancer recovery, long-term recovery, needs to be focused on "healing the whole person." Cancer isn't over when treatment is done. The healing process must continue after a person has "rung the bell" heralding their last chemo session and be valued as an important part of survivorship.

How have you used your experience to bring goodness to the world?

I can sum it up in three words, Cancer Be Glammed. A year after my recovery I was still struggling with cancer created body issues like my lack of breasts and my inability to find support and recovery products that would help me to look and feel more like myself. While I had had an excellent medical team, I was ill-prepared for coping with appearance related challenges like being breastless and bald as well as lifestyle issues including being a mother with cancer.

When my treatment ended, I became determined to help other women have a better recovery experience than I had. I joined forces with a dear friend of mine, Ellen Weiss Kander and we co-founded Cancer Be Glammed, the first lifestyle company for women coping with *all* forms of cancer. Our mission—to educate and empower them to have a well-informed, better prepared, practical and fashionable recovery from diagnosis through survivorship.

Our website www.cancerbeglammed.com provides patients and survivors with easy online access to lifestyle information and solutions, practical and fashionable recovery products and gifts, helpful resources, and a dynamic international community of support from patients, survivors and relevant experts.

Of equal importance is our commitment to supporting and promoting other survivor created or inspired small businesses. These are companies that were founded by survivors who design and produce much-needed cancer recovery products.

I am thrilled to announce that we have recently launched a unique "Life & Style" Recovery Boutique on www.cancerbeglammed.com where we have partnered with 15 women-owned, survivor businesses. Their "best in class" products and thoughtful gifts are featured and sold in our Recovery Boutique.

In addition, I am immersed in the cancer world and I have become a patient advocate working with the oncology community, healthcare companies and professionals to improve the patient experience and to provide support tools to help women recover from the psychosocial effects of cancer.

What are a few of the biggest misconceptions and myths out there about fighting cancer that you would like to dispel?

• Cancer is Cancer

There is no secret sauce or one size fits all approach or treatment for coping with a cancer diagnosis. Each person's cancer is unique as is their recovery experience. Even though they may have the "same diagnosis" and similar treatment protocols to someone else.

• Once Treatment is Over—You Are Cured

Recovering from cancer is not limited to physical health. Cancer also creates mental health issues and lifelong challenges. Friends, families and strangers often feel like once treatment is completed a person's cancer experience is over and they should get on with their lives. Very often that is not true and survivorship is more complex.

• Why Do Patients and Survivors Care About Their Looks When All they Should Care About is Getting Better?

Caring about how you look while coping with hair loss, scars, weight gain/loss, body changes and other appearance-related issues from surgery and treatment is **not** about being vain. It's about trying to reclaim your dignity, confidence and self-esteem while it feels like the world is constantly shifting under your feet.

Fantastic. Here is the main question of our interview. Based on your experiences and knowledge, what advice would you give to others who have recently been diagnosed with cancer? What are your "5 Things" You Need To Beat Cancer? Please share a story or example for each.

These are the five things that helped me to survive cancer. They are:

1. Rely on The Medical Experts

It is very tempting to fall down the Google rabbit hole and read everything that you can about your diagnosis. I am guilty as charged. While there may be good advice and tips on managing treatment or surgery, there is a ton of information/misinformation on the internet as well as medical content that does not apply to you.

2. Be Well Prepared for Oncology Appointments

If you are like me, just the word oncology makes my heart beat hard and my hands sweat. Far too often I would leave an appointment and kick myself for not asking my oncologist some of the questions that I wanted him to answer. Come prepared with a written list of questions and symptom information that you would like to ask. There are treatment planners and digital Apps that can help.

3. Accept Help Gracefully

I am a private person and at first I was overwhelmed by the offers of our friends and family for help. I nicely told them that we were fine and declined. A dear friend of mine essentially said, "Stop it! These are people who love and care for you and they want and need to be included in your treatment and recovery. It's important to them, so let them help." She was absolutely right! Not only did we end up needing the support when my treatment became more involved but it was wonderful to have a surprise meal each night!

4. Seek Out Support Groups & Services

Cancer can put a strain on families, relationships, finances and careers in addition to your physical and mental health. Thankfully there are wonderful organizations and support groups founded by people who understand what you are going through and want to help. Whether they are on-line or in-person, seek them out. I have not typically been a "joiner" but when I finally went to a breast cancer support group, I felt like I could breathe again. I didn't have to say a word and everyone in the group got it.

5. Be Kind & Good to Yourself

Cancer surgery, treatment and recovery can be all consuming. Please don't compare yourself to how other survivors have handled it. Focus on being kind and good to yourself instead. When I felt too fatigued to attend a school function or didn't want to join everyone for a holiday dinner, it was tempting to feel like I was letting my family down. The truth is that I was listening to my body and it was telling me to rest. In the end, recognizing what you need to do to get better and making it a priority benefits not only your recovery but everyone in your life.

You are a person of great influence. If you could inspire a movement that would bring the most amount of good to the greatest amount of people, what would that be?

I would start a movement to create jobs and opportunities for people who have been impacted by illness, personally or by a family member and they are unable to return to traditional forms of work. This would include people who had to become caregivers. My movement would inspire more employers to find creative solutions to address illness and caregiving in the workplace and to not limit or reject the talents and skills of employees in this precarious situation.

We are very blessed that some very prominent names in Business, VC funding, Sports, and Entertainment read this column. Is there a person in the world, or in the US with whom you would love to have a private breakfast or lunch, and why?

I would love to have the opportunity to dine with Arianna Huffington (of course)! I read a quote where she said, "We encourage women to speak up, to trust their voices, and to know there are solutions to whatever it is they're experiencing. I love helping women connect with their own power." Enough said.

How can our readers further follow your work online?

Please visit my website www.cancerbeglammed.com. Find, follow and like us (please) on:

Facebook: CancerBeGlammed

Instagram: @cancerbeglammed

Twitter: @cancerbeglammed

WEGO Health: www.wegohealth.com/LisaLurie

LinkedIn: @cancerbeglammed

Scan the QR code to view my "5 Things" To Know You've Got Cancer YouTube video:

Lisa Winston of Soul Expression Coaching: I Survived (Breast) Cancer and Here Is How I Did It

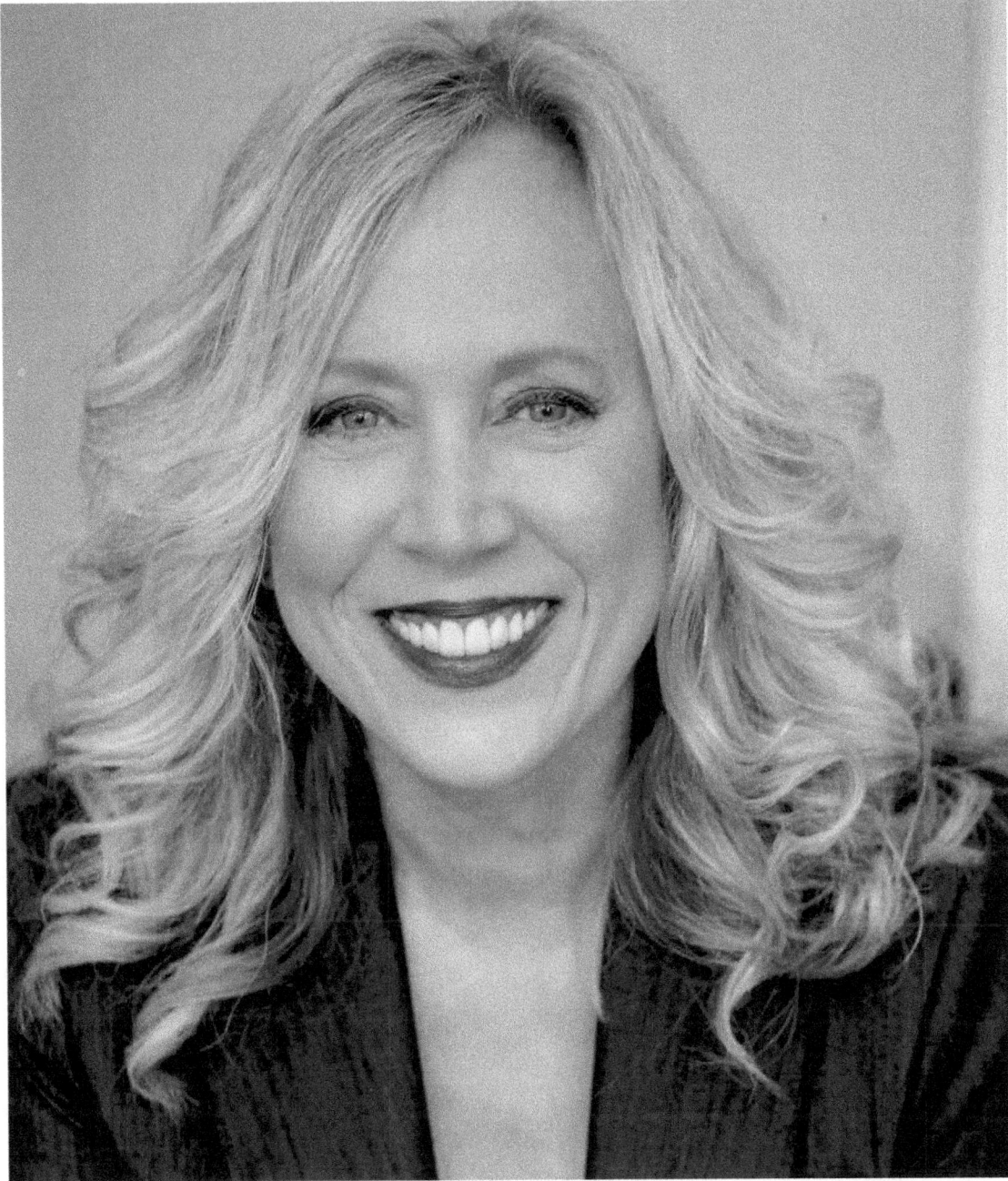

Have a consistent, loving cheerleader—The ups and downs of any devastating illness can make you feel like you're going crazy. You must have someone you can be yourself with and confide in, especially when you're at your lowest. When I was terrified and needed a shoulder, I had my cheerleader. When I had messy physical mishaps and daily treatments, I was covered. When I looked like death-warmed-over for

months, I felt safe, secure, loved, and never worried about being left alone. And my every need was taken care of so all I had to do was focus on healing. What an incredible act of love!

I had the pleasure of interviewing Lisa Winston. Lisa is a best-selling author, speaker, soul expression coach, TV host, artist, and mom. A lifetime of extreme challenges including rape, abuse, losing her home to wildfire, breast cancer and neuro-Lyme disease, made Lisa hungry to find her true-life purpose, deepen her faith, and teach others how to navigate challenges with more resiliency and joy. Today, her primary message is clear...life is happening FOR you and challenges are sent to refine, not define you.

Thank you so much for joining us in this interview series! We really appreciate the courage it takes to publicly share your story. Before we start, our readers would love to "get to know you" a bit better. Can you tell us a bit about your background and your childhood backstory?

I'm incredibly grateful to be here. Thank you for the opportunity.

I was born in the small town of York, PA, the middle of three children. I was an incredibly sensitive, anxious child who never felt like she fit in. I don't remember much of my childhood, although I vaguely remember being molested at the age of 5 by an unknown man, and again, by a neighbor boy who also threatened to kill me, years later. After that, bad experiences continued to follow me throughout my childhood into my adult years.

My only saving grace was my voice. I began singing professionally at 18 and ended up having a fulfilling music career that spanned 40 years and brought me a lot of joy. I was in two toxic marriages and had one child. I never remarried after that, but lived with someone for 14 years, during which time I lost my home to wildfire. Two months later I was diagnosed with breast cancer.

My life felt hard, but the endless exhaustion, anger, and fear eventually sent me on a spiritual journey; one that opened my eyes to the fact that "God" was gifting me with opportunities to find out who I was and what I was made of. I felt alone, yet time and time again, my family and others showed up in loving support as well as unexpected miracles in the form of earthly and heavenly angels.

Because of the challenges, my determination grew. I began to listen to, and trust that "small voice within" because I knew it was guiding me. I took big risks to "find myself" because I knew I was here for a greater purpose. And because of that, today, I'm living the life of my dreams and fulfilling my soul purpose. As I look back, it was all necessary and perfect. I'm forever grateful.

Can you please give us your favorite "Life Lesson Quote?" Can you share how that was relevant to you in your life?

I have two. Not to toot my own horn, but the first is mine. "Life is always happening FOR you and challenges are sent to refine, NOT define you." I didn't understand this until later in my life. For most of my life, I felt victimized and wondered if I was being punished for some past wrong. When we believe that, as many people do, it takes away our power. Our power to choose can change everything. We can choose to see things with a different perspective, to look for the good and take action that moves us in a better direction. We can't always understand circumstances but can learn to trust there's a bigger picture and loving energy that's orchestrating it all.

My second quote is "We can't become what we need to be by remaining what we are."—Oprah Winfrey. The "who I was" for a vast majority of my life, could never have been a light to the world, or inspired or helped others to rise. You must transform your understanding and ways of being to step into your full potential to be able to affect real change. When you say YES to life challenges, you continue to grow, gain new insights, and help others do the same.

Let's now shift to the main part of our discussion about surviving cancer. Do you feel comfortable sharing with us the story surrounding how you found out that you had cancer?

Absolutely!

What was the scariest part of that event? What did you think was the worst thing that could happen to you?

In October 2007, the San Diego wildfires took our home and everything in it. We had 10 minutes to get out with 100 mph winds and a 100 ft. wall of flames surrounding us on all sides. The fire was a monster. My daughter's dad had lost his home four years previous in the Cedar fires, so my daughter was massively traumatized that night. About three weeks and three moves after the fires, we had to find a rental home, deal with insurance agents, school, and rebuilding. It was a stressful time. I remember noticing a small dimpling in my right breast a short time later. It was new and I was uneasy about it, but put it aside for a short time. I finally scheduled a mammogram, had a biopsy, and was diagnosed with infiltrating lobular carcinoma. What? The fires and now, this? My cancer surgeon had zero bedside manner and told me in no uncertain terms I needed to have a double mastectomy, as "my" cancer was rare and tends to mirror in the other breast. My head was spinning and I felt like I was in a dream. The fire was bad enough, but this was my life, and I knew I might lose it. The biopsy was brutal, but I was more afraid than I've ever been going into surgery, not knowing if the cancer had spread to my lymph nodes.

How did you react in the short term?

The fire and cancer gave me a good deal of PTSD, but a kind of miracle happened as well.

Although I experienced very human emotions from time to time, having to deal with two crises daily forced me into present moment living. I was so busy rebuilding my life; I didn't have much time to think about dying. Oh, it crept in sometimes, but having to raise a child, treat cancer and rebuild my home all at the same time, held most of my attention. One of the San Diego news stations started following our progress and featured us regularly, which brought a sense of fun into our lives. My treatment went on for months, but each day brought a new set of things to do. Honestly, having it all happen at the same time was a gift. It really pulled me through.

After the dust settled, what coping mechanisms did you use? What did you do to cope physically, mentally, emotionally, and spiritually?

I spent hours doing Qigong and reading spiritual books and saw a therapist for a short time. I had lost all my artwork and musical equipment in the fire, and at the prompting of my daughter, began to paint and sing again. Most of my friends disappeared during that time; however, I made new friends, and reconnected with some old friends who showed up bearing gifts and hugs. And my family, most especially my dear sister, who had her own set of serious health issues at the time, showed up with unwavering love and support.

Is there a particular person you are grateful towards who helped you learn to cope and heal? Can you share a story about that?

The year I was treated for cancer and rebuilding remains mostly a blur, so there are things I don't remember. Some of my musician friends did a benefit for me, which was incredibly loving and generous. I also had more than several angels show up unexpectedly, who cooked meals for my family and gave support. But I have to say that my precious mother (who is now gone) and sister, were the two people who held my hand through it all. They lived on the east coast, so visits were few. We spent hours on the phone together. My sister, who suffered several strokes the June before the fires, flew to CA to be with me during and after my cancer surgery. I remember her "bagging" me (cutting a hole in a large garbage bag and putting it over my head) so I could take a shower. She held me when I cried, made me giggle, and was my rock. She was unbelievably selfless, and I am forever grateful to her.

In my own cancer struggle, I sometimes used the idea of embodiment to help me cope. Let's take a minute to look at cancer from an embodiment perspective. If your cancer had a message for you, what do you think it would want or say?

The cancer (it's not mine, just an experience) would want me to stop being angry and resentful toward the bad things that happened in the past. It would have me love myself and my body just as it is and, have me immerse myself in the practice of forgiveness of self and all others. It would also say, "Stop taking yourself and everything that happens so seriously. Go have some FUN! You are valuable and have nothing to prove to anyone, so, enjoy and be grateful for every precious second you're given on this earth."

I believe most dis-ease is energy and emotion stuck in the body. When we don't cope with or heal past traumas, our miraculous bodies, which we take for granted, carry that pain, which eventually manifests as disease. I thank the cancer for reminding me that I needed to let go!

What did you learn about yourself from this very difficult experience? How has cancer shaped your worldview? What has it taught you that you might never have considered before? Can you please explain with a story or example?

My cancer experience taught me that no disease can define me. It was an experience, but not who I am. And getting a cancer diagnosis is not necessarily a death sentence. Tons of people survive cancer and go on to live long, healthy lives. Early on, my doctors showered me with gloom and doom, so I chose to ignore the dark, foreboding messages and create positivity around my situation. And why wouldn't I? No one knew the outcome. I know from experience if we stay in a good place and focus on good things, we have a better chance of a good outcome. Cancer also taught me that we are stronger than we know. If we can muster just enough courage to get through one moment at a time while navigating a devastating disease, we learn to be humble, strong, and confident. It also teaches us gratitude for our precious life and loved ones, and compassion for those who suffer.

How have you used your experience to bring goodness to the world?

Before I had cancer, my life was a mess. My vibrations were incredibly low. My relationship was a disaster, and I was very unhappy. After cancer, I woke up and turned my life around. I left that relationship *and* my music career to go in search of my life mission. I realized that time is short, and NOW is all we have to enjoy life and make a difference. I'm grateful for my experience because it helped shape me into who I am today. It's also given me insights and wisdom I'm able to share with others.

What are a few of the biggest misconceptions and myths out there about fighting cancer that you would like to dispel?

1. Cancer is an automatic death sentence—Millions of people have beat cancer and continue to; early detection improves the odds, and treatments are getting better and better. Even late-stage cancers are more curable, and life expectancies, longer.
2. Cancer is something you have to "fight"—Some people use the word fight to summon stamina and strength for the journey. I get it. But for me, fighting against anything usually means resistance, stress, or violent struggle. I believe finding acceptance on some level, doing things that create laughter and joy, having a consistent, loving support system, and loving self-care are a few things that calm and heal the body and make the journey more tolerable.
3. The cancer will come back—I've been cancer-free for 14 years and hope to be for life. Many people never have another recurrence. I believe focusing on gratitude and what and whom you love is a better way to spend your time, as opposed to fearing it will come back. Get your yearly exams but don't give cancer any more attention than it deserves.
4. Losing your breast makes you less of a woman—I experienced this feeling for a long time, and I know post-surgery is a big adjustment for most woman. However, being an amazing woman involves way more than your body parts! After my surgery, I felt unwhole and ugly. I felt my partner would be turned off by what he saw, but he wasn't. And four years ago, I attracted the most amazing man into my life at 59, who loves me just the way I am. I

still struggle at times, but in no way am I less than a woman.

Fantastic. Here is the main question of our interview. Based on your experiences and knowledge, what advice would you give to others who have recently been diagnosed with cancer? What are your "5 Things" You Need To Beat Cancer? Please share a story or example for each.

1. Have a consistent, loving cheerleader—The ups and downs of any devastating illness can make you feel like you're going crazy. You *must h*ave someone you can be yourself with and confide in, especially when you're at your lowest. When I was terrified and needed a shoulder, I had my cheerleader. When I had messy physical mishaps and daily treatments, I was covered. When I looked like death-warmed-over for months, I felt safe, secure, loved, and never worried about being left alone. And my every need was taken care of so all I had to do was focus on healing. What an incredible act of love!

2. Raise your vibes—Science shows that negative emotions hinder the body's ability to heal. So, why not at least *try t*o be more positive? Believe me; I understand a cancer diagnosis is a terrifying slap in the face. I've been there and encourage anyone fighting cancer to be a "fighter" of a different sort. Whether it was cancer or collapsing with neuro-Lyme disease and 12 co-infections, I only allowed myself a little time to feel sorry for my situation and then I got to work. I danced to Jason Mraz, stuck post-it notes with positive messages all over my apartment, wrote in my gratitude journal (even when I didn't feel grateful), did Donna Eden's energy medicine and Qigong in small bursts, meditated, took walks and more. If there was a chance it would make me feel better or even heal me, I was going to do whatever it took. And it DID. It raised my vibes, brought bursts of laughter, and gave me the strength to go the distance.

3. Look for what's working—When we're scared and don't feel well, we tend to complain and focus on what hurts or what's wrong. I was a complainer. One day my partner asked me, "What's right with your body? What's working?" I looked down and noticed my nails were growing! Small potatoes to healthy people, but a big deal when your body feels terrible. It was a wonderful shift out of the darkness into light. It brought a sense of play to my days. And helped me feel gratitude for the many blessings I had in the moment. When you focus on what's wrong and what's bad, it lowers your vibes. It makes everything bleak. When you choose to look for body parts that work, as well as things that are good in your daily life, it's a game changer.

4. Go easy on yourself—There's nothing you did to create the cancer. You're not being punished for anything and there's no perfect way to handle this very bumpy journey. So go easy on yourself. Give yourself love, compassion, grace, and space. Honor your feelings. Love and nurture your body. Find your center with breathwork or meditation. And don't allow anyone to bring disrespect or negativity into your life. This is *your* life, *your* path, and *your* time to heal. You get to choose how you want to walk it and with whom. Surround yourself with loving supporters. Honor yourself and demand others do so, too.

5. Have faith—I've always had a strong faith, but early on in my cancer and Lyme journey, I lost it for a time. After all I had been through; I couldn't believe I was getting hit again. I knew God (Spirit, the Universe) was always with me throughout my life and trials—

through synchronicities, people, and Divine timing. So why did I feel so alone? At one point, I screamed and shook my fist at the ceiling, "I hate you and don't believe in you anymore!" I felt more and more distant from what I once believed. After about a month of this behavior, I started thinking about what it would feel like to live in a world without a God or guiding energy. It was then I realized if I gave up my faith, I would have nothing. As I looked back over my life again, all I could see was the love of the Divine. And so, with outstretched arms and hands I said, "I surrender."

We humans want our lives to be perfect. We want wealth, health, love, money, joy, and only good things. But we forget that challenges are part of our existence. Without them, we don't have the opportunity to refine who we are, or to know the depth of our love or strengths. Without them, we don't often get to experience the deep goodness and love of others and we easily take everything and everyone for granted. Faith is remembering there's a much bigger picture we can't possibly see or understand that's being orchestrated by something much bigger than us. We can trust it. Let's face it—we live on a ball revolving in outer space. Our hearts beat without a battery and our lungs are breathed without our help. When I look at the miracles all around me, I can't help but choose to have faith.

You are a person of great influence. If you could inspire a movement that would bring the most amount of good to the greatest amount of people, what would that be?

I'd love to inspire a movement where everyone who has any kind of devastating diagnosis would have total access to loving counselors for support, access to any kind of treatment they desired, a network of professionals and volunteers who would answer questions and hold their hands and hearts from start to finish. Too many people are without support and health insurance. I wasn't even given the opportunity to have breast reconstruction. My insurance barely gave me enough money to buy a prosthesis. After treatment was over, I was kicked to the curb. Too many people get lost in the shuffle. To carry the burden of a terrifying diagnosis along with not having the ability to be cared for on all levels is a crime.

We are very blessed that some very prominent names in Business, VC funding, Sports, and Entertainment read this column. Is there a person in the world, or in the US with whom you would love to have a private breakfast or lunch, and why?

There are so many amazing beings I respect, honor, and cherish. However, the one woman I'd love to say thank you to is, Oprah Winfrey. She is an incredibly strong, resilient, powerful woman, a beacon of love, light and hope to many. I'm blown away by how she overcame so many significant challenges and yet, held her vision and stayed on course to achieve her dreams ultimately, impact the world. What an inspiration. I think we deeply connect with her because she's incredibly genuine, warm, and knows, first-hand, the struggles people face. Two of my favorite quotes by her are: "Where there is no struggle, there is no strength," and "True forgiveness is when you can say, 'Thank you for that experience.'" These quotes speak great truth into what we're talking about in this interview. Thank you, Goddess. You are a gift.

How can our readers further follow your work online?

Thank you for asking! Readers can find more of my story, what I do, TV episodes and more here. My website: www.LisaAWinston.com. My show: www.MindsetResetTV.com. Social Media: www.facebook.com/lisa.winston.501, www.facebook.com/lisawinstoncoach, Instagram: @LisaAWinston and my email: thebeautyofauthenticity@gmail.com

Scan the QR code to view my "5 Things" To Beat Cancer YouTube video:

Liz Benditt of The Balm Box: I Survived (Breast) Cancer and Here Is How I Did It

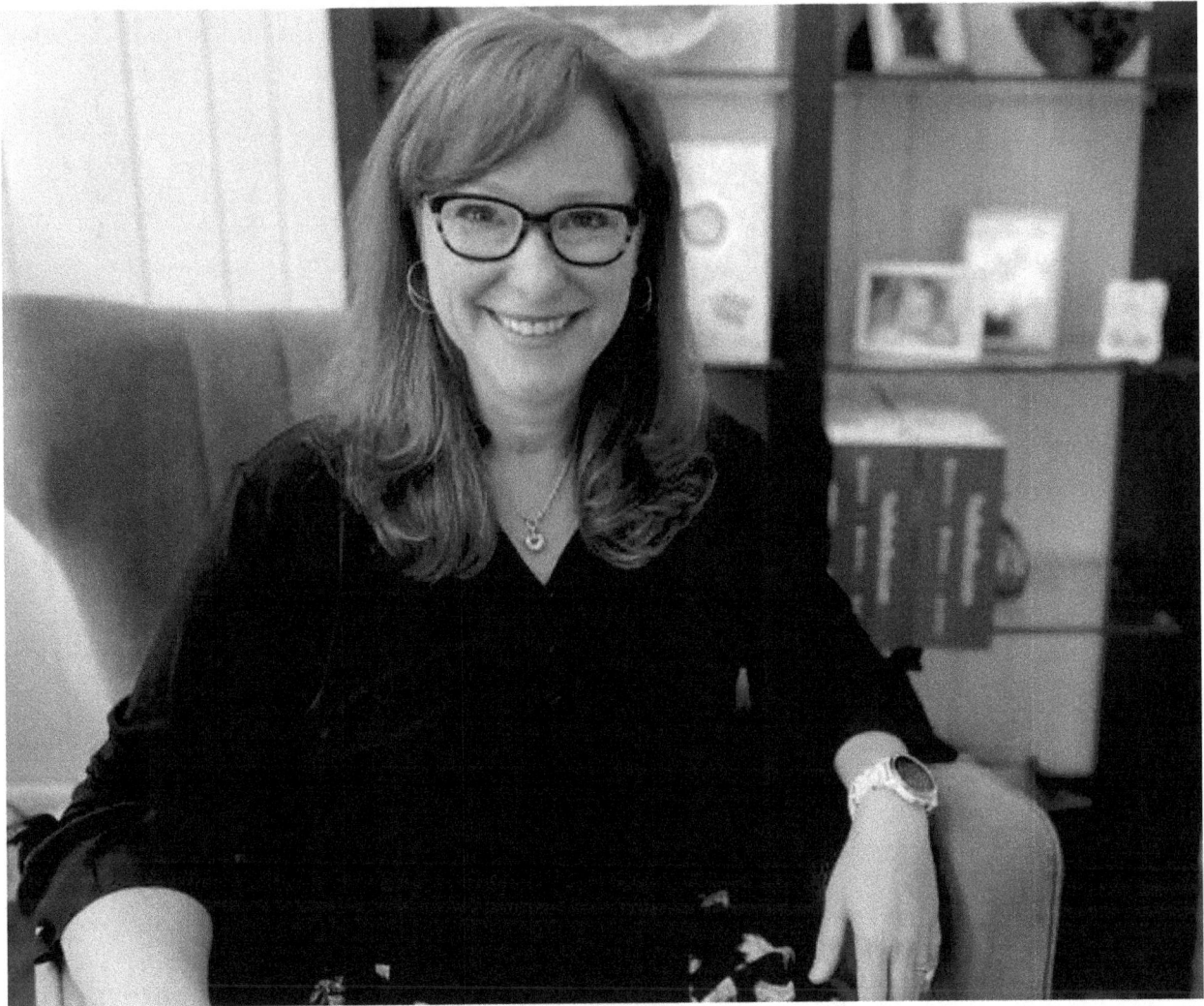

Interview doctors who are willing partners, not dictators—Cancer treatments are brutal and unpleasant—for me, actively participating in my treatment plans helped me feel like I had a wee bit of control over my situation. Especially during the dark times, when I was so very tired, in pain, and emotionally spent; knowing that I CHOSE this treatment, that I was not a nameless, faceless, powerless patient lost among the whims of an oppressive medical establishment, was genuinely helpful.

I had the pleasure of interviewing Liz Benditt. Liz is a four-time cancer survivor. She is President and CEO of The Balm Box, a self-care and gifting site for breast cancer patients. In addition to teaching undergraduate business marketing courses at University of Kansas, Benditt also serves on the Education First Shawnee Mission board of directors, and volunteers with The Mainstream Coalition and National Charity League. She lives in the Kansas City suburbs with her husband and two children.

Thank you so much for joining us in this interview series! We really appreciate the courage it takes to publicly share your story. Before we start, our readers would love to "get to know you" a bit better. Can you tell us a bit about your background and your childhood backstory?

I was born in Southern California but moved around a lot as a kid—we lived in San Diego, Los Angeles, Chicago, and State College Pennsylvania by the time I graduated from high school. I earned my bachelor's degree at Boston University, moved to Orlando Florida to work for Disney for a few years before heading back to California to earn my master's degree at University of Southern California. While I was earning my MBA, my parents relocated to the Kansas City metro area and my mother was diagnosed with Breast Cancer. I wanted to be closer to her, so after graduation I accepted a position at Hallmark.com and moved to Kansas City. My friends in Los Angeles thought I was crazy to move to "flyover" country—but within a few years of moving to the Midwest I met my husband, bought a house and had a few kids. I adore our community and cannot imagine living anywhere else.

Can you please give us your favorite "Life Lesson Quote?" Can you share how that was relevant to you in your life?

I love this quote from Zig Ziglar, "F-E-A-R has two meanings—Forget Everything And Run, or Face Everything And Rise." I actually jotted it down on a sticky note for my office and look at it daily. I am at a crossroads in my life and career, taking a huge leap of faith based on an idea that I could fundamentally change "get well soon" gifting, making it better for patients and gift buyers alike. Leaving the security of full-time employment, cutting our household income in half, with two kids still in the house who will eventually need college tuition, in the middle of a global pandemic...it is A LOT to take on. It is terrifying and exhilarating. Run or Rise—those are the options—and every day, I proactively choose to Rise.

Let's now shift to the main part of our discussion about surviving cancer. Do you feel comfortable sharing with us the story surrounding how you found out that you had cancer?

Well, I've had cancer FOUR TIMES, and the diagnosis was different each time. The FIRST time I was diagnosed with cancer was in 2009. I was at the pool with my family and my baby son was napping while lying on my chest. Because of my unique position, cradling my son on my chest with my legs bent to hold him in place my mother had a clear view of a mole on my upper thigh.

She didn't like the look of it and nagged me for weeks to have it checked out. I finally succumbed and made an appointment with her dermatologist. It turned out to be melanoma. Because melanoma is a fast-moving cancer, I went from diagnosis to surgery in 4 days' time. I was told that if the cancer spread, I'd have about 1 year to live. If it hadn't spread, no big deal. Lucky for me, it had NOT spread—we stocked up on sunscreen, wide brimmed hats and SPF swim shirts and tried to get back to "normal."

Eleven months later in 2010, a routine breast cancer screening required a biopsy. While the surgeon was feeling my breast her fingers traveled up to my neck—she found a lump on the side of my neck and booked a biopsy for both breast and neck. At that time the breast biopsy was negative, but the neck biopsy turned out to be thyroid cancer. I fell into a teeny-tiny category of patients with a rare surgical side effect called "hypoparathyroidism." That side effect landed me back in the hospital for a few weeks and was (and still is) very tricky to manage. I'm lucky to work with a phenomenal endocrinologist who is open to a combination of traditional and non-traditional treatments to keep me healthy. By 2012, I was back to "normal"—I ran my first half-marathon, started a new job, drove carpool, and volunteered in my kids' classrooms. Cancer was in the rear-view mirror.

Fast forward to 2015—in a routine bi-annual skin cancer screening the dermatologist biopsied a questionable piece of skin on my nose. It was basal cell carcinoma. While not life threatening, the size and placement on my face made for a complex 2-part plastic surgery to remove the infected skin while maintaining the integrity of my nose and face shape.

About 18 months later my annual mammogram showed some pre-cancerous cells. Rather than biopsy them immediately, the doctor waited another 6 months to check again. The cells had multiplied so I went forward with a biopsy—which brings us to my last (hopefully!) cancer diagnosis—breast cancer in Fall 2017. I had a lumpectomy followed by 35 radiation sessions in late 2017 and spent much of 2018 recovering from severe skin damage caused by radiation treatment.

What was the scariest part of that event? What did you think was the worst thing that could happen to you?

My reactions to my diagnoses have evolved over time. Certainly, being diagnosed with melanoma skin cancer when my children were 3 and 1 years old was absolutely terrifying. I had an agonizing weekend, waiting for the call to let us know if the cancer had spread or if it was contained. I'm a planner by nature, so I definitely thought about how I would spend my last year with my family and mourned what my children's lives would be like without their mother. The best part about overcoming surgery at home with oblivious and demanding toddlers is that there was not a ton of time to ruminate on "worst case scenarios" between diapers, stories, snacks, playtime, and baths. I do recall feeling my lungs expand when we got the "all clear" call from the surgeon. I think I had been partially holding my breath all weekend. That call cut off the melodrama playing out in my head and allowed me to snap right back into the daily grind of being a working parent.

The next time I thought about dying was when I went into hypocalcemic shock post-thyroidectomy. I couldn't feel the muscles in my hands, arms, or face and couldn't speak or move.

I was very, very scared that I was going to be "stuck" that way forever. That took me to a very dark place. Again, luckily, it was not long until the medical team started an IV calcium drip and I immediately started feeling better. Once I knew there was a treatment for the side effect, I was able to manage the recurrences more calmly, with more confidence that it was only temporary.

After overcoming the terrors of melanoma and hypocalcemia, I was far calmer about my basal cell and breast cancer diagnoses. The experience and knowledge that I made it through two prior medical dramas gave me tons of confidence that I would persevere. By the time I was diagnosed with breast cancer in 2017 I was angrier and more annoyed than scared. I was confident the surgeries and treatments were going to stink, but that I would eventually be okay.

How did you react in the short term?

My immediate response to ALL of my diagnoses has been to track down DATA and INFORMATION. What are the key markers of my diagnosis? Where does my tumor fall on the scale of "small/no biggie...to...huge/dead woman walking?" What are the different treatment options? Are there holistic alternatives to surgery and/or medications? What are the medical outcomes and odds of recurrence for people following different treatment paths and do those paths differ by patient age, gender, and relative health of the patient at diagnosis? I found myself reading a ton of scholarly articles not meant for people without medical degrees and typed up pages and pages of notes and questions.

For me, information was comforting—knowing what to expect and having a prepared list of questions gave me a sense of CONTROL over my situations. I'm not sure that all that research really made a significant difference in my medical outcomes, but it certainly was helpful to me mentally and emotionally.

After the dust settled, what coping mechanisms did you use? What did you do to cope physically, mentally, emotionally, and spiritually?

I am a PLANNER and a bit of a control freak. So once my treatment plans were locked in and I exhausted my need for information—I spent a lot of time preparing for surgery and recovery. I shopped, arranged childcare, cooked meals, got ahead on work projects—basically I stayed very busy. In the moment, I did not do anything in particular to prepare myself mentally, emotionally or spiritually. Those emotions snuck up on me in the years post-surgery.

Is there a particular person you are grateful towards who helped you learn to cope and heal? Can you share a story about that?

My mother is a rock star—her grace under pressure, ability to know when to listen or lecture, to fill in all the little life-gaps that happened when I was suddenly down for the count—all of that. She is my touchstone and pillar of support.

I got the melanoma phone call on my way to work on a Tuesday morning. This was the cancer diagnosis that very well could have been a death sentence. We wouldn't know whether I was a goner until after the lymph node biopsy taken on the same day as the surgery which would confirm if the cancer had or had not spread.

At the time, my father was working on a long-term project in Asia and my mother was LITERALLY boarding a plane headed for China to reunite with my dad, who she hadn't seen in a month. I told her about the diagnosis and that the doctor wanted to schedule the surgery no later than Friday. She hung up the phone, turned to the flight attendant, and demanded they let her off the plane. The gate was closed, and they were about to pull away from the gate—to this day, I'm not sure what my mother said or did—after all, this was after 9/11 when security was heavily enforced. But she was able to get off the plane and come home. She was with me for all the pre-op consultations and surgery, at my side during post-op, and once home, hovered near the sofa to fetch me drinks and ice while I recovered from surgery and waited for the Monday phone call that would tell us if the cancer spread and if I was going to die.

To this day, I am so phenomenally grateful for her presence that week and weekend. She was so calm, held my hand, and regularly reassured my husband who was barely able to contain his panic. She was the voice of reason, the adult in the room, while staying warm and compassionate and comforting.

I think I learned how to face my fears with calm and grace through her example. That week where she talked her way off a plane en route to China, to skip a much-anticipated trip to stay home and be a nursemaid, to quietly support me and my family—there are no words to convey my gratitude.

In my own cancer struggle, I sometimes used the idea of embodiment to help me cope. Let's take a minute to look at cancer from an embodiment perspective. If your cancer had a message for you, what do you think it would want or say?

I'd like to think my cancers taught me to slooooooow down. There is no rushing through recovery—you must wade through it slowly, with patience. I am pretty much the least patient person on the planet. Once I make a decision—whether it's a meal plan for family dinner, how to attend three events in one night, or booking a beach vacation, I'm ready to GO FORWARD FULL STEAM AHEAD. I plan out the most efficient route and MAKE IT HAPPEN.

Cancer taught me that sometimes the most efficient routes cut out necessary rest stops. Skipping those rest stops makes the route longer, more miserable, and difficult for me and everyone around me.

Slowing down meant leaning into self-care and allowing myself to be less efficient with my limited time and resources. It meant learning how to say, "no" I cannot take on that project or "sure" I can take that on, but it will take me twice as long as normal to complete it. Pre-cancer, admitting to needing time for rest and recovery was unthinkable. Post-cancer, it's a learned life habit.

What did you learn about yourself from this very difficult experience? How has cancer shaped your worldview? What has it taught you that you might never have considered before? Can you please explain with a story or example?

I learned the discipline of gratitude.

Despite having had cancer 4 times in 10 years I remain grateful—I genuinely see myself as lucky! I see the hardships that so many go through because of even a single cancer diagnosis—from losing jobs, to bankruptcy, to crumbling marriages and unsupportive friends and family. All four times, in every way, I was SO lucky, and ergo SO grateful.

- I was never at the risk of losing my job(s)—I worked with phenomenally kind and generous leaders that gave me enormous grace to take time for treatments and recovery without penalizing my career trajectory or income.
- I had comprehensive insurance coverage—our out-of-pocket costs were affordable. Cancer did not come close to bankrupting our family.
- My marriage is rock solid—never once did my illnesses crack our relationship. My husband was and is my #1 fan, and firmly supported every one of my treatment decisions—even those I chose not to pursue. He came to all my consultation appointments, asked thoughtful questions, and made goofy dad jokes to lighten the mood in the room. We were (and are!) a team.
- My support system is amazing—I have an incredible network of girlfriends that rose to the occasion again and again to support me and my family. From meals, to carpools, to chatty visits, I felt supported and cared for—all four times.
- As mentioned above, my mother is a rock star—her stalwart support and ability to stay calm under pressure have made ALL the cancer treatments so much more bearable.

How have you used your experience to bring goodness to the world?

I launched www.TheBalmBox.com in Fall 2020 to support cancer patients and caregivers with "functional" self-care and gift boxes for breast cancer patients!

The idea for The Balm Box started when I was undergoing radiation treatment for breast cancer. It was incredibly difficult to predict what tools I would need to go through and recover from radiation until I was in the middle of it, scrambling for bra-alternatives, aluminum-free deodorant, and burn salves. A nurse made me a mini-pillow to hold between my seatbelt and breast so that the belt wouldn't chafe. There was no central resource, website, or retailer known for all this "stuff" and I found myself up late at night researching page 20 searches on Google and Amazon looking for solutions. Most of the cancer-treatments and gifts online were pink ribboned cute/sassy t-shirts and mugs—I wanted relief not stuff.

The challenge with most cancer treatments is that patients do not know what they are going to need to help them self-soothe until they need it RIGHT AWAY. I wondered—where is the resource for cancer patients to proactively plan for treatment and recovery side effects?

It didn't exist.

It wasn't until 2020 that the moons aligned and gave me a quiet few months at my desk at home during the pandemic to really build out the idea into a legitimate business plan. I started by sending out a survey to friends and family to validate the idea—the survey went viral and collected almost 600 responses.

My market research revealed that I was most definitely NOT alone in my frustrations and there was a huge level of interest from both cancer patients and caregivers. I was not the only person frustrated by the total lack of functional self-care and gifting options.

The Balm Box launched in Fall 2020 and has grown so much in the past year! We've helped HUNDREDS of patients so far, and I am so thrilled with the market response to the business!

What are a few of the biggest misconceptions and myths out there about fighting cancer that you would like to dispel?

1. Cancer is so very often TREATABLE—it is not always an automatic death sentence. So many folks FREAK OUT after being diagnosed with cancer. But not all cancers are alike, and certainly many are more fatal than others. Just the single word "cancer" does not ALWAYS equate to DOOM AND GLOOM. After surviving four cancers—I'm still very much alive and well!

2. "Kicking cancer" tote bags and coffee mugs are great for folks once they are DONE with their treatments and on the road to recovery. But when patients are in the middle of treatment, hurting, exhausted, and mentally drained—those t-shirts and tote bags are not always inspirational. In fact, they can be the opposite—like pressure filled pointer fingers, making patients feel the need to appear sunny and cheerful when they feel anything but. Don't pressure patients to be a picture perfect rock star spouting motivational quotes and dancing to TikTok videos. Sure, there will certainly be a small portion of patients who love that stuff and genuinely find it meaningful—but be careful—most of us do not. Our TheBalmBox.com market research backs this up.

Fantastic. Here is the main question of our interview. Based on your experiences and knowledge, what advice would you give to others who have recently been diagnosed with cancer? What are your "5 Things" You Need To Beat Cancer? Please share a story or example for each.

1. Treatment Plans are up for discussion—they are not a directive. Given my age and general good health, Doctors almost always recommended the MOST aggressive treatment plans for me—but ultimately, I was the one who made the decision regarding what I was willing to put my body through. I focused on the odds. We are lucky to live in the age of information. There is great research and data on a patient's odds of a recurrence or complication for most standard cancer treatments like surgery, radiation, chemotherapy, and hormone therapy. This is SO subjective! For example: for me, engaging in hormone therapy post-breast cancer would reduce my odds of recurrence by 50%. That sounds high, right? But in reality, post-lumpectomy and radiation treatment, my odds of recurrence were about 15%. Ten years of hormone therapy would take my odds of a breast cancer recurrence down to 8%. This is such a personal and subjective decision—are the side effects of hormone therapy worth an 8% reduction? Some women would say YES, absolutely! Others say, NO, not worth it!

2. Information is power and gave me more confidence in my choices. To actively participate in my treatment plans, I needed a care team willing to include me in the upfront planning.

I interviewed and selected doctors who were willing to collaborate with me as a partner—I did not want a medical overlord. In my ongoing cancer journey I have met some brilliant, skilled medical professionals that were horribly arrogant and dismissive. One made me cry in his office. No matter their stellar credentials, I refuse to work with other humans that are mean, rude, or downright creepy. I am incredibly fortunate that I live in a major metropolitan city and could choose from a variety of doctors, all covered by my health insurance. Learning to actively interview and select care teams that aligned with my values and personality has been a game changer.

3. Nurse Navigators are worth their weight in gold. Inevitably, most cancer patients will work with more than one doctor at a time, and sometimes it is not clear when to call which doctor with a question or issue—enter the Nurse Navigator. Not all medical centers keep Nurse Navigators on staff, but I was lucky that my local hospital includes a small team of Nurse Navigators. These professionals have been a phenomenal resource. Especially during my breast cancer treatments, my nurse navigator acted like a neutral third party who helped answer questions, made recommendations on the timing between appointments and guided me to the right specialists for my specific diagnosis and medical history. She was warm, smart, resourceful, and sympathetic. Having a medical professional who was only accountable to ME, not one of my doctors, who would listen to my concerns and provide thoughtful insights and suggestions, was invaluable.

4. Self-care is not selfish. As a working mother during all four of my cancer diagnoses, I was so much more attuned to taking care of others before myself. My personal time was never a priority, smooshed into the edges of the day before anyone woke up or after everyone was asleep. Cancer treatments are almost always exhausting—I found myself needing to rest at least 2–3x more than pre-cancer. That leaves a lot fewer waking hours to squeeze everything else in. The reality is that some things must go—whether it's early morning workouts, making homemade dinners, attending every kid's orchestra concert or soccer game, finishing the laundry or all the above—you will not be able to do it all and will have to prioritize where to spend your finite time. Taking care of YOU, prioritizing YOU while undergoing treatment is the fastest path to recovery. One of my favorite items in some of The Balm Box packages is a literal credit card entitled, "The Cancer Card: The Exclusive Membership you always never wanted." I encourage all cancer patients to flash that card at will—use it to skip the dishes, retain control of the TV remote, order pizza, or have your teenager fold the laundry. (It builds character—I promise!) It may seem anathema—but prioritizing yourself in the short-term will ensure you are around to prioritize others in the long term. That's not selfish—it's practical.

5. Saying thank you goes a long way. Do you know how often your radiation tech or oncologist is asked about THEIR day? (I actually don't know for sure, but I'm guessing not a lot!) We are all humans—medical personnel included—and human beings appreciate being appreciated. Aside from simply being kind, showing appreciation for your care team is the very best way to ensure you get the best care. Want that ideal early morning appointment slot? Need an extra tub of free lotion? Want a hospital bed next to the window? People bend over backwards to help patients that are personable and gracious. Seriously—being kind, saying thank you and asking people about themselves is one of THE best ways to help yourself! Win-Win!

You are a person of great influence. If you could inspire a movement that would bring the most amount of good to the greatest amount of people, what would that be?

Education is power! I am a hu-uuuuge advocate for the importance of supporting public education in our country. Learning how to learn and cultivating critical thinking skills are essential tools for productive adulting. Supporting public schools should be a non-partisan issue. There is no better investment than our children's education.

I leaned on my education as a patient, parent, and now small business owner. I am grateful for the teachers who invested their time and energies in me, who cultivated a lifelong love of reading and encouraged me to keep asking questions. Through my advocacy work with Education First Shawnee Mission and Mainstream Coalition in Kansas, I hope to continue to grow support for further investments in public education and would love to see more grassroots organizations around the country follow suit.

We are very blessed that some very prominent names in Business, VC funding, Sports, and Entertainment read this column. Is there a person in the world, or in the US with whom you would love to have a private breakfast or lunch, and why?

I am a huuuuge fan of Hoda Kotb, the NBC Today Show anchor. I could not agree more with her perspective about cancer—she's quoted as saying, "Cancer survivors are blessed with two lives. There is your life before cancer, and your life after. I am here to tell you your second life is going to be so much better than the first." She's talked about how overcoming cancer gave her the confidence to fight for her dream job at NBC. It's been so very true for me, as my cancers gave me the confidence to leave my corporate career and become an entrepreneur. She is whip smart, passionate, funny, and sassy—I am a total fangirl and would LOVE to take her out to lunch!

How can our readers further follow your work online?

Check out The Balm Box at www.TheBalmBox.com, or on our socials, Facebook: TheBalmBox, Instagram: @BalmBox, Twitter: @BoxBalm

Lou Torres of LUNGevity Foundation: I Survived (Lung) Cancer and Here Is How I Did It

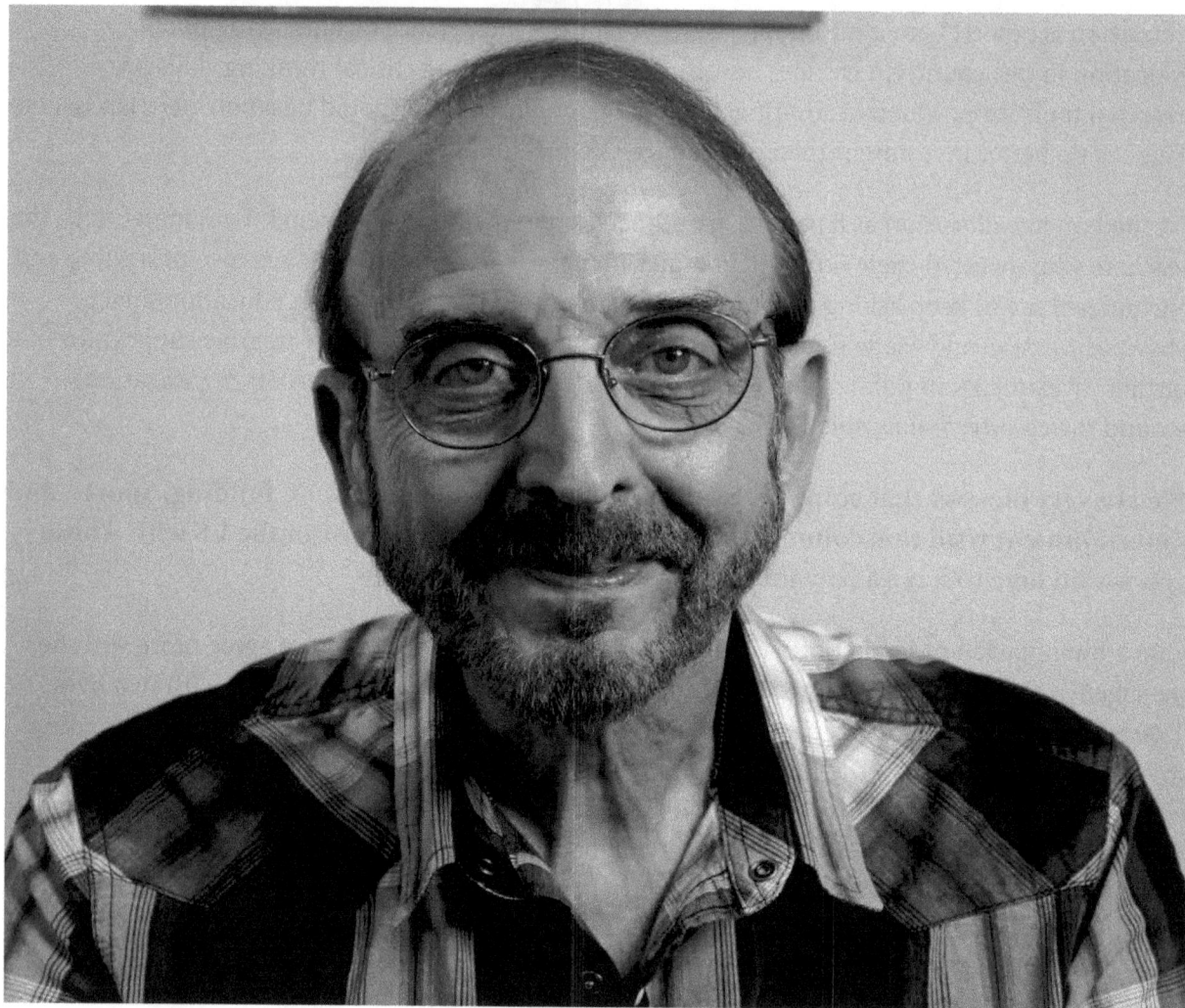

Don't be a "tough guy or gal." This is a hard road to walk alone, and your family can only help you so much. They try to empathize, and we appreciate their efforts, but at the end of the day, they can't fathom what we're going through. It makes a world of difference to engage in conversations with people who are in the midst of their own battle with cancer or have survived the disease and can impart their knowledge of how to get the most out of your treatment with the least amount of side effects.

I had the pleasure of interviewing Luis (Lou) Torres. Luis (Lou) is a former musician who "got a real job" to marry his wife but has returned to writing and recording his own music. Since his retirement in 2017, Lou enjoys spending his time helping others through community service. He currently lives in North Carolina.

Thank you so much for joining us in this interview series! We really appreciate the courage it takes to publicly share your story. Before we start, our readers would love to "get to know you" a bit better. Can you tell us a bit about your background and your childhood backstory?

I was born in New Jersey but grew up in a small town in Long Island, NY. As the third oldest of four children, I witnessed my parents work tirelessly to provide for us until their divorce when I was 9 years old. At age 11, I experienced a life-changing injury when I plunged 65-feet to the ground while swinging out over a high ledge. I crushed my left arm, broke my back and my leg, and was forced into a full body cast for one year. Unfortunately for me, my accident occurred in the 1960s which meant I couldn't prop up an iPad and attend virtual class from a hospital bed, so I missed an entire year of instruction. By the time I returned the following year, I'd fallen so far behind my peers and had to spend the rest of my school years catching up until high school graduation. I left home at the age of 17 and supported myself through college by working several jobs along the way (musician, carpenter, electrician, hospital worker and more.) In short, my childhood was challenging, but it helped me understand how to manage life and depend on myself and those around me to survive.

Can you please give us your favorite "Life Lesson Quote?" Can you share how that was relevant to you in your life?

My favorite quote is from Ralph Waldo Emerson, it follows:

"Finish each day and be done with it. You have done what you could. Some blunders and absurdities no doubt crept in; forget them as soon as you can. Tomorrow is a new day; begin it well and serenely and with too high a spirit to be encumbered with your old nonsense." My entire life into my early adult years, I operated out of fear. I had an unhealthy desire to always be perfect in whatever I was doing and if I wasn't, I immediately felt shame. After high school, I began working under a psychiatrist at a local hospital, who put things into perspective for me one day: "Humans, on average, perform 1,400 actions each day," he said, "Yet so often, we'll focus on the one or two mistakes we made that day instead of the 1,399 things we did right." From then on, I made the conscious effort to live my life freely and appreciate all the positives I have going on in my life instead of concentrating on what isn't right or out of my control.

Let's now shift to the main part of our discussion about surviving cancer. Do you feel comfortable sharing with us the story surrounding how you found out that you had cancer?

Yes, of course.

What was the scariest part of that event? What did you think was the worst thing that could happen to you?

It took a few months to receive a definitive diagnosis, but when you're waiting to find out if you have CANCER or not, a few months can feel like *years*. Once I was diagnosed with stage 1a lung cancer, my mind immediately went to the worst outcome: dying.

How did you react in the short term?

Once I understood that there was a great chance that I had lung cancer, I began to "catastrophize" and went into a state of anxiety and depression.

After the dust settled, what coping mechanisms did you use? What did you do to cope physically, mentally, emotionally, and spiritually?

I jumped online and started researching everything about my form of cancer but most of the information online was either too general or too specific, so it wasn't very helpful. In addition, many of the statistics about survival and prognosis are based on multi-year averages and don't reflect the present state of treatment and patients' response to it. It was a tough time for me as I was also a full-time caregiver to my wife of 42 years who suffered from early onset dementia. I constantly worried about her care and what would be needed for her future. I kept the news mostly to myself before finding the LUNGevity Foundation forums which instantly changed my life. Through LUNGevity and their Lung Cancer Support Community (LCSC), I had a team, a "tribe," if you will, of people who understood exactly what I was going through and could reassure me that my life wasn't over. For the first time since my diagnosis, I finally felt hopeful that there could be life after lung cancer. With the support of my LUNGevity "tribe" I had a restored sense of faith and determined that I could improve the chances of my outcome if I could lose the negative attitude. I even increased my workouts to better recover from the surgery I was told I would need.

Is there a particular person you are grateful towards who helped you learn to cope and heal? Can you share a story about that?

I'm fortunate enough to have a small, yet impactful network of people who have helped me along this journey—Curt, Lexie, Michelle, Tom and several others all come to mind. Around the same time, I connected with another survivor via the LUNGevity patient forums by the name of Eric Byrne, who shared a rather inspirational story about a man named Robert who, despite his symptoms and the harshness of his treatments, never let his will to *thrive* with cancer waver. Here I was—no symptoms, doctors telling me they could only see a single nodule and I had a great potential for a good outcome, but I was mired down in fear, doubt, and anxiety for what would happen if I didn't survive. Robert died in 2012 due to complications from a severe chest infection but was cancer-free at the time of his death and is regarded as the longest surviving dual lung cancer patient in the UK, having survived both SCLC and NSCLC for almost 20 years. His story prompted me to change my perspective on life and be grateful for every day I have on this earth. That along with the people I now consider family prepared me to face this challenge with knowledge and a sense of empowerment I had lost during the original diagnosis.

In my own cancer struggle, I sometimes used the idea of embodiment to help me cope. Let's take a minute to look at cancer from an embodiment perspective. If your cancer had a message for you, what do you think it would want or say?

I would say that my cancer's message would be that life can change in a minute and forever. Therefore, I try to live every day as someone who looks out for others who need help. We'd all like to leave our mark on this life and we never know when that door might close.

What did you learn about yourself from this very difficult experience? How has cancer shaped your worldview? What has it taught you that you might never have considered before? Can you please explain with a story or example?

Through this process, I've learned the importance of helping others in need. My worldview has always been flexible and developing but now I try to be one who does as much as I can for others. In the past I would shun "support groups." I felt very independent and had handled anything that came at me with courage (maybe bravado) and strength. But my LUNGevity support family has taught me that a group of like-minded people can come together and do amazing things for one another.

How have you used your experience to bring goodness to the world?

Prior to finding LUNGevity, I didn't know how I would survive this harrowing experience. Through the organization, I gained a strong support system of lifelong friends on similar journeys and felt empowered to become an active decision-maker in my treatment process by utilizing LUNGevity's educational patient resources and participating in survivorship programs. I found the peer-to-peer support to be most valuable in my process, so I now moderate the online LUNGevity message boards, constantly looking for newcomers who are seeking answers or, in some cases, support. When I'm not scouring the LUNGevity message boards, I donate my time, and sometimes money, to various food pantries and women's shelters while also being an active member of an Alzheimer's Caregiver Support Group and Al-Anon.

What are a few of the biggest misconceptions and myths out there about fighting cancer that you would like to dispel?

In my case, for people I support, it is that lung cancer (like many cancers) is no longer an automatic death sentence. Treatments are advancing so rapidly that "Dr. Google statistics" do not reflect what is happening today with the ever-evolving treatments. The most important rule to remember is to get appropriate cancer checks (breast, lung, colon, etc.) because early detection improves your chances of survival and provides the best options for treatments.

Based on your experiences and knowledge, what advice would you give to others who have recently been diagnosed with cancer? What are your "5 Things" You Need To Beat Cancer? Please share a story or example for each.

1. Get appropriate checks before you're diagnosed with cancer. You won't develop cancer from a scan, but that scan can save your life. My cancer was found from a kidney stone CT

scan. I was diagnosed as Stage 1a, went through surgery and have been cancer-free or NED (No Evidence of Disease) for over two years.

2. Learn about your disease. I'm not saying to look for prognosis or longevity statistics as they are almost always averages and not the best data. Rather, you should learn about the disease; what is it, what causes it, what protocols are considered "gold standard" as well as the testing that should occur during your diagnostic phase. In my case, I gained a lot of valuable knowledge from my LUNGevity peers that helped me to be a better advocate in my diagnosis and treatment.

3. Make sure that your Primary Care Physician (PCP) is a good one. Some folks only see their PCP now and then and may not have a great relationship or trust in their judgment. This is the person who will likely help you to put together your cancer team (oncologist, surgeon, pulmonologist, etc.) In my case I had a pulmonologist and surgeon, but no oncologist. My "tribe" at LUNGevity helped me to understand the importance of a full team and I made a change that helped significantly going forward. The oncologist was more specific and detailed in the testing he required during my post-surgery period.

4. Don't be a "tough guy or gal." This is a hard road to walk alone, and your family can only help you so much. They try to empathize, and we appreciate their efforts, but at the end of the day, they can't fathom what we're going through. It makes a world of difference to engage in conversations with people who are in the midst of their own battle with cancer or have survived the disease and can impart their knowledge of how to get the most out of your treatment with the least amount of side effects.

5. Choose to live (something one of my LUNGevity brothers preaches). We all know that attitude is key in how our bodies resist disease and heal from injuries—and cancer is no different. You need to be determined to live. It may sound basic, but my initial reaction was to plan for my demise. After I found a support system, my pessimistic attitude changed and I increased my workouts to gain more strength, opened myself up to others about my disease so they would better understand, and started looking for ways to improve my overall health. All this before I even had a final diagnosis.

You are a person of great influence. If you could inspire a movement that would bring the most amount of good to the greatest amount of people, what would that be?

If I had the power, I would love to show people that our differences are normal, and we should judge ideas based on their merit instead of judging each other. In my view, we've become like human bear traps; always ready to spring with steel teeth if we hear or see something we don't agree with. Heck, I grew up in a family where folks would even debate during dinner and then all went out together to have some fun. No harsh judgments or hard feelings. I miss those days.

We are very blessed that some very prominent names in Business, VC funding, Sports, and Entertainment read this column. Is there a person in the world, or in the US with whom you would love to have a private breakfast or lunch, and why?

He's neither a business, financial nor sports figure... but, as a musician, I'd like to have a lunch with Yusuf Islam (a.k.a. Cat Stevens). His music influenced much of what I did and still do. I'd welcome the opportunity to talk about what influenced his music to be so creative and real.

How can our readers further follow your work online?

While I don't operate a personal website and interact with family and friends only via social channels, I'm constantly searching the LUNGevity Lung Cancer Support Community message boards for new members to embrace. Joining a community of people who knew exactly what I was going through and could provide advice to help me along my journey was instrumental in pulling through my anxious state. Nowadays, I pay it forward and do the same for others who—if they're anything like me—fear what the future holds and are uncertain of where to start in making their next health decisions.

Scan the QR code to view my "5 Things" To Beat Cancer YouTube video:

Marianne Sarcich: I Survived (Breast) Cancer and Here Is How I Did It

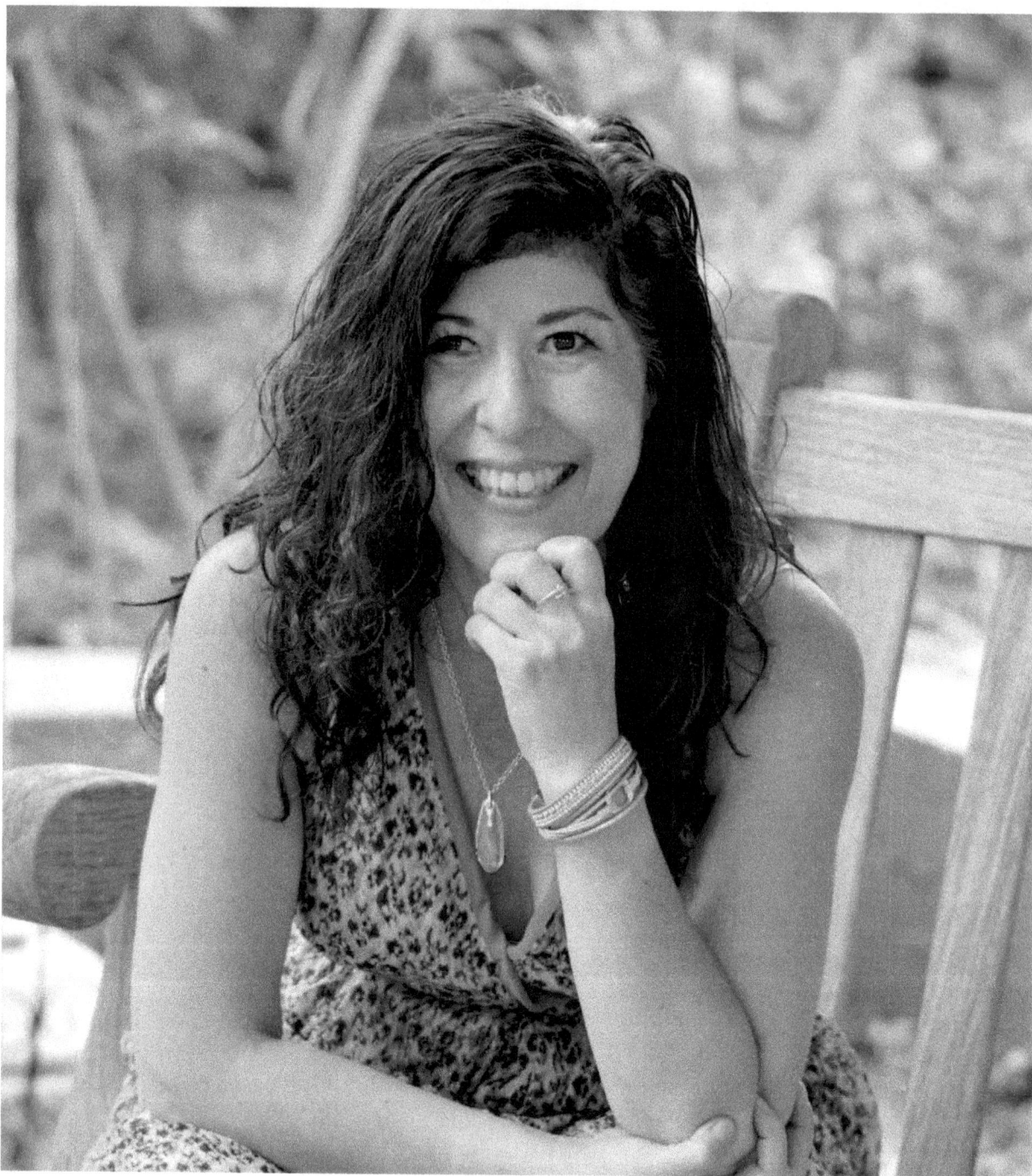

Take time to learn what is okay with you and what is not. And keep checking in with yourself because things can change by the second. It's all new and sometimes very overwhelming. This is your breast cancer experience, and no one else's. There is no wrong way to respond to it. There is just your way. So, for instance, if you don't want to tell anyone outside of your immediate family, that is your right. Set that boundary

and protect it. If that upsets other people, that is their response to deal with.

I had the pleasure of interviewing Marianne Sarcich. Marianne, a breast cancer survivor and advocate, is the founder of the breast cancer peer support group In This Together Philly Wilmington, where she helps patients and survivors in Eastern Pennsylvania, New Jersey and Delaware. She advocates locally and nationally creating programming and awareness for the breast cancer community, with a focus on metastatic breast cancer. Her affiliations include Living Beyond Breast Cancer, National Coalition for Cancer Survivorship, WEGO Health, Sharsheret, Society for Integrative Oncology, AnaOno, Young Survival Coalition, Triage Cancer, The Grace Project, Outcomes4Me and MBC Travelers.

Thank you so much for joining us in this interview series! We really appreciate the courage it takes to publicly share your story. Before we start, our readers would love to "get to know you" a bit better. Can you tell us a bit about your background and your childhood backstory?

Of course. I'm a mother of two incredible daughters, Elise and Anna, and I'm married to a wonderful husband, Paul. And now, I have a son, Alex, who joined the family this summer when he and Elise married. I love to start my day with a run outdoors, sometimes with our rescue dog, Poppy. I lived and worked in New York City before I had kids and to this day I miss living there. I'm a NYC city cat at heart.

Now, I live in the very caring community of Wilmington, Delaware, although I didn't realize the depth of their care until I got my breast cancer diagnosis.

Can you please give us your favorite "Life Lesson Quote?" Can you share how that was relevant to you in your life?

The one that speaks to me the most right now is this...

"Be a blessing to somebody." — Maya Angelou

What it has brought to me, I believe, is more than what I have brought to others. I discovered that being that blessing is so emotionally healing for me. I still deal with anxiety from my breast cancer. And helping others has become one of the ways I manage it. It's extraordinary how very healing it can be.

Listen to Maya say these words yourself. Because then you will learn another powerful perspective from her that can become a self-care tool to comfort yourself in frightening times.

"I bring everyone who has ever been kind to me with me…Come with me, I need you now…So I don't ever feel I have no help. I've had rainbows in my clouds."

That resonates so much with me. Rainbows in my clouds. You can hear her for yourself at this link:

vm.tiktok.com/ZMRSg1Ve7

Let's now shift to the main part of our discussion about surviving cancer. Do you feel comfortable sharing with us the story surrounding how you found out that you had cancer?

I'm happy to. One of the things I've discovered is that sharing my story is healing for me. So I've become very transparent with my breast cancer experience.

My cancer story began Wednesday evening, July 28, 2016. My hand accidentally brushed down my chest, and I felt a lump. My breath stopped. I froze. I was afraid to even bring my hand back up to that lump. My first acquaintance with my now constant companion — cancer fear — was that moment.

I was diagnosed on August 19, 2016 and declared no evidence of disease (NED) the first week of November. Today, I am still NED. In between August 19th and today were many surgeries, a second biopsy, monstrous anxiety and oh so much living.

What was the scariest part of that event? What did you think was the worst thing that could happen to you?

I remember being in such an emotional spin when I got my diagnosis. My biggest fear that rose above them all — including the fear for myself — was who would take care of my family, our then 10-year-old Anna, and our college senior Elise? That's my job.

Who would keep their childhood on track and normal? Of all the things not okay with me about what cancer could and would do to our lives, disrupting their childhood was what upset me the most.

How did you react in the short term?

So I went into what I call "Marianne Mode." My inner control freak took over, and I left no virtual stone unturned in my desperate quest to learn what I had to do, where I should be treated and who should be treating me. All in order to live. My small yellow notepad and pen together with my laptop and phone became my makeshift breast cancer war room in my dining room. I worked every connection I had. And soon that yellow pad was filled with a long list of potential breast surgeons.

While I was doing that, I was also planning support for my husband and children. And this is where I hit a personal wall. I discovered my immense fear of saying the words, "I have breast cancer" out loud. But, if I didn't tell people, how could I get support for my family?

Remember, however, I was in "Marianne Mode." That meant, no time for obstacles, including my own. So I shifted my perspective and told myself I was asking for help for my family, not me. That and a huge emotional shove by my inner control freak got me over that wall. Although, the only way I could tell people was by text, and writing those texts made me cry.

The time between learning about my diagnosis in August and going into my mastectomy on September 26th was jammed with pure panic and frantic, non-stop work. I had to find transportation for Anna to and from school for weeks while I recovered. I had to arrange meals for the family to lift the burden off my husband. I had to make sure Elise had the support she needed at college and ask for additional financial aid. I had to help my husband learn how I managed Anna's asthma care, something that was always my responsibility. And I distinctly remember writing up some notes for him on this and breaking down. Because, I thought, *I am writing myself out of my own life.*

I also had to find ways to lift the financial burden off my family. I spent an enormous amount of time researching financial grants only to discover that as soon as I was rolled out of the OR, I would no longer be eligible for any of them. You have to be in treatment to be considered. And the mastectomy was my only treatment. That meant that I had to complete all financial grant applications before I went into surgery. The pressure was enormous.

After the dust settled, what coping mechanisms did you use? What did you do to cope physically, mentally, emotionally, and spiritually?

Recovery right after my mastectomy became my full-time job. I loaded it with some fairly good coping tools, mostly new to me. I replaced my early morning run with a meditation from www.calm.com, which was something new. I went for mini walks several times a day; literally just back and forth in front of my house and then back to the couch.

And I spent time every day on finding the good in the day because I knew this much about myself. I'm the person that usually is overcome by negative thoughts. So I forced myself to look for the good. Literally. Looking for the good was an activity on my daily to-do list. And I created a note in my Google Keep app, a note which I still have today, where I jotted down my findings. It could be the littlest things. That was okay because at least it got me focused on something good and took me out of dark thoughts. What I discovered was doing this brought on a feeling of calm. Even reading over my notes triggered that calm feeling. It wasn't until much, much later that I discovered that gratitude work is actually an evidence-based therapeutic tool.

However, a few weeks later I was hit with a tsunami of emotional upheaval when my oncologist told me I was no evidence of disease or NED at our first meeting. Doesn't make sense, right? Agreed. I never saw it coming, and yet now, I know. It's fairly common.

Is there a particular person you are grateful towards who helped you learn to cope and heal? Can you share a story about that?

If I have to single out one person, then it's my husband. There is an image of him I will never forget. Paul coming home from work and me watching from my spot lying on the couch after my mastectomy. Without taking off his coat, he quickly checked on me and then went right into the kitchen to get dinner ready, still with his coat on. Eventually he sat down to eat, yes, with his coat off finally. He repeated all of that for weeks. The circles under his eyes broke my heart. I hated the burden I had become. Yet how he showed up for me and our family was so beautiful. I will never forget it.

I do have to say, however, it's difficult to single out one person. There is no way I would have gotten through my breast cancer without my children, my friends, and my local community. Things like Elise, who was studying at Arcadia University, finding a friend to drive her to the Hospital of the University of Pennsylvania to visit me after my mastectomy, and Anna, who made me a flower out of pipe cleaners to brighten my day. And the moms in my community who brought me dinner even though they didn't know me; or even sent their husbands to my door with things like a memory foam pillow because as one husband told me, "My wife says your ass hurts, so here's a pillow." He wasn't wrong, I had said that.

In my own cancer struggle, I sometimes used the idea of embodiment to help me cope. Let's take a minute to look at cancer from an embodiment perspective. If your cancer had a message for you, what do you think it would want or say?

This is a tough one for me. Whenever I have visualized my cancer, I have seen it as a parasite with not a single human trait. No compassion. No empathy. No mercy —simply a parasite looking for a host to survive. And that host is me. Whether or not I survived was irrelevant to this parasite.

So on the same vein, my takeaway from my cancer is I too want to survive. And if the choice is you or me, cancer, it will be me. I will do as you do. I will do what it takes to live.

What did you learn about yourself from this very difficult experience? How has cancer shaped your worldview? What has it taught you that you might never have considered before? Can you please explain with a story or example?

What I discovered is how little I knew myself. I mean, really knew myself. With cancer, things get real really quickly. And what would be best for me? Well, I didn't always know. I know now, for the most part. And if I don't know, I know to take the time and ask myself is this okay with me. Something I never would have done before breast cancer. In fact, that simple question is in my self-care tool kit. And just the fact that I have a self-care tool kit is something new since breast cancer. I now consider self-care medicinal.

Because of breast cancer, I now understand community and how pivotal it is—to receive care and love from the community, and to give it. My breast cancer was the first time I was on the receiving end from my community. A meal train was started and strangers came to my house every night for weeks with home cooked meals. Gifts were given to our daughters to comfort them on the day of my mastectomy. Even a stand-alone freezer was found and delivered so we could freeze the many meals we were given. All of this was humbling and beautiful. And taught me so much about what it means to be part of a community. And now, because of that, I'm a very active member of my community. Not just with my breast cancer group.

How have you used your experience to bring goodness to the world?

The breast cancer peer support group I started, quite honestly, I started for selfish reasons. My anxiety was still not managed well despite all my efforts. And I realized that I needed to spend time with people from the breast cancer community in person. So I launched that group to help myself. We had about 10 of us initially.

As membership began to grow, I realized I needed to do more than just create in person get-togethers. And here's where I think my story of bringing goodness to the world really begins. There were so many unmet needs among the members. So I expanded the mission and kept expanding the mission to fill the needs as best I could.

For instance, I created resource lists on everything from financial grants to free travel and lodging for out of town treatment. Because I never forgot the panic and effort I went through to do that research myself before my mastectomy, I launched a card writing program and rallied volunteers from within the group and the local community to send inspirational and supportive cards to members each month. I started a second Facebook group to gather community volunteers to help me support the group. And then I started a third group for the members to exchange items with each other, like wigs and drain holders. And I launched a recovery recliner program with power lift recliners I gathered from the community and loaned out to group members for them to recover in after surgery. Anything to help ease the burden of the diagnosis and to help the members become informed patients who are confident in self-advocating.

Now I've become known in my local community for my breast cancer advocacy. And I often get messages from strangers asking for advice or information. And I get tagged in Facebook posts regarding breast concerns.

And, to support my local community, at the beginning of the pandemic, I launched a Facebook group and partnered with a friend of mine, Chryssa Cohen, to deliver meals and snacks to the Delaware frontline workers. Through our group, called To Our Helpers with Love, we rallied the local community and ended up delivering just over a thousand meals. I did what I could to get some press coverage in the hopes of generating additional donations.

What are a few of the biggest misconceptions and myths out there about fighting cancer that you would like to dispel?

I'm so glad you're asking this. There are several. The first one is we may be feeling very physically ill and emotionally wrung out while still looking fairly healthy. And that makes the disease invisible at times and tricky for people to know what's truly going on with us. Just remember, how we look has nothing to do with how we actually feel.

Another one is metastatic breast cancer is incurable. These patients are in forever treatment. But they are often asked by friends, family and even the medical community questions like, when will you finish treatment? Questions like these can be very painful to hear and make the patient feel so misunderstood and alone.

And for those of us like me who are early-stagers, the effects of the diagnosis and treatment can linger sometimes for a lifetime. Treatment can cause permanent heart damage; it can cause dental issues that don't pop up until years later. Memory issues, joint pain, and some of us, me included, are on a daily med for years after diagnosis that causes constant side effects.

There's more. The color pink and that pink ribbon? It's not embraced by the entire breast cancer community. It can actually trigger quite a bit of anxiety for some of us. The response to that ribbon and that color is a full spectrum from joy to hatred and everything in between. So please be mindful and understanding if a breast cancer patient or survivor in your life doesn't respond positively to a pink ribbon or the color pink. They will appreciate your intention. And, no, they may not realize until they see it what their response might be.

Here's some insights into why. Just because an item being sold has a pink ribbon doesn't mean the retailer is making a donation to a breast cancer nonprofit. Often times it's being sold purely for profit. But we are so trained to believe and rightly so that pink ribbon items are fundraisers for the breast cancer community. And that's just not the case. We call this pinkwashing. If you do want to support the breast cancer community by purchasing a pink ribbon item — and thank you for your support — we ask you think before you pink. Simply ask before you buy. Will you be making a donation from the sale of this item? And then ask how much and where will this donation go? If it's not going to a reputable nonprofit, save your dollars for another pink ribbon item.

And there's more. The pink ribbon is synonymous with breast cancer and breast cancer fundraising, and billions of dollars have been raised because of it. All of which is beyond wonderful. What most people don't realize, however, is less than 7% of those dollars annually goes to research for metastatic breast cancer, even though that is the only way to find a cure. To this day, researchers do not know why breast cancer metastasizes. Once it does metastasize, or spreads outside of the breast, it becomes incurable. And if only more of the breast cancer research dollars would go toward metastatic breast cancer research, perhaps we could stop it from metastasizing and even eventually find a cure.

Fantastic. Here is the main question of our interview. Based on your experiences and knowledge, what advice would you give to others who have recently been diagnosed with cancer? What are your "5 Things" You Need To Beat Cancer? Please share a story or example for each.

Community... Gather your family and friends so that they can support you and your immediate family as you move through treatment and recovery. And remember, it is okay to ask for help. Allow others to help you. Lift the burden off your family. And off of yourself.

Boundaries... Take time to learn what is okay with you and what is not. And keep checking in with yourself because things can change by the second. It's all new and sometimes very overwhelming. This is your breast cancer experience, and no one else's. There is no wrong way to respond to it. There is just your way. So, for instance, if you don't want to tell anyone outside of your immediate family, that is your right. Set that boundary and protect it. If that upsets other people, that is their response to deal with.

Your voice... Raise your voice. Those boundaries we just talked about—use your voice to set them and protect them. And feel the strength flow through you as you do it. Hearing your own voice speaking up for yourself will empower you. Because I know that a breast cancer diagnosis can make you feel powerless. But you're not. You have your voice. So if you have questions but your oncologist is walking out of the room headed to the next appointment, raise your voice. If you're headed into radiation and you're petrified, say something. Talk it through with your loved ones and with your radiation oncologist. What exactly has you frightened, and what can they do to help ease your fear?

Expand your cancer team... Go beyond creating a core team of oncologist, breast surgeon and radiologist. Add professionals who will help you maintain a quality of life during and after treatment. This includes a social worker, an oncology dietitian, a counselor and a supportive care (also known as palliative care) doctor. Supportive care is one of the best things you can give yourself at diagnosis. And it's so misunderstood. It is all about providing patients the best quality of life as defined by that patient. That's you. It encompasses care of the family too. In fact, studies show supportive care not only can significantly increase quality of life but also improve the efficacy of treatment. And, the American Society of Clinical Oncologists recommends in its guidelines that supportive care be given early on.

Self-care... Rethink self-care and consider it now medicinal. It is how you will restore yourself emotionally as you move through treatment and recovery. Create a self-care toolkit. What goes in it? Whatever speaks to you. Spend time thinking about it. You are worth it. In my tool kit, you will find running outdoors in the early morning, spending time with my family, mindfulness, meditation and having alone time.

You are a person of great influence. If you could inspire a movement that would bring the most amount of good to the greatest amount of people, what would that be?

There is a love/pain relationship between some of us in the breast cancer community and how breast cancer awareness is currently depicted in what we call the mainstream; anyone who has not had a breast cancer diagnosis. Why? Because many of us don't feel included and heard in the current breast cancer narrative believed by the mainstream. What they don't know hurts us.

Like breast cancer is incurable. When you become metastatic, you will die. That's not pretty. That's not pink, but that's the reality. Like men get breast cancer too. And yet they are severely underrepresented in breast cancer research. The disparities in treatment that cause not only physical and emotional fallout, but even death among minority communities like Black/African-Americans. And they too are sorely underrepresented in the research. The young can get breast cancer, even in their twenties, even while pregnant, and yet they are frequently dismissed when they bring breast concerns to medical professionals; too often hearing the words "you're too young to have breast cancer."

Imagine just the emotional healing that could happen if the entire breast cancer community felt heard for who we truly are and not for who the mainstream have been taught we are. And then imagine the strides we could make together, breast cancer and mainstream communities, with this new understanding.

Reshaping that narrative to make it inclusive of us all — that is a movement that would impact countless people now and in the future. And that is a movement worth launching and getting behind.

We are very blessed that some very prominent names in Business, VC funding, Sports, and Entertainment read this column. Is there a person in the world, or in the US with whom you would love to have a private breakfast or lunch, and why?

What comes to mind are memories from the pandemic of spending time with my family, all of us sitting on the couch, eating dinner and having a great time watching a movie. And it's hard to find something that we all truly enjoy. That movie was *Zombieland,* and then we watched the sequel. So, with those memories in my heart, I would love to hang out with Emma Stone. I've enjoyed her performances for years. But now that she has gifted our family with such wonderful memories during such a difficult time, I want to say thank you.

And, honestly, I would also love to say thank you to Taylor Swift. That's whose music fills the kitchen as we get dinner ready, and fills the car as I drive my daughter to and from school and around town. She's been a family favorite for years, and we have countless beautiful memories thanks to her.

How can our readers further follow your work online?

I use my personal Facebook page for my breast cancer advocacy. And I post many things publicly on that page. In fact, last year during breast cancer awareness month, I created a post everyday on a different topic I wanted people outside of the breast cancer community to know. And I plan on doing the same this year. If someone has had a breast cancer diagnosis and lives in Eastern Pennsylvania or New Jersey or Delaware, they are more than welcome to join the peer support group that I run. Here is the link for it:

www.facebook.com/groups/2006782929610286

Scan the QR code to view my "5 Strategies" For Moving Through Cancer YouTube video:

Former Comcast & AT&T CEO Mike Armstrong: I Survived (Prostate) Cancer and Here Is How I Did It

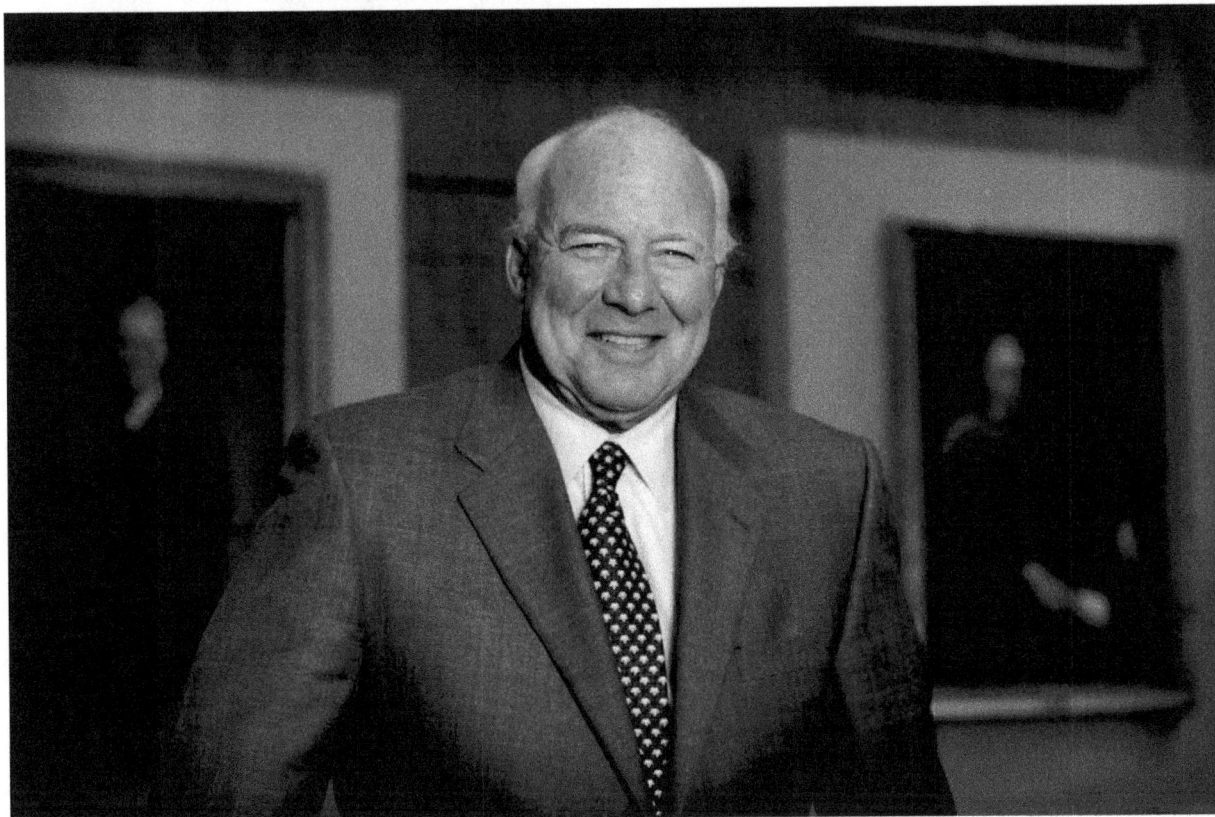

Find others with cancer or those who have had cancer, especially the type you are facing. You can learn from and get much-needed support from these folks as you make your trip through "recovery."

I had the pleasure of interviewing Mike Armstrong. Mike is the former Chairman and CEO of Comcast, AT&T and Hughes Electronics. He began his career at IBM where he spent more than three decades rising through the ranks to become chairman of the IBM World Trade Corporation. Having battled leukemia and prostate cancer as well as serious illness throughout the 1990s and early 2000s, he became an active supporter of Johns Hopkins Medical School and its hospitals after retiring from the corporate world in 2002. In 2005, he was named chairman of the Board of Trustees of Johns Hopkins Medicine. Now fully retired, Armstrong is on a mission to share his story as a two-time cancer survivor to help others on the cancer journey find hope. He and his wife Anne are donating most of their net worth to projects that advance medicine, help the disadvantaged, and make this world a better place.

Thank you so much for joining us in this interview series! We really appreciate the courage it takes to publicly share your story. Before we start, our readers would love to "get to know you" a bit better. Can you tell us a bit about your background and your childhood backstory?

I was born in Detroit, Michigan to wonderful, hard working parents. I was raised during WWII, and we all learned the value and importance of hard work and sacrifice. I got my first job at age 11 doing lawn work in my neighborhood and then at 15 got a special drivers' permit to drive a truck to pick up and deliver abandoned railroad ties for a landscaping company. During college, I worked as a bartender and also worked six days a week summers at a flour mill, loading/unloading 100/140-pound flour bags to and from box cars.

Can you please give us your favorite "Life Lesson Quote?" Can you share how that was relevant to you in your life?

"Never Give Up"

Let's now shift to the main part of our discussion about surviving cancer. Do you feel comfortable sharing with us the story surrounding how you found out that you had cancer?

I found out about my first cancer (hairy cell leukemia) from a phone call. After 31 years with IBM, I took the CEO job at Hughes Electronics in Los Angeles. Right after I moved to California, during my second week at this new and demanding position, I got a call from my doctor back East, who had recently given me a very complete physical exam. Instead of telling me I was healthy and all is well, he told me I had leukemia, that it was serious, and had had gone undetected for some time. He referred me to one of the Los Angeles' top leukemia experts at the UCLA Cancer Center. That's a tough way to start a new career!

I learned I had my second cancer (prostate cancer) after my PSA numbers started rising mysteriously. I say mysteriously because a series of biopsies showed no evidence of cancer. As it turned out, the cancer was in the front of my prostate, making it hard to detect. When they finally detected it, it had gone unnoticed for a long time (like my first cancer). We did not know how serious it was until they opened me up and saw that my cancer had expanded out of my prostate and into my abdomen. A quick surgery turned into an extended procedure, and I went from expecting to be cancer-free post-surgery to being told I had a 50% chance of living cancer-free for five years.

In addition, both of these cancers gave me serious additional illnesses that each had the potential to also take my life. With my leukemia, I got a blood infection that turned into sepsis and put me in an ICU for a harrowing week of uncertainty. With my prostate cancer I developed Parsonage-Turners Syndrome (PTS) which damaged my phrenic nerves and reduced my ability to breathe to 20% of capacity.

What was the scariest part of that event? What did you think was the worst thing that could happen to you?

Like many other cancer patients, the worst possible outcome is death, which I faced numerous times with both my cancers and the associated diseases I suffered. Short of death, probably my worst outcomes were the sepsis I encountered after my treatment for leukemia and the PTS I suffered with my prostate cancer. Likely the most difficult news I ever received was that when the first-time cancer (leukemia) entered my life, which was a phone call from my doctor that I got during my first weeks as CEO of Hughes Electronics, it was both the worst day of my life and the most memorable. In essence, this doctor was telling me that I might die! That is something that is very hard to forget.

After the dust settled, what coping mechanisms did you use? What did you do to cope physically, mentally, emotionally, and spiritually?

In both cases, my leukemia and prostate cancer, when I learned that my cancer had gone undetected for too long, I knew I was in a fight for my life. My first imperative was to seek out and secure the best medical care and advice. In both instances I was able to locate a specialist in my particular type of cancer. Both of these physicians worked at NCI-designated cancer, so I knew they were connected to the most up-to-date research and data on cancer diagnosis and treatment. With my leukemia, my doctor enrolled me in a clinical trial of a new drug that literally saved my life.

Regarding my career, I had to do a lot to manage my work schedule. Since I was CEO, this involved a much higher level of assessment and action. My final decision on how to deal with my cancer was not just mine to make. I had to answer to and consult with both board of directors at Hughes and also the board at General Motors, which had a controlling share of Hughes. Collectively, we agreed that it would be best not to share my cancer with the general public. The risk was that it might erode confidence both from employees and shareholders. We decided to wait 30 days, which was the length of time I was scheduled to be receiving chemotherapy. After that, we would have more information about my chances of survival. If the chemo worked, if I was cancer-free, there was no reason to raise concern among shareholders and company employees. If the chemo didn't work, we would consider how and when to break the news about my cancer.

That did not mean that it was business as usual. I had a chemo pack strapped to my waist with a tube going into my arm feeding chemo 24–7 that was hard to hide at work. So I told co-workers that my doctor was monitoring my health and that was enough to assuage curiosity. However, chemo and the low blood counts from my leukemia drained my energy. So I had to cut back on my long workdays and travel. In addition, I suspended my regular workout routine, something that I depended on to help me relax. The good news was my treatment was aggressive and only lasted 30 days. After that, if I was still battling cancer, I would be able to share the news with a larger group of supporters. Luckily, in 30 days, I was cancer-free!

Is there a particular person you are grateful towards who helped you learn to cope and heal? Can you share a story about that?

Having a high-profile job as CEO for a major US corporation meant I could not share my illness with anyone except for my wife, secretary, and doctor. As such, that was my "support group." My wife, Anne, of course, was my biggest supporter. We met while in high school and have supported each other throughout the many ups and downs of our lives together. And while I was on my own in California (my wife was still back East settling our affairs), Anne and I had regular daily phone calls that were an essential component of my wellness and treatment regime.

In my own cancer struggle, I sometimes used the idea of embodiment to help me cope. Let's take a minute to look at cancer from an embodiment perspective. If your cancer had a message for you, what do you think it would want or say?

The biggest message cancer brings is that it can kill you. And while this was always on my mind, I was determined not to let it kill me. I knew I had one primary goal, and that was to eliminate the cancer from the rest of my life. This was so different from other challenges I had faced in my life, both physical and medical. This was truly the "fight of my life;" it was a fight that had but one winner, the cancer or me.

Another message this disease taught me was how precious life was and how it important it was to appreciate it and make the most of it, and give back for all that life had given me.

What did you learn about yourself from this very difficult experience? How has cancer shaped your worldview? What has it taught you that you might never have considered before? Can you please explain with a story or example?

I learned that when life throws challenges your way, you need to do your best to meet these challenges. I also learned that this is not easy. Cancer is one of the toughest challenges anyone faces in this life. Most of us struggle to keep positive in the face of all this uncertainty and continuous bad news. Still I believe one needs to do their best to try to keep hope. Hope alone won't cure cancer, but combined with good treatments and great medical advice, it is a powerful strategy to keep you on course, fighting your disease with all you've got.

How have you used your experience to bring goodness to the world?

After living through the advanced leukemia and prostate cancer, my wife and I felt as though we needed to have a clear purpose in life, something that made a difference making this world a better place. In essence, we wanted to do what we could to help others who were less fortunate than us. So, we decided to give away the majority of our life savings to worthwhile causes and medical research.

What are a few of the biggest misconceptions and myths out there about fighting cancer that you would like to dispel?

Cancer is death. Just not true. Cancer is an illness, often a serious illness. But increasingly medicine and therapy are controlling and/or eliminating cancer.

Can cancer come back? Yes, I had three different cancers and all serious. I fought them with excellent doctors, the right medications and necessary recovery timeframes. Once cancer comes into your life, it seems to be always lurking over your shoulder.

Your cancer doctor. Cancer demands not just a doctor, but the right doctor for your disease. I had the right doctors. My leukemia doctor was a cancer specialist at the UCLA Cancer Center, my prostate cancer doctor at Johns Hopkins Medicine and my carcinoma doctor was also a renowned specialist. My advice is look for an academic research center and/or and National Cancer Institute designated cancer center. These are the hospitals that have the most up-to-date information about cancer. And if they don't know about your type of cancer, they can find someone who does. That does not mean that you can't also be treated by a local oncologist, but just make sure you get a consultation at one of these major cancer centers. It cannot hurt, and in many cases it helps a lot.

Also make sure you explore the possibility of clinical trials. Important to note, clinical trials are not designed to save cancer patients but to learn about new drugs and treatment, so there are no guarantees. But it is just one more tool in the cancer tool shed that you should be aware of and explore.

Fantastic. Here is the main question of our interview. Based on your experiences and knowledge, what advice would you give to others who have recently been diagnosed with cancer? What are your "5 Things" You Need To Beat Cancer? Please share a story or example for each.

1. The right doctor for your cancer.

2. The right medicine for both your cancer and your medical condition.

3. A fighting attitude. Cancer is a tough disease that is tough on you and demands a fighting, determined, and sustaining patient to prevail.

4. Make room in your job and life to fight your cancer. I cancelled all travel and significantly reduced my long workdays.

5. Bouncing Boards. Find others with cancer or those who have had cancer, especially the type

you are facing. You can learn from and get much-needed support from these folks as you make your trip through "recovery."

You are a person of great influence. If you could inspire a movement that would bring the most amount of good to the greatest amount of people, what would that be?

I wanted to inspire hope in cancer patients and encourage them to never give up. Part of this was by sharing my story and the stories of other who have faced difficult cancer challenges. In addition, I wanted to provide guidance and advice from cancer experts on how to select an appropriate/effective doctor, learn about treatment options, and how to generally navigate the difficult, confusing and circuitous path through the cancer journey. "Cancer with Hope" is meant to help the cancer patients though this journey wherever it might take them and to remind them to appreciate life and try to make the most of it, no matter what challenges lie ahead.

Nick Lynch of Collidescope: I Survived (Kidney) Cancer and Here Is How I Did It

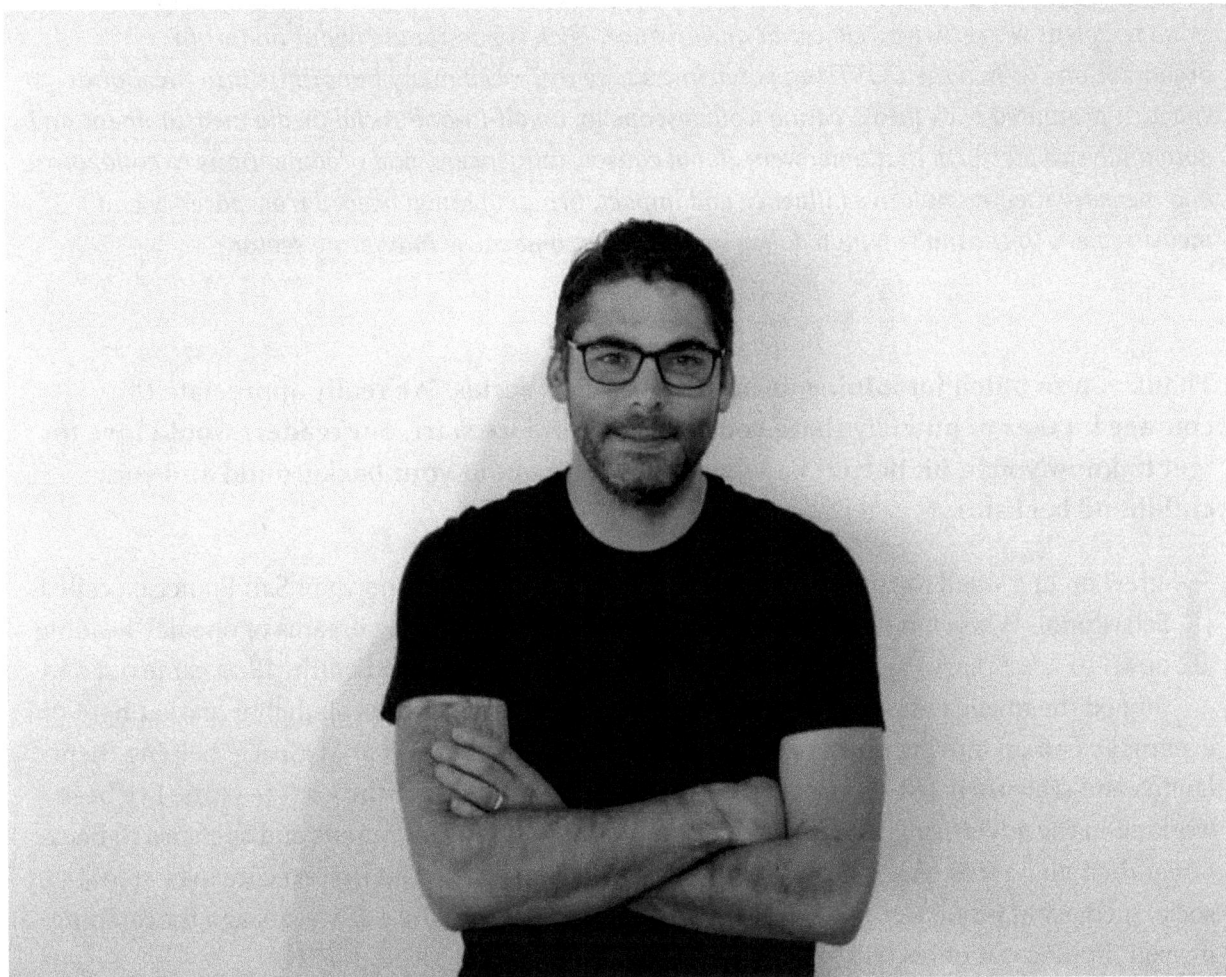

Seek "normalcy"—The minute you hear your cancer diagnosis, nothing is the same. You feel that people treat you differently, the things you do on a daily basis change, and it's easy to feel that the life you had before is gone. Find places, people, or even things that make you feel "normal." These moments helped me recharge and reminded me that there are things to look forward to after the surgeries and treatments.

I had the pleasure of interviewing Nick Lynch. In an ever-changing and evolving digital world, Nick has spent his professional career building solutions for brands to better identify and target their audiences online. Nick is more than a businessman: from personal experience as a former Make-A-Wish recipient who survived cancer at an early age, Nick is passionate about nonprofit organizations. When the COVID-19 pandemic suddenly forced many nonprofits into the digital space, it prompted Nick into creating Collidescope.io, an all-in-one social media measurement and data analytics platform that empowers global causes, influencers, and organizations to collaborate and measure their cumulative influence and impact, bringing much needed transparency and measurement to the multi-billion dollar social impact and cause marketing sector.

Thank you so much for joining us in this interview series! We really appreciate the courage it takes to publicly share your story. Before we start, our readers would love to "get to know you" a bit better. Can you tell us a bit about your background and your childhood backstory?

I grew up in a small town in northern California about 60 miles north of San Francisco called Sebastopol. When I moved to San Francisco for college, I had big dreams of one day heading down to Los Angeles and becoming a famous music producer. When the iPod came out and flipped the music industry upside down, I quickly pivoted to focus on digital marketing. I did eventually end up moving down to Los Angeles, but instead to work at MySpace, helping them launch and scale their self-serve advertising business—MyAds. For the last 15+ years, I've been working in the advertising technology space building solutions for brands and agencies to better target their audiences on social and digital media. I've helped sell and/or execute over $100M+ in social media and influencer marketing campaigns. I also went viral a few years ago for catching my son flipping out of his crib—www.youtube.com/watch?v=_UCRI4bJeMs

Can you please give us your favorite "Life Lesson Quote?" Can you share how that was relevant to you in your life?

"Be faithful in small things because it is in them that your strength lies." —*Mother Teresa*

Growing up, I'd watch my dad make a list of all the small details required to accomplish the various projects he'd be working on. The running family joke has always been about his lists. I never understood how important those lists were until I started using them. They help you spend time focusing on the small things, stacking the small wins, and creating momentum for larger outcomes. It's a repeatable formula that allows me to confidently tackle any challenge.

Let's now shift to the main part of our discussion about surviving cancer. Do you feel comfortable sharing with us the story surrounding how you found out that you had cancer?

When I was three, I was diagnosed with a stage 3 Wilms Tumor in my kidney. Before my diagnosis, I had seen several doctors who continuously misdiagnosed me. The diagnostics always seemed to be the same vague "stomach issue" following with the same prescriptions to alleviate the pain and symptoms.

My mom truly never believed these doctors and would not stop searching for answers on her own. Finally, we found a doctor who recognized the symptoms and suggested we go to Oakland Children's Hospital right away. By the time they had found the cancer, it had spread from my kidney into the main vein of my heart. At that point, the cancer was most likely weeks away from going into my heart and completely stopping it.

What was the scariest part of that event? What did you think was the worst thing that could happen to you?

About 7 years ago, I ordered all of my medical records from my cancer diagnosis and treatment. This included the operation report and all of the subsequent chemotherapy and radiation treatments. As a kid, especially as young as I was, it was difficult to grasp the gravity and seriousness of cancer. As you grow older, you piece things together based on the memories and reactions of the people around you. Reading these reports provided better context into my cancer, my treatments, and the various medical, physical, and emotional reactions. Reading these detailed doctors notes transported me back and I began feeling what my family probably felt; immense anxiety and fear. It wasn't until I read these notes that the prospect of me dying became very real.

How did you react in the short term?

My cancer experience up until I reviewed my reports would probably be considered atypical. Growing up, I never felt like I had limits. My parents made sure I was active and never let my cancer history be an excuse to not try or do anything. If you didn't see my scars, you'd never know I was a cancer survivor. But, when I was reading through my medical records and reports, I cried. It became very real in ways that I had never felt before.

After the dust settled, what coping mechanisms did you use? What did you do to cope physically, mentally, emotionally, and spiritually?

After reading through the hundred or so pages of my medical records, and reliving this childhood experience, I moved from sadness to immediate gratitude. Rehashing these emotions enhanced the level of gratitude I had for my doctors and family. Thinking about the consistency and strength it took for other people to support me allowed the focus to be taken off of the cancer and more on the amazing people in my life. This created the space for gratitude as well as mental and emotional healing.

Is there a particular person you are grateful towards who helped you learn to cope and heal? Can you share a story about that?

I cannot imagine how hard it must have been for my parents to hold it together, stay strong, and never show me how dire the situation actually was. It's a true miracle that I had not known how bad my cancer was until reviewing the reports. They shouldered the entire burden of my illness, allowing me to heal and grow into a mentally and emotionally strong adult. For that, I am deeply and forever grateful.

In my own cancer struggle, I sometimes used the idea of embodiment to help me cope. Let's take a minute to look at cancer from an embodiment perspective. If your cancer had a message for you, what do you think it would want or say?

Since my cancer, my mom has survived breast cancer and my dad is now in remission for prostate cancer. Cancer is the unfortunate, recurring theme in my life. However, I also look at it as a reminder of how strong we are individually as well as collectively. I never once doubted that either one of them would beat it. I *knew* they would beat it. Strength is made perfect in weakness, so for me, cancer would want me to know that I am strong.

What did you learn about yourself from this very difficult experience? How has cancer shaped your worldview? What has it taught you that you might never have considered before? Can you please explain with a story or example?

I have turned my cancer into a mantra. Whenever I am up against a huge hurdle or challenge, or when fear creeps into a decision I have to make, I remind myself, *you beat cancer to make a difference*. It's an affirmation I use to help me push through, stay motivated, and get me to where I need to be in this life.

How have you used your experience to bring goodness to the world?

As part of my recovery, I was granted a wish through the Make-A-Wish foundation to go to Disneyland. I credit that experience as "the great equalizer" for my family and I. The power of a wish is very real, and it's those moments I remember most; not my treatments. For the last six years, I have been deeply involved with the LA Chapter of Make-A-Wish and was even able to grant my first wish a few years ago.

It's through my work with Make-A-Wish and my professional experiences in digital advertising and marketing that I saw a tremendous need for better marketing solutions and technology for brands and advertisers to better work with nonprofits and causes. Then, when COVID-19 shut down all in person events, that need was only amplified. That is the inspiration behind why I co-founded Collidescope.io.

Collidescope.io is a social media analytics and measurement SaaS platform that allows brands, global causes, and influencers to collaborate and measure their cumulative influence and impact.

We provide third party validation and transparency into how a brands social impact marketing dollars are being spent, provide marketing and mission impact measurement, and identify campaign optimizations that increase donations and decrease costs. We also utilize the insights from those campaigns to build scoring that informs how they contribute to a company's environmental, social, and governance (ESG) efforts.

As consumers demand brands to be more aligned with causes that positively impact the world, we aim to provide a solution that allows brands to scale these initiatives while ensuring value and especially, transparency.

What are a few of the biggest misconceptions and myths out there about fighting cancer that you would like to dispel?

When people hear, "cancer," they immediately think the worst. There is no doubt that any cancer is serious, but it is by no means the beginning of the end. It's important to remember the world is full of fighters and survivors. Reinforcing the reality that there are paths forward and past cancer will help to dispel the doom and gloom myth.

Fantastic. Here is the main question of our interview. Based on your experiences and knowledge, what advice would you give to others who have recently been diagnosed with cancer? What are your "5 Things" You Need To Beat Cancer? Please share a story or example for each.

1. Breathe—Cancer turns people's worlds upside down. It's disorienting. Center yourself and seek techniques to silence your mind. Meditation can help guide you in finding this stillness. Don't forget to breathe.
2. Acknowledgement—It is okay to admit that you are scared. It is okay to admit that, "this sucks." Acknowledging your feelings and confronting them will help you identify and communicate your needs whether that be to other people, your doctors, or yourself.
3. Seek "normalcy"—The minute you hear your cancer diagnosis, nothing is the same. You feel that people treat you differently, the things you do on a daily basis change, and it's easy to feel that the life you had before is gone. Find places, people, or even things that make you feel "normal." These moments helped me recharge and reminded me that there are things to look forward to after the surgeries and treatments.
4. Build routine—No matter the size or kind of routine, it's important to have them. It allows you to feel a bit of control, during a time when you can feel helpless. This could be a daily walk, 10 minutes a day to journal, or a weekly call with your friend to talk about the football games over the weekend. Routines become a foundation and a pillar to lean on when things feel out of control.
5. Give yourself permission—Give yourself permission to have a bad day, ask for help, be vulnerable, happy, excited, sad, love, and be loved. Be kind to yourself.

You are a person of great influence. If you could inspire a movement that would bring the most amount of good to the greatest amount of people, what would that be?

I hope to inspire the 3 "T" movement. Getting people to understand that they all have the gift of 3 "T's:" time, talent, and treasure. I believe that most people get stuck at the start; they want to do great things but don't know how, where, or when to start. If more people realized that all they had to do was think about their own 3 "T's," it would get them off the starting block and progressing toward something amazing. The great part about activating our 3 "T's" is that there is no minimum or maximum requirement—just give any amount of one or all and positive change will happen.

We are very blessed that some very prominent names in Business, VC funding, Sports, and Entertainment read this column. Is there a person in the world, or in the US with whom you would love to have a private breakfast or lunch, and why?

The Obamas! But if I had to only pick one it would be the former First Lady, Michelle Obama. As an entrepreneur, I seek out origin stories of companies, but mostly find true inspiration from female founders; primarily because the challenges these amazing women overcome to build successful companies are exponentially greater than what men face. Reading both *Becoming* and *A Promised Land*, provided additional context into just how special she is. It would be an honor to meet her.

How can our readers further follow your work online?

For more information about how we are helping brands better measure and scale their social impact and cause marketing efforts while supporting nonprofits build their digital and social media presence, check out www.collidescope.io

Parul Somani: I Survived (Breast) Cancer and Here Is How I Did It

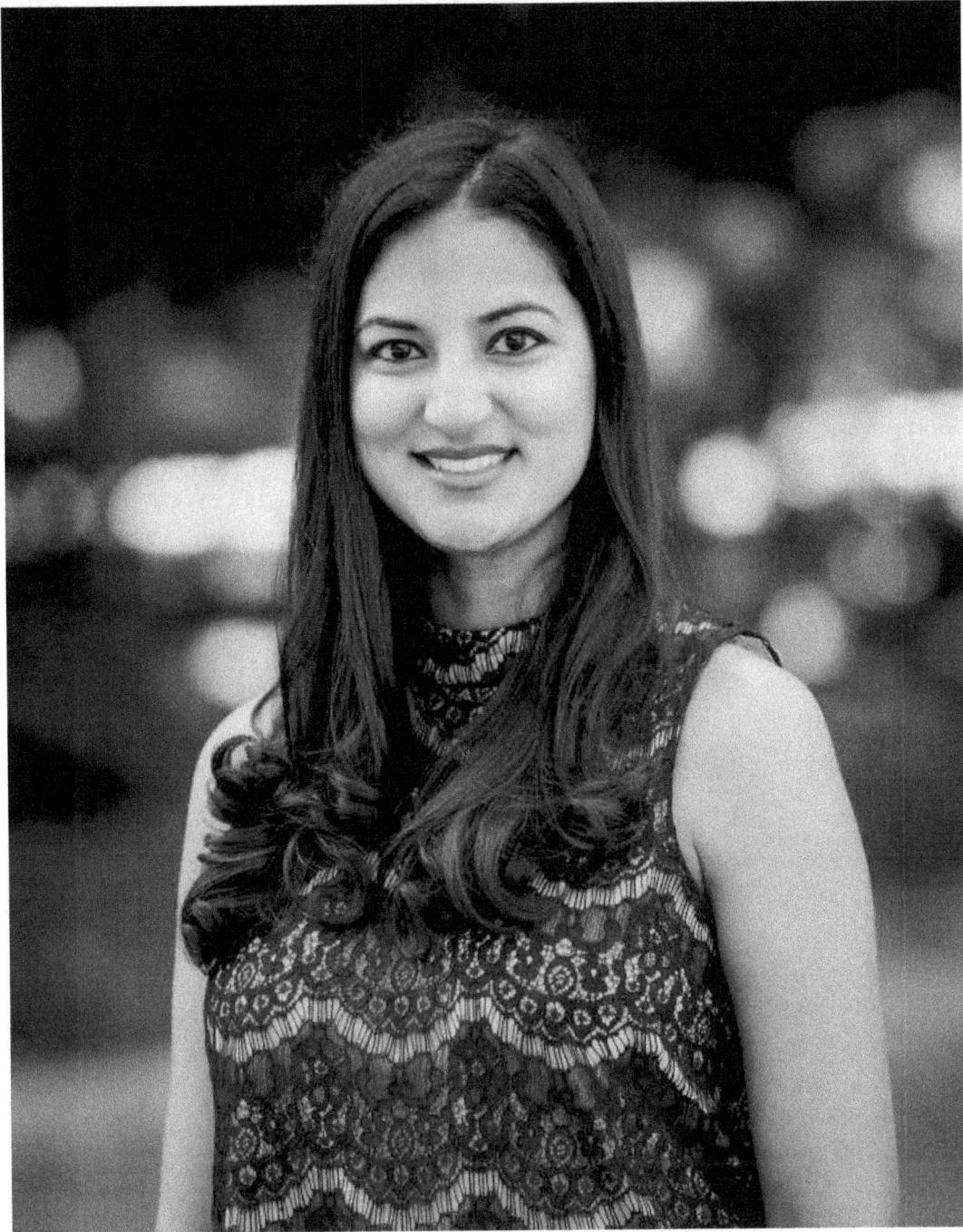

Compassion for yourself: The emotions will come in waves, and are sometimes triggered when you least expect it. Be kind to yourself during this roller coaster and protect your mental well-being by reminding yourself all for which you have to be thankful and maintaining faith that you will emerge stronger from the experience.

I had the pleasure of interviewing Parul Somani. Parul is an inspirational speaker promoting resilience and self-advocacy to help strengthen mental well-being, navigate life's challenges, and live an authentic life. She has presented keynotes and facilitated seminars for global employers, conferences, and nonprofits, authored a cancer blog which has been read in 85 countries, and been awarded honors by the American Cancer Society and others for her patient leadership. Parul holds degrees from MIT and the Harvard Business School, and previously had a 15+ year career in management consulting in Silicon Valley.

Thank you so much for joining us in this interview series! We really appreciate the courage it takes to publicly share your story. Before we start, our readers would love to "get to know you" a bit better. Can you tell us a bit about your background and your childhood backstory?

I'm an immigrant living the American dream. I was born in India, but my parents moved my sister and me to the States when I was three years old for a better education and future. Growing up in the 1980s-1990s in the Pacific Northwest, my childhood was a story of two cultures. While one day I might have been playing basketball, competing in a debate tournament, or performing a drum solo, the other I might have been training in Indian classical dance, learning Hindi, or watching Bollywood movies. Seeing my parents juggle multiple jobs and entrepreneurial ventures to support us and persevere through their own hardships, I learned the value of work ethic and grit. My parents established a high bar for academic excellence early on, but raised me with the freedom and independence of defining my own dreams.

While I don't remember when I first learned the word, "cancer" had a presence throughout my childhood. I was still playing with dolls when my mother wore a wig due to her treatment for early onset breast cancer. Whether it be cultural norms or other constraints, we never discussed my mother's diagnosis outside of our immediate family — for decades. Not even years later, when I was a teenager, when my mother spent months living in India to care for my grandfather after his late stage cancer diagnosis. As much as I was shaped by what I experienced in childhood, I was equally shaped by what I did not. By not seeing open and honest discussion about the diagnosis, I learned how important it is to be willing to share and show vulnerability. I always knew that if I were to ever be diagnosed with something like cancer, I would share it with the world.

Can you please give us your favorite "Life Lesson Quote?" Can you share how that was relevant to you in your life?

A quote that has been very relevant in my recent life is, "Tell your story of how you've overcome what you're going through now, and it will become part of someone else's survival guide." A friend of mine shared this saying with me when I announced my pivot to become an inspirational speaker, and I love it because it perfectly captures my belief that I can help others navigate their challenges by openly sharing how I faced my own.

Let's now shift to the main part of our discussion about surviving cancer. Do you feel

comfortable sharing with us the story surrounding how you found out that you had cancer?

I was holding my newborn in bed, still struggling to walk from my C-section, when I received the call. Not long before, I had been at a 38 week ultrasound for my baby when I felt a lump in my chest. Despite being told it was likely a clogged milk duct since I was only 31 years old and pregnant, I insisted on a referral for an ultrasound and biopsy. I never made it to that appointment though because my water broke soon after and my newborn arrived 2 weeks early. If that wasn't chaotic enough, she had breathing problems soon after delivery, had to be intubated, and we had to be transported by ambulance to another hospital with an acute NICU. Armed with the knowledge that I carry a *BRCA1* mutation, resulting in a high risk of breast cancer, we coordinated our own appointment for a biopsy at the new hospital. My husband wheeled me from the NICU to the breast clinic, where the breast surgeon also assured us that the tissue felt soft and was "likely just a clogged milk duct." Relieved, we headed back to the NICU after receiving frantic calls from my mother wondering where we were since it was time for the baby's feeding. Days later, my daughter was thankfully discharged with a clean bill of health and we were able to go home.

I knew it was a bad sign as soon as I saw that the breast surgeon was calling on a Saturday. I handed my baby to my mother and answered the call, learning that "the mass is malignant after all." I had triple-negative breast cancer (TNBC), one of the most aggressive types, and would require (at minimum) chemotherapy, a bilateral mastectomy, and breast reconstruction. I only began to tear up when she said, "Obviously, this means you will need to stop breastfeeding soon." It was only after I got off the phone that I dropped my head in my hands and started bawling.

What was the scariest part of that event? What did you think was the worst thing that could happen to you?

The scariest part was the uncertainty. While the breast surgeon believed the cancer to be early stage, we wouldn't really know until we assessed if it had spread to the lymph nodes or not. The biopsies of my lymph nodes were inconclusive, however, and the doctors didn't know if the suspicious swelling was due to the cancer spreading or my lymphatic system's response to my recent C-section and other biopsies. They wouldn't know for sure until surgery, which would be month's later after chemotherapy. I got my PET scan results a couple of weeks after my initial diagnosis, confirming the cancer had not spread elsewhere in the body. It was only then that we had comfort in knowing the cancer was not Stage 4. I still remember how overwhelming that relief felt, and the realization of how much my life had changed when the definition of "good news" was to find out that I'm not dying after all.

Despite how long it took to understand the full scope of the diagnosis, I remained steadfast in my view that I would ultimately be fine. Even when I had to share the news with my husband that his wife had been diagnosed with breast cancer at the same age his birth mother passed away from the same disease, my response to his distressed reaction was, "It's going to be fine—you won't need to do anything without me. The next few months will be tough, but I'm going to be fine." You can call it hope, optimism, denial, or delusion, but envisioning any other outcome was simply unimaginable.

How did you react in the short term?

My initial response was to go into warrior mode. My husband and I often talk about how "hope is not a course of action," and we found it empowering to do what we could: researching the diagnosis, lining up 2nd opinions, figuring out what questions to ask, understanding our insurance and employer benefits, etc. One could drown under the weight of the uncertainty and fear, so it was more energizing to focus on what we could control.

After the dust settled, what coping mechanisms did you use? What did you do to cope physically, mentally, emotionally, and spiritually?

The first month was pure survival mode. It took that long to understand the scope of the diagnosis, identify my care team, and align on a treatment plan. It was only once that was done that I was able to think about how to cope with this new reality. To maintain my physical health, I went on walks with my dad (when the fatigue wasn't so strong that I felt like I'd been hit by a truck) and only ate the healthy food that my mom prepared for me. When it came to coping mentally, emotionally, and spiritually, what I found most helpful were: remaining connected with friends and family to fuel the natural extrovert within me; sharing my experience real-time in a blog titled "New Job. New Baby. New Cancer." with the intention of being candid and raw, but also positive and uplifting; and practicing gratitude for all that I had to be thankful for despite the diagnosis.

Is there a particular person you are grateful towards who helped you learn to cope and heal? Can you share a story about that?

One of my hardest parts of treatment was the realization that I couldn't be there for my newborn in her early months the way I had been for her older sister. I wouldn't be able to continue nursing her. I wouldn't be able to take her to mommy and me music classes. I wouldn't even be able to lift her up for weeks after each surgery. Fortunately, my parents were visiting for the baby's delivery when I received my diagnosis, and their trip turned into a one-way ticket for the next six months. Along with my husband, my mother not only helped care for me throughout treatment, but she was also the mother to my newborn that I just couldn't be at that time. Knowing my young baby, who had just given us such a huge scare after her own birth, would be surrounded by love, allowed me the freedom to focus on my own healing.

In my own cancer struggle, I sometimes used the idea of embodiment to help me cope. Let's take a minute to look at cancer from an embodiment perspective. If your cancer had a message for you, what do you think it would want or say?

It would want me to remember the power of self-advocacy. What if I hadn't gotten genetic testing and learned of my *BRCA1* mutation? What if I had dismissed the lump as a clogged milk duct? Given I couldn't even feel the lump anymore once my milk came in after the delivery, what if I hadn't gotten a biopsy done until I felt the lump again when I stopped nursing a year later? Just how different would my prognosis have been then? My cancer diagnosis wasn't a dark cloud — catching it early was the silver lining. My cancer will always be a reminder that our intentions, our actions, and our self-agency can make all the difference.

What did you learn about yourself from this very difficult experience? How has cancer shaped your worldview? What has it taught you that you might never have considered before? Can you please explain with a story or example?

My cancer helped me find my way back to myself again. I was 14 years old when I wrote a paper on my "life philosophy" covering my views on everything from family and career to love and aging. Even then, I wrote, "By sharing my life stories and lessons with others, I can prevent them from making any of the mistakes I did." I had always wanted to make a difference in the world by helping and inspiring others. By the time of my diagnosis, however, I had spent years on the corporate career track, neglecting my health and working too many long hours on projects for which I had no passion. We often talk about how chemotherapy ages the body, but I believe it also matures the mind. My cancer gave me a revelation in my 30s that people don't often experience until their 60s—an awareness, if not reminder, of my priorities and the legacy I want to leave in this world. This realization drove me to pivot my career, become an inspirational speaker, and chart a path to sharing my life stories and lessons with others.

How have you used your experience to bring goodness to the world?

As a patient, I shared my experiences in my blog, as well as in films on survivorship and mindset. As a survivor and caregiver, I have counseled dozens of people through their own cancer diagnoses, sharing my experiences and helping them understand what questions to ask and how to best advocate for themselves. As a *BRCA1* carrier and former genomics executive, I champion the power of actionable genomics and precision medicine, as well as how the healthcare system needs to be improved to support it, by speaking at events for organizations like the World Economic Forum's Global Precision Medicine Initiative, the HLTH conference, and the American Cancer Society. As a business leader, I serve on the advisory board for the Stanford Health Communication Initiative and healthcare companies, bringing a unique perspective as a strategist, operator, patient, and caregiver. Lastly, I work with employers and organizations to empower their members to build their resilience and strengthen their mental well-being.

What are a few of the biggest misconceptions and myths out there about fighting cancer that you would like to dispel?

There is so much I've learned about cancer, but a few of the biggest misconceptions are that:

1. "I'm too young to get cancer:" My prognosis, and life story, would be entirely different had I believed the guidance that my lump was likely a clogged milk duct since I was "too young and pregnant." In the years since, I've met countless women who have been diagnosed with breast cancer in their 30s and early 40s—earlier than when annual mammograms are recommended. Some of the most painful stories are of the women who received Stage 3 diagnoses because they (and sometimes their doctors!) dismissed the lump as nothing to worry about for more than a year. Be aware of changes in your body and advocate for yourself if you believe something could be wrong.
2. "Cancer is cancer:" There is no one type of cancer or one way to treat it. There are critical differences in facing an early stage diagnosis vs. a late stage one, physically, mentally, and

emotionally. Similarly, even within the same category of cancers, the sub-types are not all created equally. The clinical trials, the recommended therapies, etc. all differ based on the characteristics of the tumor. Seeking out an oncologist who specializes in my specific sub-type, a triple-negative breast cancer was key in ensuring my treatment plan would have a higher likelihood of success.

3. "It's a fight:" People often talk about "fighting cancer" as if it were a battle, that we can win as long as we're strong enough, positive enough, and fight hard enough. We don't "fight" cancer, we "face" it. We recognize how scary it can be, we do our best to navigate the healthcare system to treat it, and if we're lucky, we have the opportunity to learn from it.

Fantastic. Here is the main question of our interview. Based on your experiences and knowledge, what advice would you give to others who have recently been diagnosed with cancer? What are your "5 Things" You Need To Beat Cancer? Please share a story or example for each.

The five things you need to navigate cancer after a recent diagnosis are:

1. A bias towards action: It's perfectly normal to be shocked, to cry, and to wonder how life can be so unfair. These feelings are natural and important to process. It is empowering, however, to focus energy towards action. By focusing on understanding the diagnosis, learning from others familiar with such situations, and identifying what questions to ask, I felt like I was able to maintain some control, in an otherwise very uncontrollable situation.

2. The time to find the right care team for you and your diagnosis: It was exactly one month from the time I learned of my diagnosis to when I began neoadjuvant chemotherapy, and that was the longest month of my life. Knowing that this fatal thing was growing inside me, all I wanted to do was get it out. I had been advised, however, that months matter, but days do not. Taking the time to do the research and get multiple opinions to find an oncologist with a deep expertise for my specific tumor type, helped me identify the treatment center and care team that felt most right for me. Given how much trust I would be putting into those providers, and time I would be spending at the clinic, these were critical decisions.

3. A treatment plan that is your "path of least regret:" The problem with being comfortable with data is that we got caught up in a never-ending cycle of research and second-guessing. We reached a point where we were reading and comparing the details of clinical trials to essentially identify our own treatment plan, only to further confuse ourselves since no perfect data exists for what we need to know. I soon realized that determining a treatment plan was more art than science. Not only did different oncologists have different recommendations, but I was being asked what I prefer! After days of debate and research, I realized my decision came down to one powerful question: What would be my path of least regret? Specifically, if the cancer were to recur in 5 years, what course of action would I least regret given the information at hand? Working with my care team to develop a treatment plan that was my "path of least regret" gave me the peace of mind I was seeking going into treatment.

4. A helping hand: Navigating a cancer diagnosis is overwhelming for both the patient and their family, and it truly takes a village. This is the time to be willing to ask for help, and

accept the help and support that is offered to you. Oftentimes, people want to help, but just don't know how. Turn to your friends and family and let them know what you need — whether it be groceries and meals, transportation to appointments, childcare help, a shoulder to cry on, or even just a welcome distraction.

5. Compassion for yourself: The emotions will come in waves, and are sometimes triggered when you least expect it. Be kind to yourself during this rollercoaster and protect your mental well-being by reminding yourself all for whom you have to be thankful and maintain faith that you will emerge stronger from the experience.

You are a person of great influence. If you could inspire a movement that would bring the most amount of good to the greatest amount of people, what would that be?

The movement I want to inspire is one where resilience and self-advocacy are better understood, valued, and instilled in people of all ages. Challenges and hardships will be inevitable, but the more people who can face those with learned resilience and a sense of agency, the stronger the mental well-being of our collective society will be.

We are very blessed that some very prominent names in Business, VC funding, Sports, and Entertainment read this column. Is there a person in the world, or in the US with whom you would love to have a private breakfast or lunch, and why?

I would love to meet with Brené Brown! In her book, *Rising Strong*, Brené shared that her vision for her career was to "start a global conversation about vulnerability and shame." I would like to do the same for resilience and self-advocacy, not just due to the role they played in my cancer journey, but because of how they have helped me face and navigate everything from daily stress to unexpected curveballs throughout my life.

How can our readers further follow your work online?

Readers can check out my website: www.parulsomani.com to learn more about my mission and work, to subscribe to my newsletter for updates and educational content relating to resilience, self-advocacy, and more, or to contact me regarding a speaking engagement. I look forward to hearing from them!

I'm also on social media:

LinkedIn: @Parul Somani

Instagram: @pdsomani

Facebook: DesigningSilverLinings

Twitter: @pdsomani

Scan the QR code to view my "5 Things" To Navigate Cancer YouTube video:

Rob Paulsen of 'Animaniacs' & 'Pinky and the Brain:' I Survived (Throat) Cancer and Here Is How I Did It

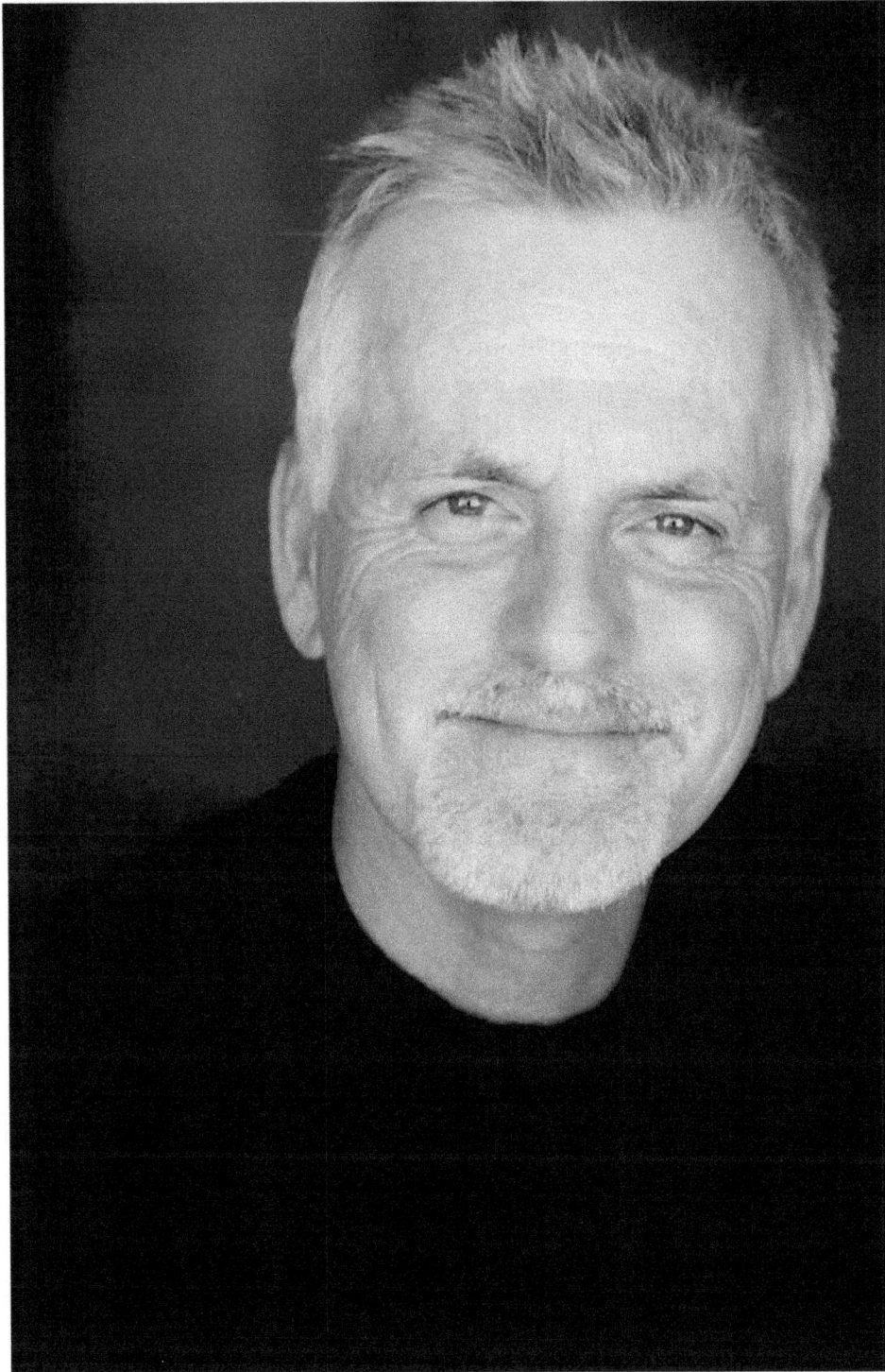

I believe that laughter is the best medicine. You can't O.D. on it. Whether you're dealing with typical things that people have: cancer, divorce, being broke, or going through all sorts of financial issues; losing a job, losing a loved one...whatever it is, I have found that laughter is a profoundly

powerful bit of medicine.

I had the pleasure of interviewing Rob Paulsen. You probably grew up with Rob. Your kids are growing up with Rob. Name not familiar? What about Pinky from 'Pinky and the Brain?' Yakko from 'Animaniacs?' A martial arts expert turtle named Raphael? That's Rob Paulsen, one of Hollywood's busiest, most talented, and most passionate performers who specializes in the art of voice acting, a career that has earned him a Daytime Emmy, three Annie Awards, and a Peabody.

Thank you so much for joining us in this interview series! We really appreciate the courage it takes to publicly share your story. Before we start, our readers would love to "get to know you" a bit better. Can you tell us a bit about your background and your childhood backstory?

I grew up in Michigan. I wanted to be a professional hockey player. Thankfully, I learned early on I had neither the talent, temperament, nor dental insurance to be a hockey player. Because I'm a very rational man, I moved to California in 1978, 43 years ago this year to apply my trade.

I was a singer who became an actor. I moved out to LA to do that sort of thing and appeared on TV shows like *MacGyver* and *St. Elsewhere*. I happened to be in some features and a bunch of on-camera commercials.

It was about the mid-'80s. I got a call from my agent who said, "Have you ever thought about doing animation?" I said, "Oh my God! Are you kidding me? Every, every kid with a pulse wants to work on cartoons!" I just wanted to work. So I said, "Of course."

The first thing I noticed when I got to my first recording session, which by the way, was for *The Transformers* and nobody knew it would become what it has; I thought, *oh my gosh! I recognize many of these actors from episodic television growing up in the '70s, and none of them are limited by the way they look. I love that!*

I jumped at the chance and I lived the axiom: Luck is when opportunity meets preparation. I had no idea that by picking up everything I owned and driving out to California, it would put me in a position to get lucky because I was prepared. I've since had the opportunity to do all these animated character voices just to make my soul happy. I didn't really think about making a living in this business.

I have done two *Teenage Mutant Ninja Turtles* movies, Rafael from when you were a little guy and on another iteration from 2012 to 2016 on Nickelodeon, I was 'Donatello'. If I live to be 100, maybe I can knock out all four turtles. And speaking of Nickelodeon, I finished another show there called *Jimmy Neutron: Boy Genius* in which I played a character called 'Carl Wheezer' who is enjoying some sort of Renaissance. Don't ask me why. People just like the little fellow.

So that's what I do and get paid to do.

Can you please give us your favorite "Life Lesson Quote?" Can you share how that was relevant to you in your life?

My favorite life lesson quote is one I kind of appropriated and added my own stuff to it.

When I was a young fellow, my grandparents and my aunts and uncles used to have a copy of Reader's Digest Magazine. At the end of every issue was a segment in which jokes were told. It was called "Laughter's the Best Medicine"—my ethos. The way I've lived my life, both pre and post-cancer is I believe that laughter is the best medicine. You can't O.D. on it. Whether you're dealing with typical things that people have: cancer, divorce, being broke, or going through all sorts of financial issues; losing a job, losing a loved one...whatever it is, I have found that laughter is a profoundly powerful bit of medicine, and that's why I use that particular quote.

Let's now shift to the main part of our discussion about surviving cancer. Do you feel comfortable sharing with us the story surrounding how you found out you had cancer?

I absolutely do. As I mentioned, I am a hockey player, and while I'm not good enough to make any money at it, I am good enough to play with a couple of buddies out here in Burbank. There are a couple of nice hockey rinks out of here.

Being a typical "weekend warrior" athlete, a typical guy, unless I can't feel a limb or I'm bleeding profusely, I go to my doctor once a year for my physical.

One morning about five years ago, I was shaving and noticed a lump on the left side of my neck. I make my living with my voice, and was able to work. I didn't have any pain or precipitous weight loss. I did a little bit of research on the internet. It could have been throat cancer. It also could have been a low-grade infection, and I chose to believe that.

This was in the middle of the year. About six months after that I was at my physical, maybe January or February of 2016, and the lump was still there. It didn't feel any larger, but it was significant. You could see it if I pointed it out, so I said to my doctor, "What do you think about this doc?" And within seconds he said, "Not good." I thought he was messing with me. He said, "No, seriously if this were a low-grade infection, it would be soft. This is like a knot. We don't want a lump in this part of your body. This is not a good sign."

It turned out to be Stage 3 Metastatic Squamous Cell Carcinoma. The primary tumor was at the base of my tongue, deep in my throat tissue. This area on my neck was the spot to which the cancer had already spread. After a bunch of punching, they found it. It was not very comfortable, but they did find it. And that is how it was discovered.

One of the most miraculous things—in addition to recovery and surviving—is the fact that there are world-class therapists, oncologists, radiation oncologists, and nutritionists—people who, overnight, take you under their respective professional wings and do everything in their power to give you the best shot. People I didn't know 20 minutes before that diagnosis are now people I've come to know very well for the past five and a half years. I hope they are in my life forever because even though I'm cured, these people have become part of my extended family.

This is only one of the glorious side effects, if I may, of my cancer treatment. It has allowed me to see the silver lining, actually the platinum lining to my treatment story. Now I have connections with world-class physicians to whom I can say, "Please tell me if you have another patient who's going through the same sort of thing I was because it's very frightening."

I'm fine, but now my sense of empathy is so key. When I am either literally or figuratively holding someone's hand, I am able to say with authority, "Oh man, I get it. I really get it," that part of the experience is the best part. Obviously, I'm glad to be here, able to work, be with my family, and talk to my new friends. But, to be able to be helpful, to be able to reach out...people like you who are kind enough to give me this incredibly wonderful forum. This has given me the perspective on why we are here and I think that is something; if we're able to actually help people, great.

What was the scariest part of that event? What did you think was the worst thing that could happen to you?

Because I was diagnosed at a fairly old age, I was 59, and even if the doctors had said, "Look, we're going to keep you comfortable, but you're on your way out," I had nothing about which to be sad. Obviously, I didn't want to leave my family, but people get over stuff. They'd have insurance money and all of the typical stuff. But, that's not what they told me. The doctor said, "Rob, we're virtually sure we can cure you, but before we do, we almost have to kill you."

The treatment was brutal, for obvious reasons—through the mouth and the throat. It lit me up pretty good, but it absolutely worked like a charm. I did radiation and chemo concurrently. It was probably about a year from the time I started my treatment until I was close to a 100% or was close to Rob 2.0.

There's definitely a shift. I'm different. You're a cancer survivor, and I'm sure you understand that too. It doesn't mean it's bad. It just means it's different.

What they also said was, "Look, we know what you do for a living. We're sure we can cure you, and you'll be able to speak. Will you be able to do your job at the same level? The straight truth is we don't know." That is what frightened me because being able to be funny, creative—all the things that pay for everything in my life, comes from my voice and my ability to be creative, and that is what really scared me.

I wasn't thinking, *oh my God, I'll be suicidal,* but humor and music and joy...I mean, I'm a blue-collar worker in The Dream Factory. My job is the happy business. If I couldn't do my job, I would figure out a way to live my life, but I think that would be really tough. So for me, that was the most difficult aspect of my diagnosis—without question.

How did you react in the short term?

My first reaction... I remember clearly, and I'll never forget it. I don't think any of us forget the day that we get that phone call. My ear, nose, and throat doctor called. This was after all of the biopsy stuff. He said, "How are you feeling?" I said, "Well, I'm not sure. How am I?"

He said it was cancer as we suspected. I didn't freak out, nor did my wife, nor did my son. We were very philosophical about it. What occurred to me right away was that I live in the most populated county—in L.A. County—and at that very moment, God forbid a young mother was being diagnosed with ovarian cancer just as she and her husband were trying to get pregnant; or a young father was being diagnosed with lung cancer just six months after the birth of his first child. That was not my circumstance.

My circumstance was we just got dealt a bad hand. Everyone does. No one gets out of here without a couple of dings, whether it's cancer, divorce, car accident, you name it. None of us do. I don't care how much money you make. I don't care how famous you are. No one gets out of here without a couple of curveballs.

Also, because of this wonderful work I've been able to do, my characters 'Yakko', 'Raphael', 'Donatello', 'Pinky' have been asked more times than I can count to speak to kids in the hospital. Want to have something to prioritize and contextualize in what one considers a struggle? Talk to a young mom and dad whose child wants to hear from their favorite Ninja Turtle. Then you talk to the parents after you've had a wonderful chat with that sweet little boy or little girl, and you find out that that young man or woman is not going to make it out of that hospital until they leave in a body bag.

That happened to me a lot. I was the beneficiary of incredibly brave children and parents who taught me what real "turtle power" was—what real love, support, and profiles of courage were about. And, because I had that gift from all these people and their children, my reaction was not *OH NOO!* My reaction was: *oh well. Now it's my turn. Let's see what you're made of, hotshot.*

I'm so grateful because not everyone obviously has the benefit of seeing people in the most difficult, impossibly horrible circumstances in their lives with their children. That's how I handled it. Not only am I cured, I am doing my job and was just called in to do a new song for 'Animaniacs', so apparently I am just fine.

After the dust settled, what coping mechanisms did you use? What did you do to cope physically, mentally, emotionally, and spiritually?

My coping mechanism, as I said earlier, and I'm not trying to be coy is humor. I cultivated a keen sense of humor, even Gallows humor —if I'm on hold on the phone for too long, for example. I remember my treatment was really difficult and I'd be waiting to speak to my doctor. I was put on hold and said, "Jesus Christ! A guy could die from throat cancer waiting for you to pick up, you idiot!"

When I would mess around, they would all say, "Don't lose your sense of humor." Not everybody has that, and that's okay. Everybody has to deal with it in their own way, but if you're able to laugh while this is going on, make yourself and others laugh, and you know what it feels like to make someone else happy, that feeling is mine—to have that superpower. I fell back on that.

Some of the side effects I've had to deal with as Rob 2.0 is that I can't really taste food the way I did for the first 60 years of my life. That's been kind of disconcerting. Now food for me is just a way to keep me alive. I don't really enjoy it, but that doesn't bother me. It kind of got my goat a little bit when I was really struggling. I'd see a commercial for Jersey Mike's Subs or for a steak and thought, *oh my God. I can't wait till I can eat again.*

I lost 50 pounds. I had always been extremely athletic, so I didn't have that much weight I should lose. I started at 178 lbs. and got down to 128 lbs. I had a period of about a month and a half where I just couldn't eat at all. My mean weight now is between 139 lbs. and 143 lbs. I ate today before you were kind enough to have me on. I had a little bit of avocado and rice sushi, maybe 12 pieces, and I'm full. There was a time before my cancer when I might have had three of those and a milkshake, and I maybe would've gotten full, but I'd be ready to eat dinner in four or five hours. If I don't eat dinner tonight, I won't miss it. I've had to learn how to rethink food and what sort of place it plays in my life, if that makes any sense.

I also have to be extra careful because I now have an oncological dentist. All of the radiation to my lower jaw has exposed me to the increased risk of some dental issues if I'm not really careful. I have to use special prescription toothpaste. But all of it is utterly superseded by the joy in my ability to get back to work and still have my sense of humor intact. By and large, while I've had some serious side effects, none of them are life-changing to the extent they make my life unhappy.

Is there a particular person you are grateful towards who helped you learn to cope and heal? Can you share a story about that?

I think if I had to pick one, it would probably be a young friend of mine who's no longer living. His name was Chad Gazzola. I met Chad and his family probably 30 years ago. I was playing hockey in Calgary in a charity game to raise money for the Muscular Dystrophy Association of Southern Alberta. Chad was the poster boy. He happened to be the same age as my son. Chad had two sisters; one also had Muscular Dystrophy, which is a genetic predisposition.

Honestly, talk about getting thrown a curveball. Can you imagine having not one, but two children with Muscular Dystrophy and all of the challenges that entails? And, to my knowledge in those days, children were lucky to make it to age 13, just when you get to know them. I got to know Chad and his family intimately. They really embraced me, and Chad was a Ninja Turtle until the end.

Chad's story and seeing how he dealt with what his mom and dad had to put him through every day just to keep his lungs clear so he could breathe...it was brutal for little Chad and his sister, Mandy, the other one with Muscular Dystrophy, but never once did I hear Chad cry. I saw his mother cry a lot, but that young man, just by his example of bravery and courage changed my life so much so that at age 59, when I was diagnosed (Chad had been gone for 10 years), I thought of him immediately and more than a dozen times when I was in my Vicodin-induced stupor. I don't think I've ever felt this much pain in my life—ever. They kept telling me it's going to work, but you sure could've fooled me. I thought immediately of Chad and how tough it must've been to be born in a wheelchair and live your whole life like that with your mom having to beat the daylights out of your back to get your chest to clear up. I thought, *maybe you better suck it up.*

In my own cancer struggle, I sometimes used the idea of embodiment to help me cope. Let's take a minute to look at cancer from an embodiment perspective. If your cancer had a message for you, what do you think it would want or say?

Great question. I think what cancer taught me and continues to do is give me the opportunity to be a better man. My sense of empathy now is so very strong. And while I don't have empathy for every type of cancer or every type of physical difficulty, I have a lot more than before my cancer.

I was always sympathetic. As I said, I had these incredible teachers and these sweet kids, with different kinds of cancer or Muscular Dystrophy. Most of them didn't make it. Cancer reminds me that every single day we have a new opportunity to be better, to be more than empathic, to be more thoughtful, to be literally more human and that is not hyperbole. When you're lucky enough to have a brush with cancer that I did, where it was very clear that it was going to be uncomfortable, but by God I was going to survive, I thought, *dude, this is an incredible opportunity. You're going to be okay but just think about all the good you're going to be able to do and for yourself.*

Not only because of nice folks like you, Savio, will I be able to reach people through this lovely chat, but I get more out of it. When I am able to speak to someone with authority about their cancer struggle, and then I hear from them, or maybe I hear through their doctor, *wow that young man or that young woman was having a real hard time, and it turns out he or she really loved one of your characters. You did the characters for her and talked about your particular treatment. You were very empathic with the difficulty of her treatment, and she is just glowing and can't stop smiling.* The biggest beneficiary of that is me, and that's the damn truth.

Every day I think: *You're already a nice guy. Let's work on being a better one.* That's what cancer taught me.

How have you used your experience to bring goodness to the world?

I think my cancer—specifically because I had throat cancer—is a great help. Your kindness is no small thing. We never know when someone's going to be reading this lovely chat. With two of the shows I did, 'Animaniacs' and 'Pinky and the Brain,' both had a reboot on Hulu with Mr. Spielberg to a much larger audience, 25 years later. That alone is pretty cool, but as a result of this lovely conversation, we never know when someone is going to read it. Maybe they have a loved one who is going through the same type of cancer that I had or maybe a lung cancer or tongue cancer, something that might affect their speech or ability to speak.

But specifically, because I had throat cancer and I'm able to do my job at the highest level in Hollywood post-cancer, someone may read this chat and say, *hey uncle Bill, I know you're dealing with this really horrible treatment, but remember how you turned me on to 'Pinky and the Brain' when I was in high school and you were in college? Well, it's back on Hulu now and the guy that does 'Pinky' had precisely the kind of cancer that you have. I know you're having real trouble with treatment right now. You've got to read this guy's chat with Savio and then, let's go watch him on Hulu. That's what he sounds like after the treatment.*

That's how my cancer experience, and precisely because it affected my work, gives me an opportunity to at least bring a little bit of comfort to people. So it is I who is very grateful to you for giving me the opportunity.

What are a few of the biggest misconceptions and myths out there about fighting cancer that you would like to dispel?

I think probably the biggest was I had to let my friends know that I was fine talking about it. I had to tell them, "Look, if you guys have any questions, I am happy to answer them." They didn't ignore me, but they didn't know what to say, and I don't think that's unusual. It wasn't out of anything but ignorance. Mind you, it wasn't like anybody got pissed off. My colleague was struggling with a real health issue, and I just didn't know what to say. I didn't want to upset her.

I can tell you folks out there who love someone with cancer—a friend, maybe a relative, someone whom you care about greatly—call them up, ask them how they're doing. At least in my circumstance, I never had a problem with hearing from anyone. It made me feel great when friends of mine went out of their way to call and just say, "Hey man, I can't imagine how tough this is, or even if it is tough. I just want you to know I'm thinking about you. Is there anything you'd like to talk about?"

Put the onus on a cancer survivor. Let them say, "Let's talk about sports. Let's talk about something that isn't cancer." That way you're honoring your desire to chat with them, but you're also not leaving it up to them to say, "Well, I don't know if I want to talk about my cancer."

So the biggest myth I can dispel from my own experience was that folks who are friends or loved ones of people struggling with a serious health issue, call them up. Take the time to call them. Don't be afraid of chatting with them. They'll let you know if they're not strong enough. Just go and give it a shot.

You are a person of great influence. If you could inspire a movement that would bring the most amount of good to the greatest amount of people, what would that be?

That's very kind of you to say that. I think like most adults, I like to give to kids. In terms of influence, I'm a spokesperson for an organization called Boo2Bullying (www.boo2bullying.org). The whole idea is to get those being bullied and the players or the prospective players while they're young.

I'm involved with a number of different children's foundations because whether it's learning how to deal with problems, learning that violence is never the answer, or learning that bullying of course is never acceptable, I want to be an influence to kids because if we can find a way to get through to children about those important aspects, they will become better humans.

I reckon the best thing to do is try to get the kids while they're young. When I get a chance to have very deep discussions, I never know when parents or kids who watched my shows 20-odd or 30-odd years ago are now going to say, *I would really like to hear what that guy has to say. I'm going to turn him on to my kids. We're going to watch 'Animaniacs' together, and I think I'll read this discussion he and Savio had for my 20-year-old, or my 25-year-old.* If I'm able to essentially preach to the choir of children, I am in.

We are very blessed that some very prominent names in Business, VC funding, Sports, and Entertainment read this column. Is there a person in the world, or in the US with whom you would love to have a private breakfast or lunch, and why?

I had a private lunch with Steven Spielberg. What a great guy! I would love to have a private meeting or private lunch with Warren Buffet. I say that, not because it would be nice to be a billionaire. That's pretty much never going to happen, but Mr. Buffett is a wellspring of logical, thoughtful, articulate information that is applicable across any and all human spectrums.

It's not about money. It's not about how to make your next billion dollars in the stock market. It's sage advice. I think they call him the "Oracle of Omaha." When I read what he talks about, it's just common sense, but also out of kindness. I really don't know that there's anything more important in the human experience than human kindness. It is the basis of everything good in the world. I believe that human kindness is the best. It is literally what separates us from animals. And, I love my animals. I would seriously give up my life for my dog. I know there are a lot of people who would not.

Find the ability to actively seek out kindness and find ways to incorporate that in your daily life. As I mentioned in your last question: I believe that I'm a nice guy. I want to be a better one. To be able to speak to someone who's in their 90s, who can give me chapter and verse about how one comes from nothing, creates billions of dollars' worth of wealth for himself, his family, and for the people he hires and does it all with kindness, thoughtfulness, utter gratitude and appreciation for the finest country in the world, I can get an awful lot from Mr. Buffet. I'm already a fan, so that's why he would be my choice.

How can our readers further follow your work online?

They can follow me on Twitter: @yakkopinky. Instagram: @Rob_Paulsen. TikTok: @RobPaulsen311 and on Facebook: @Rob Paulsen — Voice Actor. Please, follow me and we'll have a blast. We'll talk all about cartoons and laugh our butts off.

Scan the QR code to view the Oral, Head and Neck Cancer Awareness Week YouTube video:

Dr. Ruby Lathon of Roadmap to Holistic Health: I Survived (Thyroid) Cancer and Here Is How I Did It

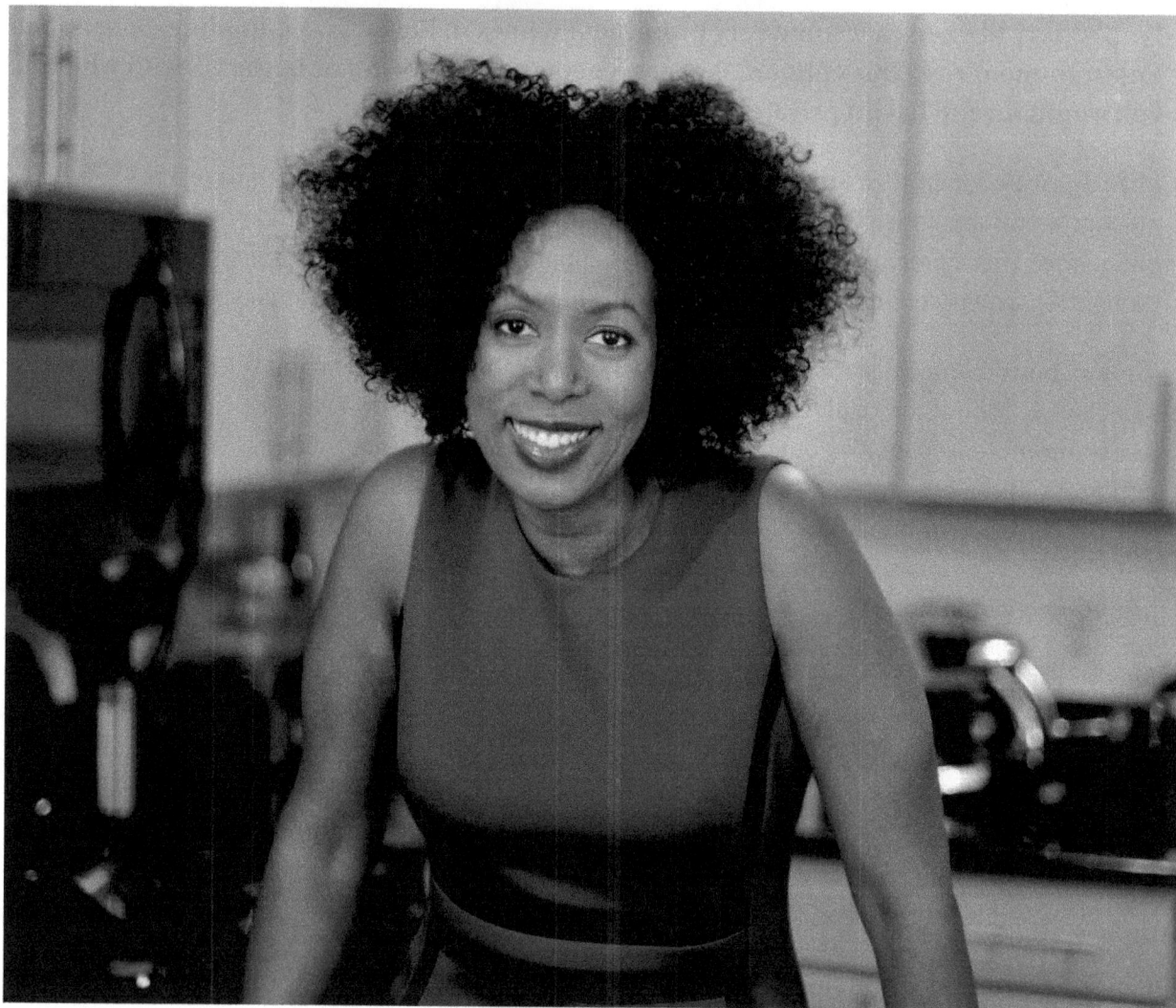

Mindset is most important, above all else. Know and believe that you can win! Your body knows how to heal. Dig your heels and be unshakeable in your resolve to live the best life you've ever had. Believing and knowing that you will not only survive, but thrive, has a different vibration than being fearful. Your body chemistry changes based on emotions; and positive, winning emotions facilitate healing.

I had the pleasure of interviewing Dr. Ruby Lathon. Ruby is a Black female engineer turned certified holistic health coach and nutritionist, after healing herself of thyroid cancer by drastically changing her lifestyle through a plant-based diet. Through her organization, Roadmap to Holistic Health, Dr. Lathon teaches others about the benefits and power of plant-based nutrition through health conferences, workshops, vegan cooking classes, consultations and coaching programs. Ruby has been featured in the hit documentary, "What the Health," and is the host of "The Veggie Chest," an online, plant-based cooking show. In addition, Ruby also lends her expertise to Body Complete Rx (BCRX), a wellness brand with a holistic approach to healthy living through a complete range of plant-based and vegan health and beauty supplements available at The Vitamin Shoppe.

Thank you so much for joining us in this interview series! We really appreciate the courage it takes to publicly share your story. Before we start, our readers would love to "get to know you" a bit better. Can you tell us a bit about your background and your childhood backstory?

My early childhood took place in Detroit and the Bahamas, hence my love of nice cars, the beach, and moving water. I'm the middle child of four kids, with an older sister and younger twin brothers. My middle school and high school years were spent in Montgomery and Huntsville, Alabama, which was a huge shift coming from the Bahamas. I grew up going to private Christian schools from elementary school through college.

Can you please give us your favorite "Life Lesson Quote?" Can you share how that was relevant to you in your life?

My favorite life quote is, "Things are always working out for me," and "If you are going to do it, do it well!" The first helps me keep a positive outlook on life and allows me to learn from mistakes without seeing them as failures or a wasted time. The second quote kind of comes from my crippling habit of perfectionism, from which I am recovering! Now it just means put your best foot forward and let your work represent you in a way that makes you proud.

Let's now shift to the main part of our discussion about surviving cancer. Do you feel comfortable sharing with us the story surrounding how you found out that you had cancer?

Sure. I found out after a routine visit with my physician. She noticed that my thyroid felt a bit larger and bumpy, so she suggested that we repeat an ultrasound that we had done a few years prior. The new ultrasound showed new nodules and that my thyroid was a bit larger. From there, the endocrinologist took over and suggested a biopsy of the suspicious nodules. That's when we detected the thyroid cancer through the biopsy. That's also how it was determined that it was gone after a year; we did another biopsy.

What was the scariest part of that event? What did you think was the worst thing that could happen to you?

The scariest part was knowing that a cancer diagnosis often means death. But I quickly dismissed that possibility and focused on how to heal. I also focused on the fact that the type of cancer that I had, thyroid cancer, had a high recovery rate. I didn't believe I would live; I knew I would live.

How did you react in the short term?

In the short-term, I shared the news with friends and family and cried a few times. Everything I was doing came to a sharp stop, and I decided to focus on the next steps to recovery. I quit my engineering job because I felt I needed to drop all stress in order to heal.

After the dust settled, what coping mechanisms did you use? What did you do to cope physically, mentally, emotionally, and spiritually?

After crying a few times, I decided I was done with the tears and that I was going to make it through this alive, period! Then I got second and third opinions on the course of treatment. And I decided that I did not like the options (remove my thyroid and start lifelong medication). I decided I wanted to heal from cancer naturally. I reached out to a friend who was versed in naturopathic medicine and got guidance on how to approach the healing process. I relied on research, my faith, prayer, and prayers of others. I also started meditating daily, which brought me a great amount of peace and inner strength.

Is there a particular person you are grateful towards who helped you learn to cope and heal? Can you share a story about that?

Yes, my friend Phyllis Hubbard was completing her studies to become a naturopathic doctor, and I became her first patient. She helped me connect to the mental and spiritual side of healing. I was an engineer at the time and this was the hardest part for me, because I couldn't see the direct connection to healing. She helped me unravel my emotions, make the mind-body connection, and tap into self-healing.

In my own cancer struggle, I sometimes used the idea of embodiment to help me cope. Let's take a minute to look at cancer from an embodiment perspective. If your cancer had a message for you, what do you think it would want or say?

Yes, I certainly tapped into embodiment as well. Ayurvedic medicine indicates that where and how you get sick can give you clues as to what you may need to examine and work on. For me, the enlargement of the thyroid, which wraps around the vocal cord, meant that I needed to find my voice and speak up for myself; it also meant that I needed to learn to establish better boundaries. I had to stop being the people pleaser and heal from childhood traumas.

What did you learn about yourself from this very difficult experience? How has cancer shaped your worldview? What has it taught you that you might never have considered before? Can you please explain with a story or example?

I learned several things. I learned of the enormous healing power of plant-based diets and natural supplementation; that was the foundation of my healing process. I also learned how much power we have within ourselves through our thoughts, emotions, and expectations. This was a huge shift for me. I changed my entire life after that bout with cancer. I changed careers from engineering to holistic nutrition; I tapped into my spiritual side and let go of so many fears. In short, I started living out loud and on purpose.

How have you used your experience to bring goodness to the world?

With my career change, I started helping others heal naturally and just live better and healthier lives, taking a holistic approach. So many people have been inspired and encouraged by my story, and it gives them the courage to listen to their intuition. I have spoken to groups around the world and inspired them to take charge of their health.

What are a few of the biggest misconceptions and myths out there about fighting cancer that you would like to dispel?

One of the biggest myths is that diet has little to no impact on cancer outcomes. I have found this to be categorically false. Eating a healthy plant-based diet is one of the most important things you can do to fight cancer and to stave off recurrence.

Fantastic. Here is the main question of our interview. Based on your experiences and knowledge, what advice would you give to others who have recently been diagnosed with cancer? What are your "5 Things" You Need To Beat Cancer? Please share a story or example for each.

Based on my personal experience, here are my "5 Things" You Need to Beat Cancer:

1. Mindset is most important, above all else. Know and believe that you can win! Your body knows how to heal. Dig your heels and be unshakeable in your resolve to live the best life you've ever had. Believing and knowing that you will not only survive, but thrive, has a different vibration than being fearful. Your body chemistry changes based on emotions; and positive, winning emotions facilitate healing.
2. Meditation is your secret power to beating fear and tapping into your inner strength. When I started meditating, I started seeing positive results like my thyroid shrinking to its normal size. When I felt fear creeping in, I'd meditate, and fear would vanish. For me, 15 minutes of meditation felt like a healing session and gave me renewed energy to keep going.
3. Trust. Trust your gut! You will have lots of decisions to make during your healing process, so learning to trust your gut will help guide you on what to do without doubt and fear. Your gut is your inner wisdom, trust it. My intuition on what to do was very strong during my healing process. When I finally stopped studying and went and relaxed at the beach, my nutrition regimen just came to me. So I went home and followed it, and it worked!
4. Eat a plant-based diet and include green juicing in your regimen. You need living food to heal. During my research on how to heal naturally, it became evident that a plant-based diet would be the optimal diet in getting cancer out of my body. Most of the cancer-fighting nutrients are found in abundance in plants, whereas cancer-causing items are found in abundance in animal products. I made the switch overnight, and I was the

healthiest that I've ever been. During my year of recovery, my skin was glowing, I had more energy, and I felt fantastic; you would never know I was fighting Cancer.

5. Get supportive and knowledgeable people around you. There are many ways to heal. Get a good team of experts that you can rely on for insight and support. I had a great support system during my recovery; I met with a myriad of traditional and holistic practitioners. It helped me be sure I was covering all of the bases, and I knew that I didn't have to know everything because I had help and support to back me up.

You are a person of great influence. If you could inspire a movement that would bring the most amount of good to the greatest amount of people, what would that be?

I would love to inspire a movement that helps people better understand the mind-body connection and how our practiced emotions can create illness or health. Secondly, I would continue to inspire the movement towards peaceful plant-based living.

We are very blessed that some very prominent names in Business, VC funding, Sports, and Entertainment read this column. Is there a person in the world, or in the US with whom you would love to have a private breakfast or lunch, and why?

I would love a private brunch with Oprah Winfrey and Leonardo DiCaprio (I know that's two!). Like so many, Oprah has been a huge inspiration to me over the years and really gets the power of thought. I'd love to share my story with her and get more wisdom-filled nuggets from her. I'm a fan of Leonardo's work, and he is a great supporter of climate change initiatives; I'd love to share my thoughts on even more aggressive earth saving initiatives and hear about his current work.

How can our readers further follow your work online?

Readers can connect with me through my website: www.RubyLathon.com where they can also sign up for my newsletter. They can also connect with on social media: @rubylathon

Selena Murphy: I Survived (Multiple Myeloma) Cancer and Here Is How I Did It

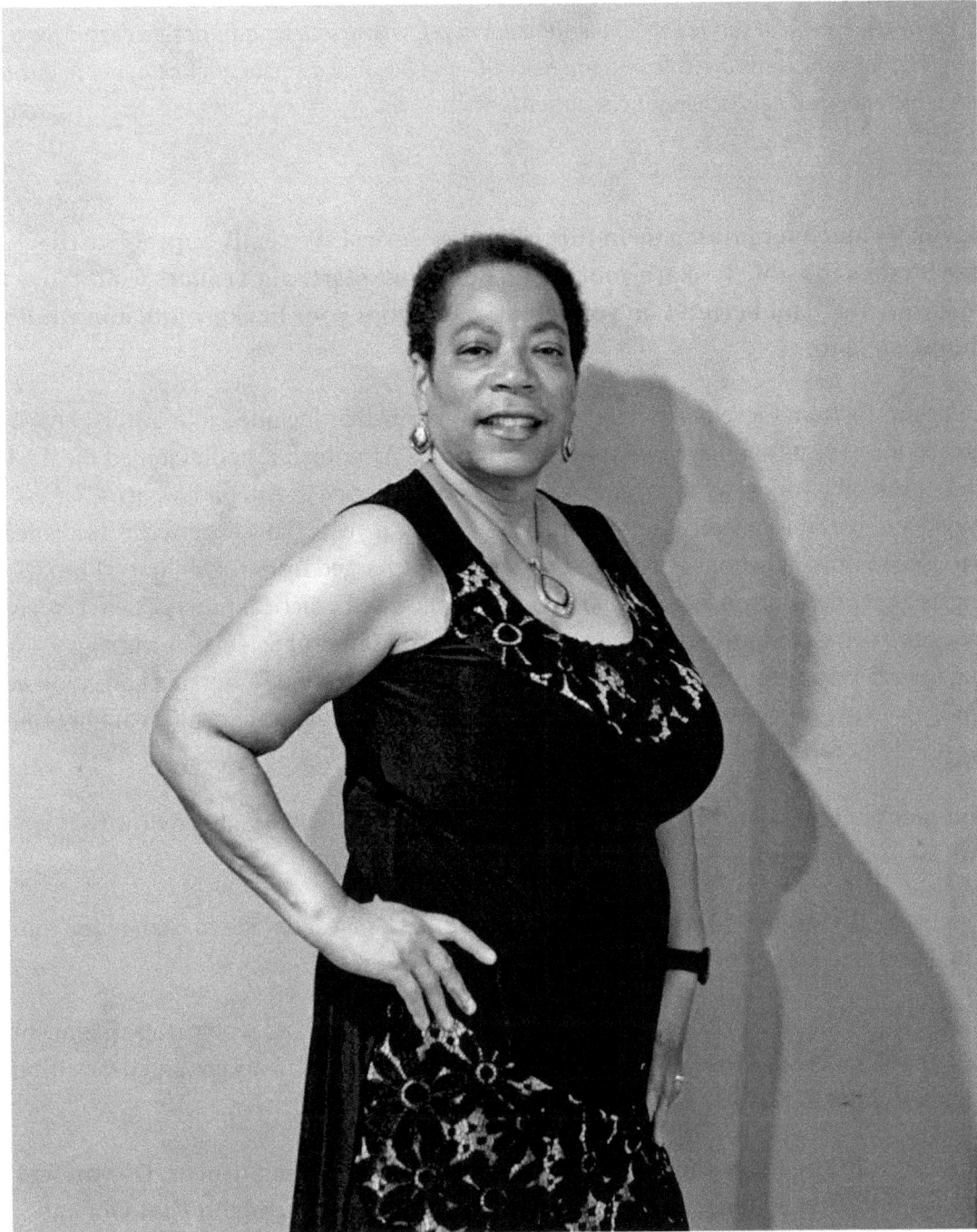

Do not be so hard on yourself. I blamed myself and was angry initially when I found out I had cancer. I had to go through some emotions to get to the point of accepting my diagnosis. Once I did that, I was able to learn more about the disease and what my options were for treatment and living with cancer.

I had the pleasure of interviewing Selena Murphy. Selena is a student in Walden University's PhD in Nursing program and works full-time as a case manager for a medical insurance company. She earned her MSN in Nursing Education from Walden in 2012. Previously, Selena served eight years in the Air Force as a medical service specialist and spent a few years as an adjunct professor for a BSN program. Her current goals are to complete her PhD and become a social change agent in a role through which she can help other cancer patients.

Thank you so much for joining us in this interview series! We really appreciate the courage it takes to publicly share your story. Before we start, our readers would love to "get to know you" a bit better. Can you tell us a bit about your background and your childhood backstory?

I am originally from Cleveland, OH. I have a large family that included four sisters. I have been married for 33 years and have two sons ages 31 and 19. After high school, I joined the Air Force, where I initially worked as an inventory management specialist. After a few years, I cross trained and became a medical service specialist for eight years. This experience awakened my desire to attend nursing school. After I was honorably discharged from the military, I began working as a certified nurse's aide, and then became a licensed practical nurse. Then, I received my associate's degree in nursing, Bachelor of Nursing and Master of Science in Nursing. I am now working toward completing my PhD in Nursing with a specialization in nursing education at Walden University. I previously worked as a staff nurse for several local hospitals and was an adjunct professor for a BSN program.

Can you please give us your favorite "Life Lesson Quote?" Can you share how that was relevant to you in your life?

"God, grant me the serenity to accept the things I cannot change, courage to change the things I can, and wisdom to know the difference." —Reinhold Niebuhr

I realize there are things that I cannot control. I cannot sit around and worry over it. I must live my life. I could not change the fact that I had cancer. I had to learn to accept and deal with the diagnosis and move forward.

Let's now shift to the main part of our discussion about surviving cancer. Do you feel comfortable sharing with us the story surrounding how you found out that you had cancer?

I fell in my driveway in early 2014. I reached my right arm out and my arm took most of the fall. I had a hairline fracture in my clavicle. Afterwards, I had pain in my right arm and shoulder for several months. I was referred to an orthopedic surgeon and started physical therapy. Before the surgeon would start injections of pain medication for relief, he ordered an MRI as part of the work up. The MRI revealed I had a tumor on my right humerus bone, and I had a biopsy done. On my birthday in 2014, I was told I had stage 3 multiple myeloma, which has an average survival rate around 29 months. I did not hear anything the doctor said after telling me I had cancer.

What was the scariest part of that event? What did you think was the worst thing that could happen to you?

For me, the scariest part was not knowing how long I would have to live and how much time I would have with my children. I did not think of myself, I just wanted to be there for them. The biggest worry I had was that the cancer may have been too far along for any treatment. I also had beautiful hair and wore braids at the time, and I was mourning the fact that I was going to lose my hair and be bald. I was also mourning myself as I was, because I knew from this point forward, I would never be the same and felt people would label me as "the one with cancer." I had also just started my PhD in Nursing program, and worried whether I would live long enough to finish it. I worried about whether I would live to see my children graduate or get married.

How did you react in the short term?

Initially, I was in shock and denial. I did not want to tell anyone unless I absolutely had to, which meant I initially only told close friends and family about my diagnosis. I did not want anyone to pity me or feel sorry for me. I wondered why this had to happen to me. How did I get this diagnosis? I was angry at myself for letting this happen, and angry at God. I felt I was not strong enough to handle it. People had always told me that God never gives you more than you can handle, but I felt very overwhelmed and at a total loss as to why this was happening.

After the dust settled, what coping mechanisms did you use? What did you do to cope physically, mentally, emotionally, and spiritually?

As I started treatment, initially getting chemotherapy twice a week, I came to the realization that I will have to fight to be here. I wanted to survive, and I realized I could not do it on my own. I realized help was available and I must accept it. I prayed that the treatment would work. I had finally to come to terms with the fact that I had cancer. I began to accept my diagnosis and the fact that I would have to have a stem cell transplant, which I had in 2015.

Mentally, I decided to have a positive mindset.

Physically, I coped by taking walks when I could. On days when I could not cook or do other chores, I had to remember not to be hard on myself, to tell myself it was okay and to accept help.

Emotionally, I coped by attending a survivorship series program where I connected with other cancer survivors.

Spiritually, I prayed and accepted my cancer diagnosis as part of God's plan for me and told myself that I was still here for a reason.

Is there a particular person you are grateful towards who helped you learn to cope and heal? Can you share a story about that?

I did not have one person who particularly helped me cope and heal more than others. My husband and two sons are the only immediate family I have nearby, and they of course supported me. I had a lot of support from several friends who provided gift cards and home cooked meals for my family while I was in the hospital and recovering from my stem cell transplant. A few friends texted or called me during this time to help lift my spirits. The one constant I had in my life was my mom, Beverly Robinson. My mom called me every day at 10:30 a.m. We talked for about 20 minutes each day about anything but cancer. This helped keep my mind off cancer and helped me to look forward to other things in life.

My student advisor and instructors in my PhD in Nursing program at Walden University were also very helpful when I had medical emergencies. They helped explain to me the different options I had and steps I could take in order to continue in the PhD in Nursing program through my illness. I was even able to take some time off to reflect and reenergize. I am grateful I was able to continue the program and look forward to being able to graduate soon.

In my own cancer struggle, I sometimes used the idea of embodiment to help me cope. Let's take a minute to look at cancer from an embodiment perspective. If your cancer had a message for you, what do you think it would want or say?

From an embodiment perspective, the cancer was telling me that this was one of toughest battles of my life. I knew I had more to give and do in life and I was not ready to give up. I have chosen to not give up and to fight to be here and be the best person I can be. I hope I can help other cancer survivors and give them hope also.

What did you learn about yourself from this very difficult experience? How has cancer shaped your worldview? What has it taught you that you might never have considered before? Can you please explain with a story or example?

One of the things I learned about myself during this experience is that I must remember to take care of myself and make time for myself. Even now, I must slow down and remind myself that I have cancer and I can't do it all. I also realize I have a lot more resilience and strength than I thought I had to survive. Cancer has changed my worldview because I feel there is no time to waste, and I should make every moment count. Cancer has taught me how to slow down and take one day at a time. Previously, I never took any time for myself. Now, I make time daily to go for a walk, take a bath or meditate.

How have you used your experience to bring goodness to the world?

I try to remind people not to sweat the small stuff. I don't get upset over things that I cannot change. I try to live my life and enjoy my time with my family and friends, and I try to encourage others to find their inner peace. As a nurse, I always had empathy for patients, but I have even more now that I have gone through this cancer journey.

What are a few of the biggest misconceptions and myths out there about fighting cancer that you would like to dispel?

The battle continues. Most of the time I feel great. Even though I look fine, there are days I have what can be considered close calls. Every new pain or symptom could mean that the cancer is back. There are times I had to have imaging, labs or other tests. Although I am in remission, there are side effects from stem cell transplant, chemotherapy and immunotherapy that have to be monitored and managed.

Fantastic. Here is the main question of our interview. Based on your experiences and knowledge, what advice would you give to others who have recently been diagnosed with cancer? What are your "5 Things" You Need To Beat Cancer? Please share a story or example for each.

1. Do not be so hard on yourself. I blamed myself and was angry initially when I found out I had cancer. I had to go through some emotions to get to the point of accepting my diagnosis. Once I did that, I was able to learn more about the disease and what my options were for treatment and living with cancer.
2. Include your village. I did not tell a lot of people about my diagnosis, and that was hard. The more support you have from family and friends, the better.
3. Accept offers of help. I initially did not want to rely on anyone for anything. I was so grateful to have support from friends who helped my family and me with meals when we needed them. I also had friends who helped with my children and attended events that I could not go to.
4. Find support. The survivor series group I attended was a great experience. I was able to talk with other cancer survivors and share my own experiences with people who understood.
5. Make time for self-care. I learned it was important to make time for myself. Learning to take care of myself has become an important part of how I deal with my diagnosis. Whether it's taking a bath, walking or reading—make time for self-care.

You are a person of great influence. If you could inspire a movement that would bring the most amount of good to the greatest amount of people, what would that be?

I want to inspire a movement of empathy and being courteous to each other. These are the moments I hope to inspire. I would encourage each person to love and cherish their family and friends and help one person they don't know. If you know someone in your community who has cancer, reach out and say hello.

We are very blessed that some very prominent names in Business, VC funding, Sports, and Entertainment read this column. Is there a person in the world, or in the US with whom you would love to have a private breakfast or lunch, and why?

My first choices would be Oprah Winfrey or Beyoncé.

A famous poet I would love to share a meal with is Amanda Gorman. Her poem that she read during the recent Presidential inauguration was inspiring and I would love to learn more about her as a person.

Locally, I would love to have a private breakfast or lunch with David Highfield, from KDKA-TV's *Your Day Pittsburgh.* He makes me laugh every morning and I know he loves food.

How can our readers further follow your work online?

www.linkedin.com/in/selena-murphy-msn-rn-ccm-8b4b1415

www.linkedin.com/in/selena-murphy-msn-rn-ccm-8b4b1415

Stephanie Scalise: I Survived (Breast) Cancer and Here Is How I Did It

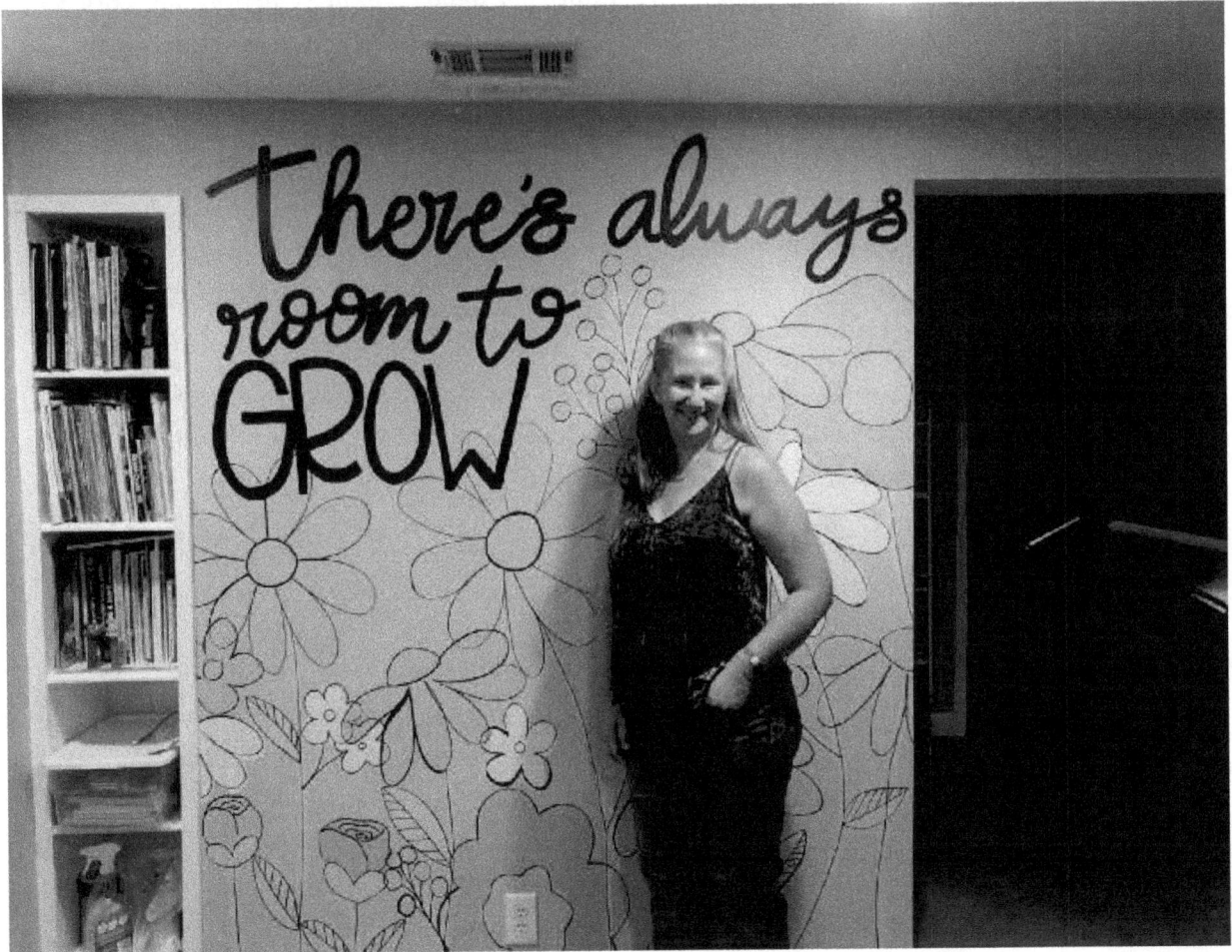

Appreciate everything you have and are given. There were days, especially after chemotherapy, that I wanted nothing to do with anyone, yet my friends and family kept visiting and sitting by my side as I slept. You can still appreciate the help, even if it's simply being physically present next to someone and keeping their spirits high.

I had the pleasure of interviewing Stephanie Scalise. Stephanie always knew she wanted to help others in some professional capacity, but it wasn't until her senior year at Syracuse University while teaching an acting class for children with Down syndrome when she decided to pursue a career in special education. She went back to graduate school and throughout her career has included stints as a substitute teacher, a vocational trainer, a reading teacher, a volunteer and a learning advocate/coach. Stephanie has worked across the country at various public schools, at elite private schools and most recently through her Atlanta-based firm SS Educational Specialists, where she focuses solely on individual learning in private practice.

Thank you so much for joining us in this interview series! We really appreciate the courage it takes to publicly share your story. Before we start, our readers would love to "get to know you" a bit better. Can you tell us a bit about your background and your childhood backstory?

I've always been a bit of a "medical misfit." If there is a one in a million chance for a side effect or reaction to occur, it is all but inevitable it will happen to me. Now two of my three daughters believe the same thing. I've always been very active. In high school it was in organized sports; in college it was family ski trips and backpacking through Europe; and in motherhood it has been joining my three daughters in their chosen sports, along with my own training and workouts. Unfortunately, that has come with way too many broken bones, strange diagnoses, and surgeries. My cancer journey started with malignant melanoma in 2000, which I had to fight to get biopsied. I always knew I'd have a lifetime of watching for cancer, but never thought it would end up being breast cancer.

I am a lifelong learner who started my professional life in fine arts, specifically advertising design, and quickly found my calling in special education and advocacy for children who learn uniquely. I had no idea until I was diagnosed with breast cancer in July 2015 how much my career path had affected my three daughters, particularly in terms of nurturing their incredible empathy for others.

Can you please give us your favorite "Life Lesson Quote?" Can you share how that was relevant to you in your life?

Shel Silverstein and Maya Angelou are my two favorites for life lessons:

"The Voice" —by Shel Silverstein

"There is a voice inside of you that whispers all day long,

'I feel that this is right for me, I know that this is wrong.'

No teacher, preacher, parent, friend or wise man can decide

what's right for you—just listen to the voice that speaks inside."

"If you don't like something, change it. If you can't change it, change your attitude."
— Maya Angelou

The Shel Silverstein quote is something I have shared regularly with my children and students. It speaks to being true to yourself no matter what is happening around you. In the end, you are accountable for your own choices and actions—and can do nothing to impact what others are going to say about you.

Maya Angelou was an exceptional person with great wisdom. She always had a smile on her face and spoke the truth. I am a true believer in the idea that if you are going to correct someone and tell them there is a better way, then you better be willing to step up and DO whatever it is in the correct way. These quotes go together quite well in that you can only control your actions, so always be true to yourself and do what is right.

Let's now shift to the main part of our discussion about surviving cancer. Do you feel comfortable sharing with us the story surrounding how you found out that you had cancer?

From day one I've been very open about my diagnosis and journey that has followed.

I knew from the moment I had my biopsy that the call was going to come back with a positive breast cancer diagnosis. And at first I was all business. The scary part occurred August 28, 2015, my initial surgery date when I was supposed to have the double mastectomy and reconstruction at the same time. They found that my lymph nodes were affected during that surgery causing them to abort the reconstruction and put in expanders instead. From October 2015 - February 2016 I had eight rounds of chemotherapy in addition to 28 doses of radiation, ending in April 2016.

What was the scariest part of that event? What did you think was the worst thing that could happen to you?

Since my mom had just gone through a double mastectomy and reconstruction, I was already familiar with the process but when I heard I had to go through both chemotherapy and radiation, I got frightened and began intense research. With my past "medical misfit" reactions, I was terrified at how my body would react to the chemotherapy drugs - and I was right in that I had an allergic reaction to my first dose.

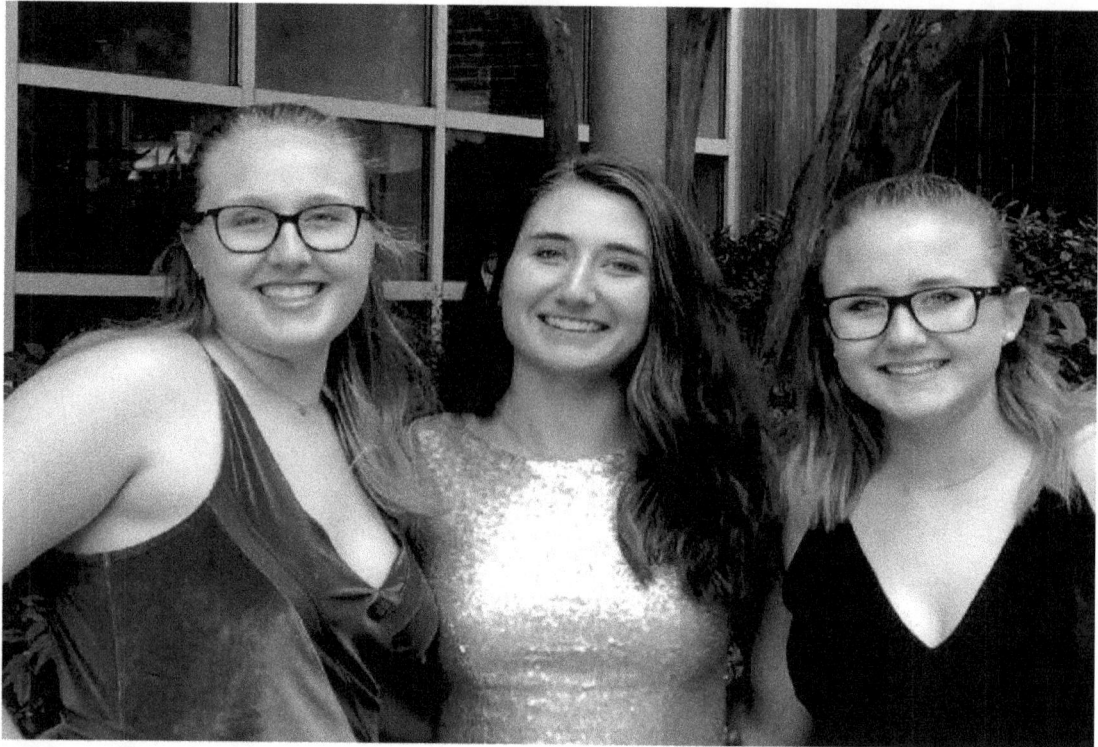

How did you react in the short term?

My first reaction was all business and self-advocacy. I told a room full of doctors and other healthcare professionals we were shifting gears and doing a double mastectomy and reconstruction instead of a lumpectomy. I was the one who led my treatment and looking back, my doctors are very happy they listened as Stage 1 quickly turned to Stage 3 during surgery with the discovery that my lymph nodes were affected.

After the dust settled, what coping mechanisms did you use? What did you do to cope physically, mentally, emotionally, and spiritually?

As previously stated, I was all business and had a "let's get this done" attitude. Before my August surgery, I got all of my volunteer and work assignments covered until October and told all of my communities why as well. I was very humbled by the outpouring of help offered by my communities and tried to defer the help, but no one let me do so. I was on multiple prayer lists from a range of religious groups, and felt the love from friends, acquaintances and even many individuals I'd never met. On the outside I stayed strong for my then 11,13 & 15-year-old daughters, but I kept asking myself, *why did it have to be breast cancer?*, and as a result, spent some time crying in the shower just so no one could hear me.

Is there a particular person you are grateful towards who helped you learn to cope and heal? Can you share a story about that?

Without question…100% my three daughters as each of them reacted in their own way. My girls are truly outstanding individuals, and I could have never imagined that this bump/challenge in our journey of life could have such a positive empowering impact on our family. The girls banded together to support themselves, me and our family as a whole. They made sure their work was done, arranged rides to and from activities, took care of me when they were home, cooked, and cleaned as needed, so all I had to do was get better. They continue to amaze me on a daily basis!!

My then oldest, 15-year-old, Samantha, took hold of the reins and made sure she and her sisters made it to every sporting and school event on time and in good spirits. She even drove me around when needed. My then 13-year-old, Lauren, was unusually quiet, but later came to find out that she was expressing herself in a personal narrative for school, which in turn was the start of Strides for Survivors, a nonprofit she and her sisters co-founded in my honor. She even slept at the foot of my bed every night to ensure I was ok. My youngest Emilie, an 11-year-old at the time, kind of shut herself off from the reality of my diagnosis and even hid in her art room in an effort to avoid anything negative. She inadvertently became a magnet for other peers going through similar family journeys and as a current high school senior, still remains a pillar for her friends in need. These girls astonish me every day, and there is no better example than through their efforts starting the aforementioned Stride for Survivors, a nonprofit organization benefiting breast cancer patients and survivors at TurningPoint Breast Cancer Rehabilitation. The fact that they do not see that raising close to $50,000 in five years as anything out of the norm is extraordinary!

In my own cancer struggle, I sometimes used the idea of embodiment to help me cope. Let's take a minute to look at cancer from an embodiment perspective. If your cancer had a message for you, what do you think it would want or say?

Wow, I've never thought of it that way. I'd have to say be true to yourself not only in the given moment but always! Live in the now and do what makes you happy, even if it is not within societal norms. Always pay it forward...leverage your knowledge and experiences to help others.

What did you learn about yourself from this very difficult experience? How has cancer shaped your worldview? What has it taught you that you might never have considered before? Can you please explain with a story or example?

Another great question. I knew I had a positive influence on my community but I never expected the amount of support I received from my clients, peers, and colleagues. I was and still am humbled by the fact that for nearly one year my family received three to five meals every week. I knew my girls gleaned empathy from my work with children with exceptional abilities (I never say disabilities), but until they managed to turn the worst experience of their lives into a phenomenal experience by starting Strides for Survivors, I did not realize how much.

How have you used your experience to bring goodness to the world?

I always shout from the rooftops about the game-changing impact TurningPoint Breast Cancer Rehabilitation has on breast cancer patients and survivors at every opportunity I get. I was so fortunate to spend time there utilizing there many resources and getting to know their very talented and compassionate staff. We as a family also show others how to turn what could have been a devastatingly awful time in our lives, into a positive opportunity to give back to the community who helped us so much.

What are a few of the biggest misconceptions and myths out there about fighting cancer

that you would like to dispel?

Just because someone is a doctor does not mean they have the final say about your body. Trust your body and react accordingly. Be your own self-advocate and get multiple opinions. Don't ever settle, fight for what you need and want for your treatment.

Fantastic. Here is the main question of our interview. Based on your experiences and knowledge, what advice would you give to others who have recently been diagnosed with cancer? What are your "5 Things" You Need To Beat Cancer? Please share a story or example for each.

1. You are not alone. There is a village of courageous women and men who have travelled this journey and emerge as thrivers on the other side. A direct quote from my girls: "When we were younger, our mom's co-teacher was diagnosed with breast cancer. At the time all we knew was that our mom was working more hours to help her friend, but never saw the impact firsthand. Another close family friend had preventative surgery 10 years ago and again our mom supported her and we've heard many stories. Our first real experience was with our grandma who had breast cancer the year before our mom. Once we became so vocal about breast cancer and started Strides for Survivors, we did not realize how many of our friends have and are currently going through this journey with their moms and/or grandmas."

2. Whether you share your diagnosis with others or chose to keep it private, pick someone to confide in and to help you along your journey. My girlfriend, who has helped three of us through each of our journeys, was just diagnosed herself. She recently mentioned how each of us got through our respective journeys differently, but knowing she has such wonderful group of women supporting her will get her through the tough times as well. Yes, she will be joining us in the distinguished club she never wanted to join, but also knows will we help her the entire way. Also, get rid of anything toxic around you—just because you are a friend or a family member, doesn't mean you can't ask them to give you space and time.

3. Take your time because if you move too fast then healing can take that much longer. You know the saying, "Two steps forward, five steps back," well; it is really magnified in your recovery. If the doctor says take two weeks of no lifting, then you do it and then take an extra few days on top of that. Your body will thank you in the end!

4. Trust your instincts/gut and speak up. Right before my double mastectomy and reconstruction, I was meeting with my plastic surgeon for my pre-op appointment. I reminded him of my "medical misfit" identity and told him if anything can go wrong/ against the plan, I would be extremely prepared. He remembers this and for the first time ever took expanders into a reconstruction surgery as well as taking a step back to wait for the biopsy results before beginning my tram reconstruction. The term tram refers to a reconstructive surgeon using your own abdominal muscles and tissues to recreate the breasts, so there is nothing foreign in your body. It was worth the wait because I could no longer have the reconstruction in the same day. I had to go through chemotherapy and radiation treatments first and would not have my reconstruction until a year later.

5. Appreciate everything you have and are given. There were days, especially after

chemotherapy, that I wanted nothing to do with anyone, yet my friends and family kept visiting and sitting by my side as I slept. You can still appreciate the help, even if it's simply being physically present next to someone and keeping their spirits high.

You are a person of great influence. If you could inspire a movement that would bring the most amount of good to the greatest amount of people, what would that be?

I think my girls have done just that. Strides for Survivors has widened the community's understanding and education of life after cancer. So many did not believe in the body's ability to heal and recover and had no idea of the support TurningPoint could bring not only to them but their families. I don't even know where to begin with my recovery. The staff at TurningPoint was not only my "go to" resource for questions that the doctors were disregarding, but they continued to be my physical therapists, my confidants, my advice nurses, my educators and ultimately, my saviors. I went in broken and confused and emerged stronger than I went in mentally and physically and also assumed the role as an outspoken advocate for breast cancer rehabilitation care. I've been a longtime member of a weekly Pilates class TurningPoint hosts, and then I've continued to leverage this remarkable organization for their tireless support, trusted massage therapy and lifelong friendships I established during my time as a patient there.

We are very blessed that some very prominent names in Business, VC funding, Sports, and Entertainment read this column. Is there a person in the world, or in the US with whom you would love to have a private breakfast or lunch, and why?

If Maya Angelou were still alive today, she would definitely be my first choice. I'm drawn to those passionate people who speak up for a cause and follow their word. Two such individuals are Spanx founder Sara Blakey and her husband/serial entrepreneur Jesse Itzler. They both talk the talk and walk the walk. I follow them on social media and absolutely love how they both put themselves and family first and yet reach so many through their philanthropic initiatives and inspirational outlooks on life. You can follow them: @jesseitzler and @sarablakely

How can our readers further follow your work online?

Instagram: @stridesforsurvivors

Facebook: Stridesforsurvivors

www.stridesforsurvivors.org

Talaya Dendy of On the Other Side: I Survived (Lymphoma) Cancer and Here Is How I Did It

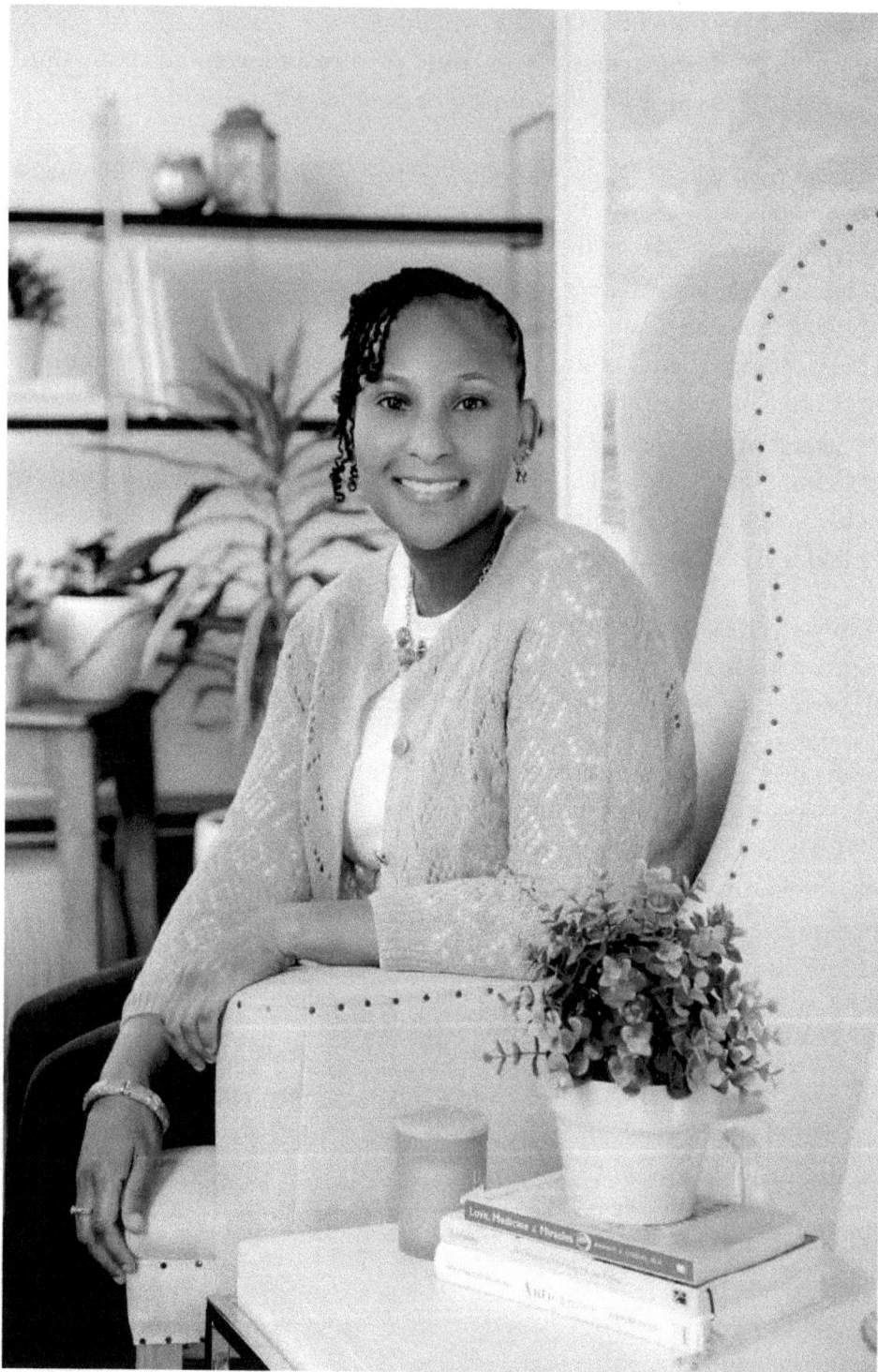

Don't be afraid to explore integrative care and complementary therapies. Those options are available to help reduce side effects, optimize conventional care, and as a whole, improve the quality of life. For example, acupuncture has helped many people that I know personally. It

helped to reduce their pain, sleep better, and reduced stress and anxiety.

I had the pleasure of interviewing Talaya Dendy. Talaya is a 10-year cancer thriver, Cancer Doula, and the founder of On the Other Side, an organization dedicated to providing personalized cancer support using a patient-centered and holistic approach.

Talaya uses her experience as a 10-year cancer thriver to serve as a partner and expert navigator by helping her clients navigate their cancer journey and ensure they are not overwhelmed, crippled by fear, discouraged, and alone. Talaya's support and guidance allow her clients to take charge of their health and focus on healing physically, emotionally, mentally, and spiritually—thereby creating a better outcome and quality of life that they desire.

Thank you so much for joining us in this interview series! We really appreciate the courage it takes to publicly share your story. Before we start, our readers would love to "get to know you" a bit better. Can you tell us a bit about your background and your childhood backstory?

As a child, I always loved to be outside playing, riding my bike, and roller skating. I grew up in St. Paul, MN, sometimes called the Twin Cities, because Minneapolis is just across the river. Winters can be long and brutal in the Twin Cities, so I always made sure to enjoy my time playing outside as much as possible.

My favorite childhood memories were when I spent the summers in Ponchatoula, LA visiting my grandma Net. Being a girl from the North, I could not get with all the bugs, wildlife, and extreme heat. However, I was fascinated by the town alligator, Ole Hardhide, and I loved spending time with my grandmother! She had so much knowledge and wisdom. She was a great cook and so much fun. Her favorite past times were playing bingo, watching the Price is Right, and the Wheel of Fortune.

I loved to listen to her talk. It seemed like there was nothing that she did not know. She seemed to have an answer for everything, whether you wanted to hear it or not. If I happened to get sick or get bad insect bites, she went to the kitchen, not the drug store. Grandma Net taught me a lot about life and how to make the best homemade pecan candy.

My grandmother showed me and taught me what unconditional love is and how it feels. She always told me that I was beautiful, smart, that I would do something with my life, and that I would do great things in this world. She would crack up when I talked because she said I was so proper and pronounced every syllable. People say that I have an old soul. I believe some of that is due to how much time I spent with her.

I remember being very uncomfortable as a child when people would stare at me. I always wondered why, what they were thinking, and what they were looking for when they stared at me. She said to me, "Don't worry about that! They are staring at you because you are so beautiful. Did you ever think of that?" Talk about a grandmother's love! Today, her words are with me. When I get that uncomfortable feeling, I think about her, I smile, and I say to myself, *she is probably right.*

She is with me in every way! One night I was really sick. All I could do was get up and pace the floor, praying for the pain to go away. She came to me and said, "Don't worry about anything. Everything is going to be alright. Don't worry." That was when I knew for sure that cancer was not going to end my life.

I can't talk about my childhood without mentioning my mother. I loved when Christmas rolled around. She made sure that we always had the best Christmas. We spent the whole day decorating the Christmas tree, watching Christmas movies, baking cookies, and laughing. My mom always made sure that I had what I needed and many of the things I wanted. She taught me the importance of having a good work ethic, taking care of myself (inside and out), and being self-sufficient. She always told me that I could do and achieve anything that I want.

Can you please give us your favorite "Life Lesson Quote?" Can you share how that was relevant to you in your life?

My favorite life lesson quote is from Lena Horne: "It's not the load that breaks you down; it's the way you carry it." This quote has been relevant to me throughout my life so far. There have been many tough times and uncertainty in my life, but I did not allow those things to lead me down the path of consistent negativity. I realized that the way I chose to look at those situations highly determined the outcome. I had to lean on my analytical skills and figure out what was really at the core of what was taking place. What, if anything, could I control? What is the lesson, and how do I use it to be stronger and better, especially if it doesn't kill me?

There is always a lesson to be learned in the things that show up in our lives. This quote spoke to me in more ways than one when I was diagnosed with cancer more than any other time in my life! I had to decide what I wanted my outcome to be and learn what I needed to do to get that outcome or get pretty close to it. I could not let cancer carry my mind away even though it was attacking my body. I learned how to let my mind lead the way. I had to learn fast *how* to properly carry the load that cancer had placed upon me. It was a time when I had to carry the load from within! There were days when the load seemed too heavy, and on those days, I had to shift the weight and take things on a minute-by-minute basis.

I learned in life that the way you carry the load might change several times in each situation, but what matters is that you carry the load in a way that benefits you and your well-being. You can use the same load that was sent to break you down, to build yourself back up.

Let's now shift to the main part of our discussion about surviving cancer. Do you feel comfortable sharing with us the story surrounding how you found out that you had cancer?

In 2010, I went in for my annual physical exam. I told my primary care doctor at the time that I had a small lump on my neck that had been there for a few weeks. She asked me if I had been sick. I told her that I had not been sick. She knew that I had been working out quite a bit, so she said it was probably just a pulled muscle. She did not look at it. She did not touch it or anything. She just blew it off as nothing to be concerned about.

Fast forward a year later. I found a new primary care doctor because the same lump was still there, only larger, and harder. Also, I did not like the lack of regard that I received from my previous doctor. I knew something was wrong. I told my new doctor about it, and she immediately looked at it, touched it, and started asking questions.

I could tell by the look in her eyes that it was not good. She told me that I needed to get an ultrasound as soon as possible. Mind you, I was about 2–3 weeks into a new job. I went in for an ultrasound and the technician had the same look. She said that everything would be reviewed, and a doctor would get in touch with me. A few days later, I got a call saying that I needed to come in for a fine needle aspiration because they were not able to determine what was going on from the ultrasound. They wanted to be sure before making a final diagnosis. I had the fine needle aspiration done and it came back inconclusive because the sample size was not large enough to make a final determination.

Finally, I went in for a full biopsy of the swollen lymph node in my neck. A couple of days later, I got the dreaded call! I found out that I had cancer on a Friday, driving home from work. I received a call from a nurse, and she informed me that the biopsy concluded that I had Hodgkin lymphoma. She told me that she could not tell me more than that, but she assured me that everything would be okay because her husband had it before and he was doing fine.

A WHOLE year later, a WHOLE year after walking around with cancer in my body, I received the news, and it was time to take action. It was time to face what I had known for a year—that something was terribly wrong.

I credit Dr. Sadia Ali Jama with HealthPartners for not blowing me off, seeing me as a human being, caring for me, and helping to save my life!

Let me make it clear, I take some responsibility in a year going by and I would never put off my health like that again! Life and fear paralyzed me and the hope that the lump would magically go away. Through this experience, I became the best self-advocate there is!

What was the scariest part of that event? What did you think was the worst thing that could happen to you?

Looking back, the scariest part of that event was the first day that I started chemotherapy. I did not know how it would affect my body. I did not know if it would work and kill the cancer.

I thought the worst thing that could happen to me was that I could die from the chemo killing my good cells as well as the bad cells. It was so unorthodox that the treatment that I was being given was keeping me alive, and in a way, killing me at the same time.

How did you react in the short term?

In the short-term, I prayed for strength every day, all day. I educated myself more on the power of mind-body connection, and I created a healing journal that consisted of healing scriptures that I read every morning. I allowed myself to feel and work through the different emotions that showed up, and I let them go so I could create space for whatever was next. I also learned as much I could about the type of chemotherapy I would be taking, the side effects, and other options.

After the dust settled, what coping mechanisms did you use? What did you do to cope physically, mentally, emotionally, and spiritually?

After the dust settled, I coped physically by continuing to exercise as much as possible. It was important to me to keep moving; even though I could not work out at the same intensity as before. I did something every day, even if it was just stretching.

I coped mentally by talking with a social worker at the hospital where I was treated. This helped me openly talk about what I had been through and start to think about how to move forward. Journaling also helped me cope.

I coped emotionally by truly acknowledging what I was feeling, the good and the bad. I needed not judge myself or my feelings. I tried to focus on things that helped me laugh and relax, like reading and watching comedy shows. I created a vision board of the hope I had for my future and what I wanted it to look like. Also, gratitude became my best friend!

I coped spiritually by continuing to read my healing scriptures daily, and I prayed and meditated. I deeply got in touch with values that were important to me and ones that I would not compromise. I envisioned a way of living that I wanted focused on and centered around peace. I realized that I was taking on too much. Everything and everyone did not deserve a place and space in my heart and head. I began to focus only on what was important to me and the things that mattered.

Is there a particular person you are grateful towards who helped you learn to cope and heal? Can you share a story about that?

I am very grateful for my mother. She was there for me throughout the entire ordeal. She went to just about every chemo infusion and would stay with me for a couple of days after to make sure that I was not alone, and I did not have any adverse reactions to the treatment.

Below is a short paragraph that I submitted for The Celebrating Moms of All Ages-Phenomenal Mother contest, which sums up how my mother helped me cope and heal.

I am nominating my mother, Lois Dendy. There are many reasons why I could nominate her, but there is one specific reason that I would like to spotlight. In 2011, I was diagnosed with Hodgkin lymphoma.

When I told my mother, she said, "I am with you until the end, baby girl." She did exactly that! My mother stood by my side the whole time and even after. She took off work and went to every chemotherapy treatment with me except for one, but even then, she made sure that I had someone to go with me.

After my treatments, she would come and stay with me for a couple of days before going back to work to make sure that I did not have any bad reactions and be there with me when I was not feeling well. She did this for six months straight! She made sure that I had what I needed.

Whenever I had an appetite, my mother would cook whatever I wanted, which usually was red beans and rice. She would come to my home and clean. She would go on different outings with me when I needed to get out of the house. She helped me to stay positive and uplifted. I knew that my mother was afraid, but she did not show it. She did not complain. She was my rock. She did not crumble.

Years later, my mother said that the hardest part was not being able to do anything. What she didn't realize is that she did everything and then some. Her actions helped to keep me alive and give me hope. Her love helped me heal!

I am very honored and happy to say that my mother was one of the winners of the contest!

In my own cancer struggle, I sometimes used the idea of embodiment to help me cope. Let's take a minute to look at cancer from an embodiment perspective. If your cancer had a message for you, what do you think it would want or say?

If my cancer had a message for me, it would say, life is too short to follow societal norms. You are put on this earth to do more! Believe in yourself and stop shrinking for others.

Your life has been about firsts, so stop putting yourself last! You spend too much time worrying about what others think, and it is time to let go, live, and go after your dreams.

I was sent to help you get moving and to get out of your comfort zone. I am here to reveal your purpose, which you have prayed for so long.

It is not pretty right now, but it gets greater later!

What did you learn about yourself from this very difficult experience? How has cancer shaped your worldview? What has it taught you that you might never have considered before? Can you please explain with a story or example?

During this difficult experience, I learned that I had blind spots when it came to how I valued myself and past traumas that I had not completely worked through. I had a lot of emotional healing that I had to do. I never had the time to sit down and think about it and heal from it. Cancer made me be still long enough to revisit and work through those things. It was a part of my total healing that had to take place at that time.

Cancer has shaped my worldview by encouraging me to look at things from multiple perspectives. Realizing that there is more detail and meaning in the bigger picture and sometimes the answers are outside of me and sometimes they are inside of me. The key is not to be afraid to look and explore.

Cancer taught me that the things that I thought were hard were actually a piece of cake. It taught me that I can do and come out on the other side of anything if I put my mind to it. It taught me to value every aspect of my life because things can change so quickly. As long as I am breathing, I am LIVING not existing!

How have you used your experience to bring goodness to the world?

I have used my experience to bring goodness to the world by volunteering with cancer organizations and serving as a mentor to those diagnosed with cancer.

I started On the Other Side to help cancer patients and their loved ones through a tough time that impacts every area of their lives.

I am also sharing my story more openly to create awareness, educate, advocate, and encourage others who have received a cancer diagnosis.

Cancer is not something that most people want to talk about or think about. However, it is necessary given the fact that more and more people are being diagnosed.

What are a few of the biggest misconceptions and myths out there about fighting cancer that you would like to dispel?

A few of the biggest misconceptions and myths about fighting cancer that I would like to dispel are that people that have cancer look a certain way. That everyone loses their hair and looks sick, and if they don't look sick, they can't be sick! Different kinds of treatment cause different side effects and everyone is not affected the same way.

When the treatment is complete, the cancer journey is over, and things will go back to normal. That is a HUGE misconception. It is not over! It means that the person is entering into a new phase. There is something called the cancer continuum, and it lasts the remainder of one's life.

Fantastic. Here is the main question of our interview. Based on your experiences and knowledge, what advice would you give to others who have recently been diagnosed with cancer? What are your "5 Things" You Need To Beat Cancer? Please share a story or example for each.

1. You must start with your mindset. I am not talking about pretending to be positive. Instead of thinking catastrophically about cancer, think about what you can control and manage. That will help you to start thinking about cancer as being manageable. This outlook is empowering. It can have a positive impact on your health, healing, and well-being.
2. Form a partnership with your oncologist and health care team. You are the captain of the team! Talk openly and honestly about your needs and what you want. It is the time to over-communicate and ask a lot of questions. Take notes, and if possible, bring someone with you to your appointments. As a team, you should be working together effectively. If you feel that is not happening, it is okay to replace or reassemble your health care team.

3. Don't be afraid to explore integrative care and complementary therapies. Those options are available to help reduce side effects, optimize conventional care, and as a whole, improve the quality of life. For example, acupuncture has helped many people that I know personally. It helped to reduce their pain, sleep better, and reduced stress and anxiety.

4. You are not a burden. Ask for help from those you trust and who are reliable. Many of your friends and family want to help. They may not know how to help or what you need. When you know, communicate that to them. If you are not sure what kind of help you need, communicate that as well and let them know that you are trying to figure it out. No one is going to have all the answers.

5. Try not to isolate yourself. I know that it can feel like no one understands what you are going through. However, it is important for your well-being and emotional and mental health to stay connected to others as much as possible. Isolation can be a result of insecurity and negative self-talk, so be mindful of your thoughts and how you are talking to yourself. This ties back to #1. Start with your mindset.

You are a person of great influence. If you could inspire a movement that would bring the most amount of good to the greatest amount of people, what would that be?

I would make sure that everyone has access to quality and equitable health care and education. When we know better, we do better.

I want to make sure that the WHOLE person is cared for. It is tough for someone to focus on their health if they are focused on finding shelter for the night. I believe that a movement focused on starting at the base of Maslow's Hierarchy of Needs (physiological and safety) and working up will bring the most amount of good to the greatest amount of people. That is where the foundation is started and built. Everyone needs that foundation.

We are very blessed that some very prominent names in Business, VC funding, Sports, and Entertainment read this column. Is there a person in the world, or in the US with whom you would love to have a private breakfast or lunch, and why?

I would love to have a private breakfast or lunch with Maya Moore for several reasons. On the court, she is my all-time favorite WNBA player on my favorite team, the MN Lynx. Off the court, her faith and strong desire to help others are commendable.

Maya received the 2021 Arthur Ashe Courage Award in July.

Her acceptance speech touched me. She urged emotional courage and using our power to empower others. She is a great example of how women can show up and serve in many different areas and have a huge, long-lasting impact. She saw a need, and she stepped out on faith to fight against injustice, and she did it at the height of her WNBA career. She is without, a doubt, a game-changer!

How can our readers further follow your work online?

Your readers can follow my work online on Facebook, Instagram, LinkedIn, and YouTube. I recently started a podcast called Navigating Cancer TOGETHER. It is on Anchor and other podcast apps.

Website: www.ontheotherside.life

Facebook: talaya.dendy.3 (personal profile)

@ontheothersidecancerdoula (business page)

Instagram: @ontheotherside17

LinkedIn: @talayadendy (personal profile)

@on-the-other-side (business page)

Podcast: www.anchor.fm/navigatingcancertogether

Text to join my email list and receive the newsletter and important information:

NAVIGATETOGETHER text to 22828

Ted Elliott of Copado: I Survived (Colon) Cancer and Here Is How I Did It

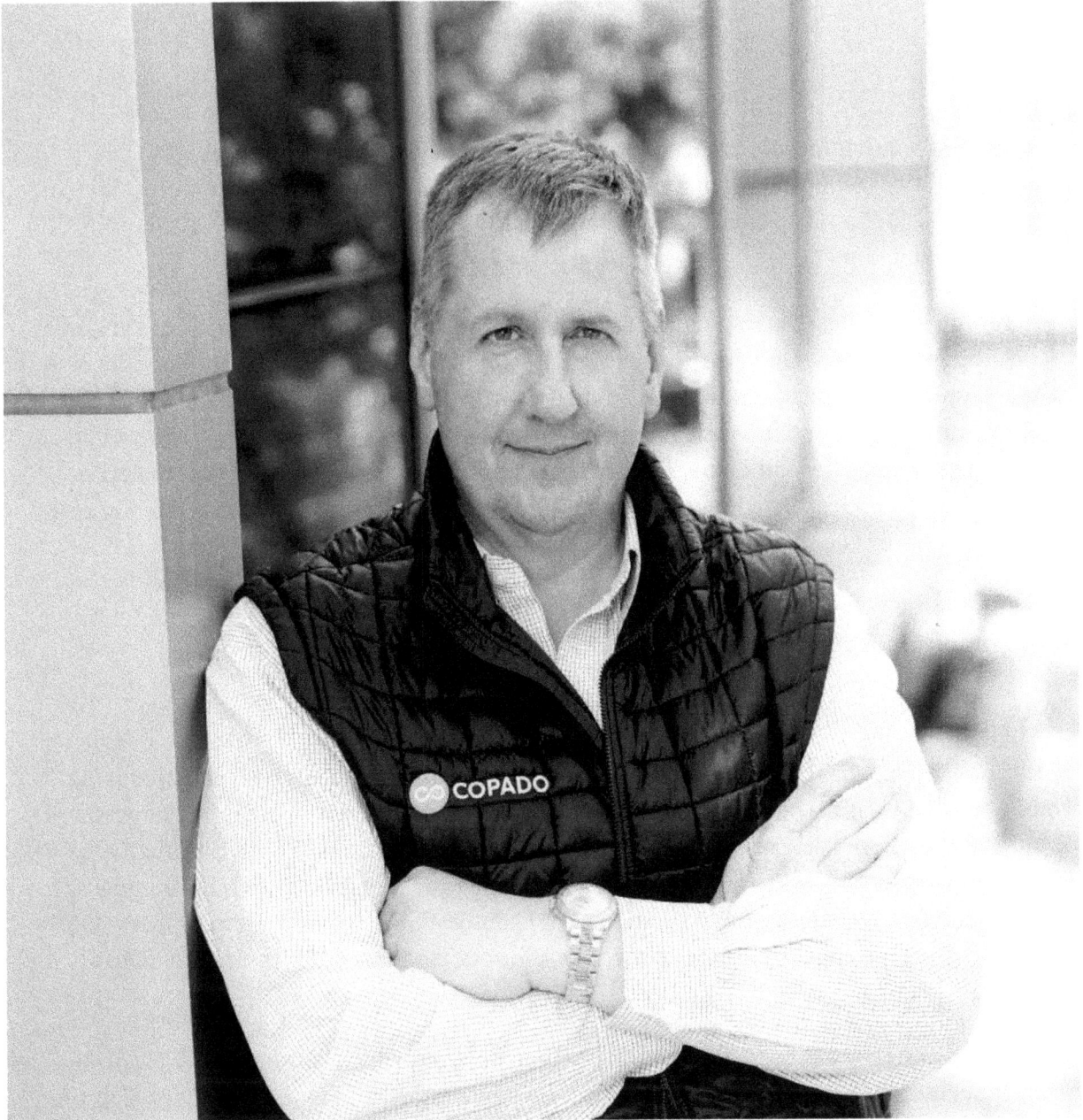

Be your own advocate. No one can advocate for you like you. At the same time, realize that your doctors treat people all the time. If they tell you to do something, listen, and respect that they are trying to save you.

I had the pleasure of interviewing Ted Elliott. Ted is the CEO of Copado, a startup unicorn on a mission to make software release days obsolete. He has a track record as an entrepreneur in software and the life sciences. Ted is committed to working on projects that will have a positive impact.

Thank you so much for joining us in this interview series! We really appreciate the courage it takes to publicly share your story. Before we start, our readers would love to "get to know you" a bit better. Can you tell us a bit about your background and your childhood backstory?

I grew up in San Francisco watching Silicon Valley scale as a center of innovation. I attended Washington and Lee University in Lexington, VA where I studied history and the University of San Francisco School of Law where I studied Venture Capital, Securities and Intellectual Property. I worked full time as a recruiter in the biotech industry to pay my way through law school and served as General Counsel for a life science business focused on cancer therapies before starting Jobscience, a software company, focused on recruitment software I sold in 2018. Since 2018, I have been serving as the CEO of Copado.

Can you please give us your favorite "Life Lesson Quote?" Can you share how that was relevant to you in your life?

"We control nothing, but we can influence anything."

Since 2018, my wife has had a heart attack and stroke, my dad was diagnosed with Hodgkin's lymphoma and I was diagnosed with an advanced rectal cancer. My family has come together through these health challenges and the COVID lockdown as a stronger unit. Copado has grown from 32 employees to more than 500 in the same time period. It has been possible to grow as a person because I am at peace understanding that I control nothing, but I can work every day to appreciate the time and people around me. I look for one thing each day to be grateful to experience.

Today, that experience is watching Copado continue to grow, which is from the efforts of so many people including our employees, customers, partners, investors, and industry leaders. Copado recently announced it raised $140 million in funding and it was a culmination of impressive work by so many people.

I look for ways to enable the people around me to look for a way to make the best of it. Ultimately we can laugh or cry at adversity, I really like to laugh.

Let's now shift to the main part of our discussion about surviving cancer. Do you feel comfortable sharing with us the story surrounding how you found out that you had cancer?

I went to the doctor, at the behest of my nine-year-old, after my wife had a heart attack. I was misdiagnosed as having fatty liver causing stomach issues. The reality was that a tumor was growing in my rectum. After a business trip, where it was obvious that I was losing blood in my stools, I decided to take a colorectal test home kit that had been sitting by my toilet for six months. I expected nothing, but was asked to have a colonoscopy where the gastroenterologist identified a 6 cm tumor in my rectum and a CT scan that found my lymph nodes in the pelvis had cancer. I was 47 and shocked.

What was the scariest part of that event? What did you think was the worst thing that could happen to you?

No one I called the first day told me I would be okay, they all told me I had a serious problem and I should get my affairs in order. I thought I was going to die; a friend of mine had just died of colon cancer in a matter of weeks, I was in shock.

How did you react in the short term?

I went for a long dog walk and cried. I kept looking for a sign that things would be ok, they were not ok. I decided to go compete in a sailboat race and came off the boat understanding I choose to live.

After the dust settled, what coping mechanisms did you use? What did you do to cope physically, mentally, emotionally, and spiritually?

Denial was my coping mechanism; I tricked myself into believing that I was just sick and used work to take my mind off my disease.

I did a lot of walking with my dog, walking was a way that I could do something to help my doctors treat me. Getting my body into the strongest position it could be came from 6,000–10,000 steps a day depending on how I felt.

I also watched a video called *Heal* that stated our mind is a powerful weapon in managing our health. It argued that if you believed you could get well and you believed you could heal, then you could influence your health with the power of positive thinking.

I deduced that we were all going to die at some point, but at least I had the luxury of accounting for what I was here to do. I sought out a daily moment of great fullness—was there a blue sky, a great phone call, a happy dog? The smallest item could bring me a sense of gratefulness and appreciation for a bigger plan that was beyond my understanding.

Is there a particular person you are grateful towards who helped you learn to cope and heal? Can you share a story about that?

My wife. She dealt with me on days where I was a pain in the neck. The days when I felt awful and had a short fuse. She took me to my appointments, she listened to my doctors, she prayed for me. She never let me know I looked bad, my hair was thinning or ever let me know anything except I would be okay and make it. My unconditional fan was essential to making it.

In my own cancer struggle, I sometimes used the idea of embodiment to help me cope.

Let's take a minute to look at cancer from an embodiment perspective. If your cancer had a message for you, what do you think it would want or say?

I think the cancer was a f@;@$,ing monster out to beat me. Its message was "you control nothing." My response was I respect that I am not in charge of the situation but I'm not going to let you define my life. The cancer forced me to evaluate who I am and why I am here and finally it brought me peace with living.

What did you learn about yourself from this very difficult experience? How has cancer shaped your worldview? What has it taught you that you might never have considered before? Can you please explain with a story or example?

Cancer is not a death sentence. How you get back up on the horse after you fall defines us. I learned what was already right in front of me but I had been blind to see. I have had a blessed life and I needed to make the most out of the people around me. If my time was up, it would have been a great ride. How could I use the extra time I was being given to make the most out of life? What was my journey and how could I contribute to the world? My thinking shifted to purpose. I decided that my first mission was to make it possible for software developers to go home for dinner with their families on release days, and make it so as many people as I could impact would have a better day at work. If I was going to get a bonus round in life, I wanted to make sure it wasn't wasted.

How have you used your experience to bring goodness to the world?

I have influenced the creation of hundreds of jobs and I am hoping to help thousands of people find purpose in their work. If people like their jobs and feel they can be successful, this is the purpose of this stage of my journey.

What are a few of the biggest misconceptions and myths out there about fighting cancer that you would like to dispel?

The biggest misconception is: You are alone. Everywhere I turned, a friend, colleague, investor, partner and customer shared their health struggles and how they or their loved ones had been impacted by cancer. We are not alone. It sucks, but if you have cancer, you are part of a big ecosystem of fighters and survivors.

Fantastic. Here is the main question of our interview. Based on your experiences and knowledge, what advice would you give to others who have recently been diagnosed with cancer? What are your "5 Things" You Need To Beat Cancer? Please share a story or example for each.

1. Speed up and don't wait to see the best doctors you can visit. I am a big advocate of finding a center of excellence that specializes in your disease. If you can get to Mayo, MD Anderson or Sloan Kettering do not pass go. Go there as quickly as possible.
2. Talk to other people who have had cancer. Listen to their experience and what worked for them; if they are there totally for you, something is working.

3. Bring a listener to all your meetings with doctors. They should also take notes. It's very hard to process conversations when you are in survival mode. Talk to your listener and see if you agree on what happened in your meetings and make sure you understand what your doctors are proposing.
4. Always go to medical records and get a copy of your MRI, PET scan, CAT scan or any other imaging. Create a binder with all your digital records, the cards of your doctors, and any information you are given. You need to always be aware of what images your doctors are looking at and comparing.
5. Be your own advocate. No one can advocate for you like you. At the same time, realize that your doctors treat people all the time. If they tell you to do something, listen, and respect that they are trying to save you.

You are a person of great influence. If you could inspire a movement that would bring the most amount of good to the greatest amount of people, what would that be?

I would like people to take pictures of their poop and show them to their doctors. I don't think most of us understand what blood looks like in your stool. When something looks wrong in the toilet, go see the doctor. Push to have a colonoscopy at a younger age; don't wait for the age of 50. Take your mortality seriously.

If you get a cancer diagnosis, get a CAT scan as soon as possible to understand how much the disease has spread. Don't accept days or weeks as an answer. I think anyone with a cancer diagnosis and the healthcare means should be able to get a scan within 24 hours to help them understand where things stand. I was told it would be 6–8 days so I went to the ER instead. Within 24 hours, I had a CAT scan. No one should have to do that.

We are very blessed that some very prominent names in Business, VC funding, Sports, and Entertainment read this column. Is there a person in the world, or in the US with whom you would love to have a private breakfast or lunch, and why?

Take a moment to figure out what you are grateful for today. If this helps anyone get perspective that will feed my journey. Actually, I'll take that back, if Marc Benioff reads this, I'd like to thank him for creating an ecosystem at Salesforce where I have met and continue to meet so many people on a journey to build the future. Copado is my second business built on the Salesforce platform, so I think Marc deserves a thank you.

How can our readers further follow your work online?

LinkedIn is the best way to follow my adventure: @tedelliott

Author Tiffany Easley: I Survived (Ovarian) Cancer and Here Is How I Did It

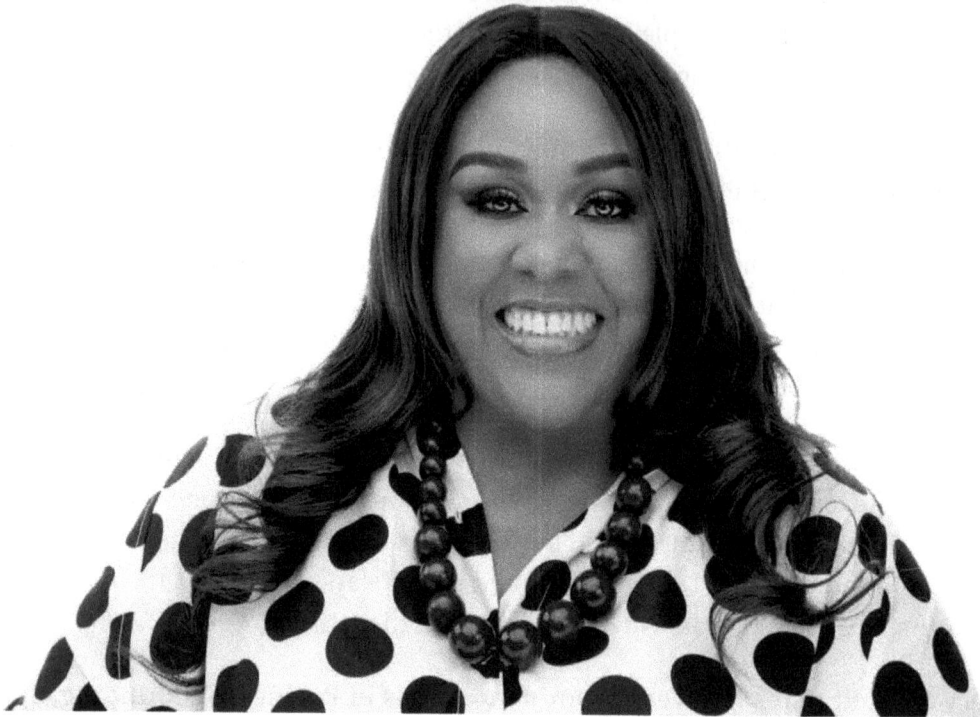

Resilience—battling cancer requires you to fight. Many times it requires you to fight the same fight over and over and over again, until you W.I.N. You must have some "bounce back" in you. You must be willing to become strong, healthy, and successful again even after something bad like cancer has happened to you. At three years of age when I faced cancer, I fought; and then at nine years of age when I thought it had returned, I fought. As I face long-term effects from chemotherapy and surgeries, I choose to remain resilient and never give up. I choose to live my best life because I beat cancer.

I had the pleasure of interviewing Tiffany R. Easley. Tiffany is an Author, Transformational Life Coach, and Speaker. Tiffany leverages her 42-year cancer survivorship to help women impacted by a chronic or terminal diagnosis navigate the trauma associated with their diagnosis in order to live a life of purpose and SOAR in their greatness. She provides resources, strategies, and tools designed to help her clients gain clarity and create a course of action to gain freedom from stagnation.

Thank you so much for joining us in this interview series! We really appreciate the courage it takes to publicly share your story. Before we start, our readers would love to "get to know you" a bit better. Can you tell us a bit about your background and your childhood backstory?

I am an accomplished Prescription Benefit Management Professional, Business and Life Coach with a solid record in driving personal/professional improvement and positive results. During my 15 years in Prescription Benefits, I have focused on client and customer relationships across multiple business segments and been responsible for over $80M in revenue. I have developed the skills and competencies—building relationships, influencing/motivating others, managing projects, presenting information in a clear and concise manner which have helped me become a successful business and brand at Tiffany R. Easley Enterprises, Inc., where I serve as the President/Director and Transformational Coach while training leaders to SOAR.

My childhood was comparable to a game of dominos. At any given moment the numbers could be against me in the form of chronic illnesses which included ovarian cancer, hydrocephalus, an inoperable cyst at the base of my brain, and infertility. It was sprinkled with several fun memories of summer camps, learning to sew and bake, and singing.

Can you please give us your favorite "Life Lesson Quote?" Can you share how that was relevant to you in your life?

My favorite "Life Lesson Quote" is by John C. Maxwell, and it says, "The greatest day in your life and mine is when we take total responsibility for our attitudes. That's the day we truly grow up." This quote is relevant to me and my life because I had to change my attitude after facing a childhood cancer diagnosis. I had to be responsible for my response to the diagnosis and how I chose to live my life after the diagnosis. My response was to never give up and always choose to W.I.N.

Let's now shift to the main part of our discussion about surviving cancer. Do you feel comfortable sharing with us the story surrounding how you found out that you had cancer?

Yes. I feel comfortable sharing the story of how I found out I had cancer. I was diagnosed with ovarian cancer in 1980 at the age of three after experiencing early onset puberty and falling off my tricycle. These sets of events prompted my mom to take me to the doctor who discovered a mass the size of a grapefruit on my right ovary. The initial treatment regimen was surgery to remove the tumor. Due to the size of the tumor, the entire right ovary also had to also be removed. After receipt of the pathology report, I was told I had Stage 1 ovarian cancer.

What was the scariest part of that event? What did you think was the worst thing that could happen to you?

My mom always shared the scariest part of that event was thinking I could die before I had a chance to enjoy life. I did not recognize or understand the vulnerability of life and death at that young age; but quickly learned after being told at the age of nine that my cancer may have returned in my left ovary. This was scary because I truly understood I could die during surgery. This was scary because the cancer I beat at the age of three may have returned and could kill me this time. This was scary because I recognized the vulnerability of life and death. I was scared and afraid because I could not control what was happening.

How did you react in the short term?

In the short-term, I lived my life as a cancer patient who would not quit and always chose to W.I.N. I chose to enjoy family, friends, school, and doing all the things I loved. I chose to fight cancer and not allow it to get the best of me.

After the dust settled, what coping mechanisms did you use? What did you do to cope physically, mentally, emotionally, and spiritually?

After the dust settled, my coping mechanism was writing. I would journal my feelings about cancer and how I felt about the disease. I journaled about all the things cancer had taken from me physically, mentally, and emotionally. As I look back on the moment the dust settled for me, I was honestly not coping but I was dealing with cancer from a very negative space. It was at that point I decided to cope with cancer through journaling. I realized cancer took my physical strength but gave me stamina to endure any difficulty I would face in life. Cancer stressed me mentally but taught me how to think outside of the box and become inspired. Cancer strained me emotionally but taught me how to appropriately channel my emotions and properly handling them. Cancer grew me spiritually. Cancer helped me embrace my call with boldness and clarity. Cancer helped me develop a deeper relationship with Jesus and love for His people. It was through journaling I was free to see all of this and begin to cope with cancer.

Is there a particular person you are grateful towards who helped you learn to cope and heal? Can you share a story about that?

My mom, Virginia Easley definitely is the embodiment of my first coach who helped me to cope and heal. She was tough but was there to make sure I never gave up. She would help me with breathing and walking exercises. She would allow me to be vulnerable and cry when I was overwhelmed from treatment or receiving bad news at a doctor's appointment. She would bathe me when I could not bathe myself, and she would pray for me when I did not know what it meant to pray. I remember at the age of nine when we thought my cancer had returned. I was so afraid leading up to the surgery. I kept asking my mom, "Am I going to die?" She would always tell me, "God will take care of you Tiffany, God loves you." As I was being wheeled down to surgery, my mom by my side, holding my hand, I looked at her with tears in my eyes and asked, "Mom, am I going to die?" My mom responded, "Tiffany, God loves you and will take good care of you, I will see you in a little while." My mom never once allowed me to believe that I would not be healed, and she always helped me to cope with my illness.

In my own cancer struggle, I sometimes used the idea of embodiment to help me cope. Let's take a minute to look at cancer from an embodiment perspective. If your cancer had a message for you, what do you think it would want or say?

Cancer doesn't just take from people, but it gives. Cancer gives strength, focus, determination, and ingenuity to those who are ready to fight and W.I.N. Yes. The battle with cancer will cause some scarring. The battle with cancer will cause some pain. The battle with cancer will cause you to enter a space you never wanted to venture into, but it will also cause you to do some phenomenal things. Cancer will give you the ability to find strength in the fight. Cancer will cause you to focus on what is truly important and not what once appeared to be. Cancer will help you embrace determination and ingenuity in giving you the victory. Cancer not only to takes, but it gives.

What did you learn about yourself from this very difficult experience? How has cancer shaped your worldview? What has it taught you that you might never have considered before? Can you please explain with a story or example?

During this very difficult experience I learned I am resilient and the power (Holy Spirit) working on the inside of me allows me to be and do exceedingly, abundantly, above all that I could ask or think (Ephesians 3:20). Cancer shaped my worldview by reminding me it has no specific race, gender, or socioeconomic status. Cancer can impact anyone.

How have you used your experience to bring goodness to the world?

I use this experience to help others SOAR Beyond trauma which has placed them at a point of stagnation due to fear, anger, disappointment, or any emotion experienced after receiving their diagnosis. I do this by providing resources, strategies, and tools for my clients and those in my sphere of influence. A few of those are—as the President and Director of Tiffany R Easley Enterprises, a business platform I use to coach women using the 5R principles of the SOAR Strategy to SOAR Beyond their place of stagnation. As the Producer and Hostess of *SOAR After A Diagnosis with Tiffany* podcast which has been created for the professional woman who desires to remain resilient while living with a diagnosis, helping women confidently step to the mic and share their survivor story with authenticity, boldness, and clarity. As the Curator, Hostess, and Producer of The Tiffany Easley Show *Soar with Tiffany* a TV show, providing our viewers with insight, inspiration, and information to assist them along their journey from trauma to triumph. We bring fun, fabulousness, and fashion to the forefront for the Survivor THRIVER to help them unleash their SOARing Lifestyle.

What are a few of the biggest misconceptions and myths out there about fighting cancer that you would like to dispel?

Misconceptions and myths about fighting cancer that I would like to dispel are:

1. Cancer is a dreadful disease; but it is not a person's destined place of residence. More often than not those who have loved ones, family, or friends who have been diagnosed with cancer or lost their battle with cancer choose to remember the disease "cancer" and not the legacy of the person. Every person diagnosed with cancer or lost a battle with cancer has a legacy, remember the legacy and not the disease.

2. Sharing your cancer story is an act of self-pity, attention seeking, or a strategy to gain popularity. Those diagnosed with cancer recognize the importance of making every moment count. Sharing their cancer story is NOT an act of self-pity, attention seeking, or a strategy to gain popularity. It is a selfless act of hope and inspiration to encourage and inspire others.

Fantastic. Here is the main question of our interview. Based on your experiences and knowledge, what advice would you give to others who have recently been diagnosed with cancer? What are your "5 Things" You Need To Beat Cancer? Please share a story or example for each.

"5 Things" You Need To Beat Cancer are:

1. Resilience—battling cancer requires you to fight. Many times it requires you to fight the same fight over and over and over again, until you W.I.N. You must have some "bounce back" in you. You must be willing to become strong, healthy, and successful again even after something bad like cancer has happened to you. At three years of age when I faced cancer I fought; and then at nine years of age when I thought it had returned, I fought. As I face long-term effects from chemotherapy and surgeries, I choose to remain resilient and never give up. I choose to live my best life because I beat cancer.

2. Strength—you must remain strong in your mind, will, and emotions as you fight against cancer. Each day you have to strengthen how you think and what you believe. You have to exert willpower and choose to live. You must make a conscious decision each day to guard your emotions and not allow them to control you. Invest in things which will strengthen your entire being. I read books, listened to songs, motivational speakers, and spiritual preachers who helped me to strengthen my mind, will, and emotions.

3. Compassion –There will be difficult moments when you may feel you can do more, feel better, or be a better version of yourself, but cancer has you feeling less than. You must extend compassion toward yourself. Give yourself permission to "just be" on the days when you need it most. I remember when I first started having days of extreme fatigue. I would be upset with myself because children my age were able to play outside for hours, and I couldn't. This is an example of why I had to learn the importance of extending compassion to myself.

4. Vision—I am speaking of foresight. You must see yourself after cancer. You must see yourself achieving your goals and reaching your dreams in spite of cancer. You must "see it" before you "see it." Growing up, I never really had an imagination, but always had vision. I always saw myself as a speaker, encouraging others to be the best version of themselves. After dealing with cancer and other chronic illness, the vision became fuel for me to make it a reality.

5. Plan—Facing a cancer diagnosis will cause you to plan. You have to plan your days around

doctor appointments, treatment sessions and when you do not feel well. I remember each day I planned for the worse and prayed for the best. On treatment days, I planned to rest more. I maintained healthy eating habits and stayed hydrated. I planned times for family and fun. I planned time for spiritual development.

You are a person of great influence. If you could inspire a movement that would bring the most amount of good to the greatest amount of people, what would that be?

I would inspire the W.I.N. Movement. I would encourage those who have or are facing cancer to Work hard, Inspire others, and Never give up.

We are very blessed that some very prominent names in Business, VC funding, Sports, and Entertainment read this column. Is there a person in the world, or in the US with whom you would love to have a private breakfast or lunch, and why?

Valisia LeKae

Instagram: @valisialekae

How can our readers further follow your work online?

Instagram: @tiffanyreasley

LinkedIn: @Tiffany R Easley

Facebook: Tiffany R Easley Enterprises

Website: www.tiffanyreasley.com

Scan the QR code to view my "5 Things" To Beat Cancer YouTube video:

Yolanda Origel of Cancer Kinship: I Survived (Breast) Cancer and Here Is How I Did It

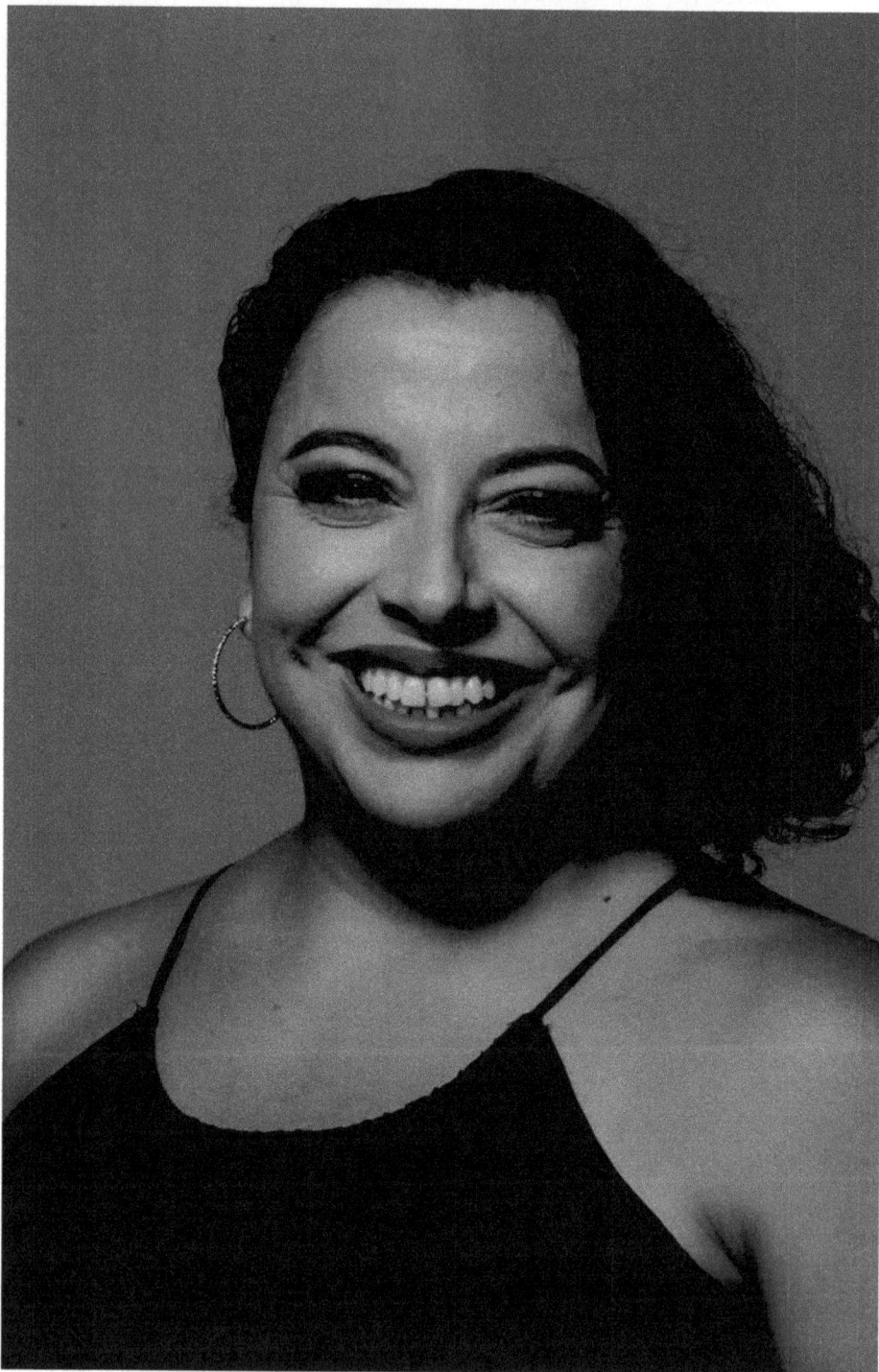

Lean on your faith and surrender your fears. I prayed a lot and asked for others to pray for me. I prayed for my family, doctors, and nurses and anyone battling cancer. I looked for stories of hope in the bible that were relevant to my current situation. I wrote down scriptures and reflected on

them often. They reminded me to be hopeful and calm during my cancer storm.

I had the pleasure of interviewing Yolanda Origel, Executive Director and Founder of Cancer Kinship. Yolanda has extensive experience working in the nonprofit sector for more than 25 years. She has served in various roles in local nonprofits where she provided direction and support in the areas of organization development, capacity-building, business development, program development, fund development and donor relations, volunteer recruitment and management, event planning, and community outreach.

Yolanda's love of nonprofit service began when she was recruited as a member of the Exeter Boys & Girls Club Youth Advisory Council member during her junior year in high school and she developed curriculum and programs for local at-risk youth. This involvement led to a program staff position which transitioned into a Program Director, and subsequently as interim Executive Director; working directly with the board, advisory board and committees, and local community leaders on strategic initiatives, fundraising activities and community outreach.

Her love for nonprofits grew even more when she began working with the YMCA in central California, which led to a position at the YMCA of Orange County when she moved to SoCal in 2004. She served as the Capital Campaign Manager of an $18M campaign for the Santa Ana YMCA. She also served as the Marketing & Communications Director for South Coast and Santa Ana YMCAs. Most recently, Yolanda served as OneOC's Nonprofit Solutions Specialist for nine years and is now the Executive Director and Founder at Cancer Kinship, a fiscally sponsored project of OneOC.

Yolanda's life's mission is to support newly diagnosed cancer patients and survivors through programs and services offered by Cancer Kinship. Being a 14-year cancer survivor has given her an incredible thirst for life, a love of extreme sports, and a very affectionate personality. Her hobbies include skydiving, photography, hiking, running, cooking, going to concerts, and spending time with friends, family and church family at Calvary Chapel Tustin.

Thank you so much for joining us in this interview series! We really appreciate the courage it takes to publicly share your story. Before we start, our readers would love to "get to know you" a bit better. Can you tell us a bit about your background and your childhood backstory?

Thanks for creating this platform to share my story!

My professional background spans more than 25 years in the nonprofit sector. I began my nonprofit career at the age of 16 when I was recruited to serve as a Youth Advisory Council member for what later became a Boys & Girls Club in my hometown of Exeter, CA. I served as Program Director and Interim Executive Director at the Club before transitioning to the YMCA and serving as the Capital Campaign Manager when I moved to

Orange County, CA, in 2004. I was working at the Y when I was diagnosed with Stage 3 Invasive Ductal Carcinoma in 2007, and I also tested positive for the BRCA1 gene. I went through 16 weeks of chemotherapy (AKA "the red devil"), had a bilateral mastectomy followed by 35 rounds of radiation and a lengthy latissimus dorsi flap reconstruction process that lasted approximately one year and required six surgical procedures. Subsequently, I had a cancer preventative hysterectomy because of my increased risk for ovarian cancer due to my BRCA1 gene. This December, I will be celebrating 15 years since my diagnosis, and I feel extremely blessed! What a wild ride it's been!

Childhood backstory: I'm the youngest of seven crazy kids born to immigrant parents from Mexico. My dad was a farm laborer, and my mother was a homemaker who was dedicated to caring for her children and home. I have three brothers and three sisters; we all grew up in a small town called Exeter in Central California—nestled between Fresno & Bakersfield near the foothills just outside of Sequoia National Park. I had a fun and normal childhood, for the most part. However, I don't recall a time in my life when cancer was not part of my vocabulary. I was introduced to the word "cancer" when I was just seven years old when my mother was diagnosed with metastatic breast cancer that took her life when she was just 42 years old.

I founded Cancer Kinship, a nonprofit organization based out of Southern CA, after losing my sister to metastatic breast cancer in 2014. My mother and sister's cancer stories are very much a part of my cancer story. All three stories bring unique perspectives and understanding of cancer survivorship issues that we, as cancer patients and survivors, have to wrestle with during our cancer battles. My hope is that Cancer Kinship can help raise awareness on the emotional impact of a diagnosis and the importance of addressing these issues as a way to reduce cancer recurrence risks and improve the quality of life of the growing cancer survivor and thriver community.

Can you please give us your favorite "Life Lesson Quote?" Can you share how that was relevant to you in your life?

I love poems by American poet E.E. Cummings, which include deep and wonderful quotes to live by; here are a few of my fav's:

"Unbeing dead isn't being alive." — A reminder that we should make the best of the days that are gifted to us; to do more than merely exist.

"We do not believe in ourselves until someone reveals that deep inside us something is valuable, worth listening to, worthy of our trust, sacred to our touch. Once we believe in ourselves we can risk curiosity, wonder, spontaneous delight or any experience that reveals the human spirit." — This speaks to my belief that there's healing power in human connection.

"The world is mud-luscious and puddle-wonderful." — This reminds me of the innocence of childhood and that we all have the ability to live in the moment just as a child plays in mud or splashes in puddles.

Let's now shift to the main part of our discussion about surviving cancer. Do you feel comfortable sharing with us the story surrounding how you found out that you had cancer?

Yes, of course. I'm an open book and very transparent about my cancer experience. I truly believe storytelling can be beneficial to the person sharing as well as those who listen, and I'm thankful for this opportunity to share mine. Here's my cancer story: I found my lump on November 22, 2007—Thanksgiving Day. I had a turkey in the oven, my family on the way, and big plans to feed my family with my home cookin.' Thanksgiving is one of my favorite holidays because I love to cook and feed my family. I often joke that I was meant to be a grandma—the kind of grandma who makes sure you never leave her home hungry.

After putting the turkey in the oven, I took a shower and was drying off with a towel when my body forced me to take notice of a sharp pain in my left breast. It happened so suddenly, and I immediately put my left hand on my breast. That's when I felt it—a very defined lump; painful, well-defined, big. I KNEW in my heart it was cancer. I just knew it. I also knew I couldn't do anything about it on Thanksgiving Day, so I just stuffed my fear down, finished getting dressed and entertained my family. Knowing that the lump was present felt like a dark shadow following me around that day and throughout the weekend.

I remember laying down for bed that night, after all was quiet and I was alone. I pressed my hand on my breast for a thorough exam. I remember thinking, *what if I die like mom? What would happen to my family?* I was the care provider for my brother, who was developmentally disabled and just received guardianship for my teenage nephew, who was now under my care. Plus, I was the sole breadwinner in my family. How would I be able to afford time off from work? What about my father? I couldn't bear the thought of my father having to bury his youngest daughter to the very disease that took the love of his life. I knew I needed to find out what I was up against. I felt like the rug had been pulled out from under me and knew in my heart that I'd be fighting the biggest battle of my life. I prayed for strength that night and cried myself to sleep.

What was the scariest part of that event? What did you think was the worst thing that could happen to you?

The scariest part was not knowing what I was up against. The waiting period, from the moment I found the lump to the moment I heard the dreaded words, "You have cancer," was the scariest for me, even though there were many scary moments sprinkled throughout my cancer battle. Not knowing if it was cancer, and if it was, what stage? Had it spread elsewhere? What's the game plan? Would I survive? How would my body handle treatment? I had so many questions that needed answers. I remembered what treatment was like for my mother. Those vivid memories I saw first-hand, through a child's eyes, of just how difficult chemotherapy and radiation were for my mother back in the 1980s. I was terrified.

Death—not because I was afraid of dying; I'm a Christian and know where I'm going when I die, so that part didn't scare me. The part that worried me the most was the impact my death would have on my family. So many people rely on me. I know I needed to fight for them.

How did you react in the short term?

The weekend before my appointment with my Primary Care Physician (PCP) was the longest weekend ever! I cried and prayed a lot during my quiet alone time. My PCP was great and referred me for my first mammogram ultrasound. I was 31 years old and hadn't had one yet. That experience is a great story in itself. I learned an important lesson on self-advocacy. Allow me to explain.

When my PCP gave me the mammogram referral, it was the first week of December. I called to schedule the appointment, and the receptionist told me that the earliest appointment available was not until the last week of January/early February. I knew that my case was urgent, and I pleaded for an earlier appointment to no avail. That's when I took the initiative to call my PCP back and asked if he'd be willing to call the imaging center on my behalf to make a case for an earlier appointment. Given my family history, the symptoms I had, and the size of the lump, it seemed extremely necessary to schedule the imaging sooner rather than later. A few minutes later, I received a call back from the imaging center informing me that they had an opening that Friday. Thank God I didn't take no for an answer and asked for help. Thank God my doctor advocated for me. That Friday, when my imaging was complete, the head radiologist came in and explained that I had a lot of cancer activity in my left breast and underarm lymph nodes and that he had taken the liberty of scheduling an appointment with a breast surgeon that afternoon.

Needless to say, I panicked. For them to take the initiative and schedule the appointment on the same day was very indicative of a serious problem. The first question out of my mouth was *am I going to die like my mom?* The drive to the surgeon's office was the longest drive ever! And the days between my biopsy and official diagnosis, and subsequent PET Scans, genetics testing, and long-awaited appointment with my oncologist, were such long and distressful days.

After the dust settled, what coping mechanisms did you use? What did you do to cope physically, mentally, emotionally, and spiritually?

I'm grateful that my breast surgeon gave me a book called, *The Breast Cancer Survival Manual* by Dr. John Link. I kept myself busy reading it from cover to cover, took lots of notes, and began writing out the many questions prompted by the manual. I wanted to become an expert in the type of cancer that I had. I wanted to understand what I could do to prepare for the biggest battle of my life. I knew that many variables were out of my control, but I wanted to be an active participant in my survival, so I changed the variables I could control.

I did a thorough inventory of my life as it related to my health and well-being. I must admit I did go a little overboard with my diet and went "cold turkey" on a lot of things, initially, such as caffeine and other foods that were staples in my kitchen. Some of the drastic dietary changes were not sustainable in the long run—however, I was able to make some wonderful changes that I am proud to say stuck—such as eating much more whole, nutritious foods, avoiding sugar and bad carbs, and basically avoiding foods found in the middle aisles of all grocery stores. I also learned about the importance of hydration, sleep and supplementation as a way to help your body heal from the aftereffects of treatment and surgery.

I also believe in the power of movement—walking, or any form of exercise is so important to your emotional and physical well-being and continued healing. Every little bit of exercise helps!

Immediately after I finished chemo, I renewed my gym membership and started working out with a trainer to help build my strength in preparation for the long road of cancer recovery. I also learned that the more I moved, the more I would reduce the risk of recurrence, which for the type of cancer I had (triple-negative stage 3 cancer) was at the highest risk within the first two years post-treatment. I had to start slow, and there were times I forced myself to get dressed and hit the gym, but I never regretted going once I was there.

Another thing I did to boost my confidence every day was forcing myself to get up, shower, get ready—which for me was putting on a little makeup, wearing a cute outfit and putting on a little perfume. There were days that I was in PJ's all throughout the day and felt like I had been hit by a bus, but dang it, I wanted to look cute! I also made my bed every day.

Another thing that helped me get through the toughest of days was music. I had several battle songs that I listened to when I was getting ready to go to chemo—to pump myself up to go. Plus, having music play in the background livened up the mood in my home for my family, especially when things were tough. (My fav bands: Dream Theater—prog rock band, and instrumentalist guitarists, Joe Satriani and Tony MacAlpine—who is also a cancer survivor)

I also captured most of my cancer experience through photo journaling. I took pictures of every stage in treatment and surgery recovery. These photos have helped me "own" my cancer story, and now that I look back at all that I've endured, I must say that I'm proud of my ability to be resilient. I've been asked why I would ever want to see those pictures, and I simply say I don't ever want to forget my struggle. It helps keep me humble, grounded, and appreciative of all that I've been able to overcome.

One last point I'd like to make related to coping is that cancer affects the family too. A few ways we managed to cope together were by going to church and having home fellowship together. We prayed together, served as volunteers for church and community, watched lots of funny movies and had mealtime together without our phones. In fact, I had a basket near the kitchen table where we placed our phones, so we wouldn't get tempted to answer texts or play with apps during meals. We also cooked a lot together. Our family became closer during my cancer battle.

Is there a particular person you are grateful towards who helped you learn to cope and heal? Can you share a story about that?

Of course, first and foremost, I'm grateful to my family and close friends who did so much to help me throughout the past 14 years. When asked this question, I also immediately think of my oncologist, Dr. David Margileth. He made me feel like the only patient in the world when we met for the first time. He took my handwritten list of questions and answered every single one. He explained the treatment plan, which alleviated much of my emotional distress. He gave me hope, and for the first time since I found the lump, I was able to sleep soundly later that night. I'm also grateful to my breast surgeon, Dr. Michele Carpenter, who gave me the opportunity to mentor her patients after I was on the other side of treatment (one-year post-diagnosis). Because of her, I learned, first-hand, the power of human connection as a way to cope and heal emotionally. I served as a patient mentor for more than 10 years, which prompted the development of my own nonprofit, Cancer Kinship, in 2018. Dr. Carpenter now serves as our Board Chair, and I'm so grateful for her belief in our mission and my ability to help others as a mentor.

In my own cancer struggle, I sometimes used the idea of embodiment to help me cope. Let's take a minute to look at cancer from an embodiment perspective. If your cancer had a message for you, what do you think it would want or say?

My cancer would say, "Your faith was bigger and stronger than me (cancer), and I didn't have a fighting chance!" Once I knew what I was up against, after receiving my diagnosis and treatment plan, I experienced a solid mindset shift that I attribute to my faith in the Lord. It was "game on," and I knew that I'd beat cancer in the end. I don't mean that smugly at all. I was often fearful and thought to myself, *what if I die fighting? What if I don't make it to next Christmas?* But even with those thoughts, as a believer, I know where I'm going when I die, so even if I die trying, I consider it a win. I became bold and have stood firm in my faith throughout the past 14 years.

What did you learn about yourself from this very difficult experience? How has cancer shaped your worldview? What has it taught you that you might never have considered before? Can you please explain with a story or example?

I learned that cancer survivorship starts from Day 1—the day a person finds a lump and/or notices symptoms and takes the necessary steps to get answers. I want to acknowledge the amount of courage it takes to get the crucial screening done, which ultimately leads to a diagnosis for many. It also takes a lot of courage to get up, get dressed and walk through the doors for the dreaded cancer treatment and/or surgery. Cancer is scary! Self-compassion is important. You don't have to be strong all the time. It's okay to say, *I'm scared,* and it's equally important to have someone or be someone who says, *I understand.*

How have you used your experience to bring goodness to the world?

My personal cancer battle didn't just end with my diagnosis. Unfortunately, when I was eight years into my cancer survival, my youngest sister was diagnosed and passed away from metastatic breast cancer that spread to her brain, just like my mother. I grieved the loss of my sister and experienced survivor's guilt and extreme sadness that prompted me to seek grief support and evaluate my life's purpose (and survivorship purpose). I wanted to make sure I used however much time I had left on this earth to raise awareness for cancer survivorship issues including, mental health, psychosocial needs, and the lack of whole-person support services required to transition cancer patients into thriving survivors. One day, while hiking and praying, I decided to begin the business planning process to develop a peer mentorship and survivor empowerment program which ultimately led to the launch of Cancer Kinship, a nonprofit agency located in Southern CA. We officially launched in November 2018 and began our programs in October of 2019. Unfortunately, COVID-19 impacted our ability to continue with our local grassroots community outreach efforts. Yet through my ongoing partnership with UHSM Health Share, our program transitioned to virtual services, and I have been able to share my services and Cancer Kinship's mission with a wider audience. It's been a blessing to have the support from our partners, which has enabled us to move our mission forward throughout the pandemic. But our work is not done. In fact, cancer patients need more help than ever before, and we are committed to meeting the unique needs of our cancer community through Cancer Kinship's core programs.

What are a few of the biggest misconceptions and myths out there about fighting cancer that you would like to dispel?

One of the comments that I heard the most during my cancer battle was, "You are so strong and inspirational." Even though I appreciated this sweet sentiment and understand why people often say that to cancer patients, it creates this expectation that cancer patients must be strong all the time. It's unfair, unrealistic, and promotes feelings of shame when cancer fighters let their walls down and express their fears and sadness. I'll never forget a sweet note I received from a colleague while battling cancer that helped me feel loved and understood. She said, "I can only imagine how hard this must be, especially during those quiet moments when you feel alone and afraid. Just know you are loved and have an army of supporters rooting for you. You are not alone." This sweet note acknowledged my fear and the difficulty of the battle. It also reminded me that I was not alone. I felt understood. A couple of other comments I heard, which I think should never be said to a cancer patient is, "Hey, at least you are getting a free boob job." Clarification: It's not a boob job. It's an amputation. And, "You didn't have a choice but to fight." Correction: All cancer patients have a voice, have a choice, and should be acknowledged for the decisions they make concerning their health. They are active participants in their battle against cancer.

Fantastic. Here is the main question of our interview. Based on your experiences and knowledge, what advice would you give to others who have recently been diagnosed with cancer? What are your "5 Things" You Need To Beat Cancer? Please share a story or example for each.

1. Inform and educate yourself on your cancer type, treatments. Read about it from credible sources, and if you don't know what things mean, or need help understanding, ask questions.
2. Lean on your faith and surrender your fears. I prayed a lot and asked for others to pray for me. I prayed for my family, doctors, and nurses and anyone battling cancer. I looked for stories of hope in the bible that were relevant to my current situation. I wrote down scriptures and reflected on them often. They reminded me to be hopeful and calm during my cancer storm.
3. Build your "tribe." Connect with cancer survivors and thrivers. They have amazing tips and stories of resiliency and can inspire hope in you. Once you are on the other side of treatment, serve as a mentor for others. Share your story; that could potentially help others going through a similar cancer battle. You will give your cancer experience a purpose, benefiting yourself and the listener. Need help connecting? Please, reach out to Cancer Kinship. We can help!
4. Don't be afraid to ask for help and accept help. I was incredibly independent and found it extremely hard to ask/accept help until one day, a dear friend called me out on my resistance. She said, "What if God put it in the heart of your friend(s) to serve in that way, and you are the barrier to the fulfillment of their purpose? Get out of the way and let them serve by helping you." Wow—talk about a reality check!

5. Take care of your mental health. Being afraid, sad, and overwhelmed are normal feelings that cancer patients experience throughout their battle and even afterward. Sometimes these feelings are directly related to treatments and are common side effects to hormone suppressive medications and other treatments. However, if you are experiencing feelings of deep despair, hopelessness, fear, panic, depressive symptoms, including suicide ideation—and these feelings won't go away—I want to urge you to talk to your doctor and seek mental health support. A cancer diagnosis is a life-altering and agonizing life experience. Don't be ashamed of seeking support that could ultimately help you live a much longer and happier life as a survivor. Self-care is important. Studies show that addressing your mental health and well-being can improve long-term health outcomes and quality of life.

You are a person of great influence. If you could inspire a movement that would bring the most amount of good to the greatest amount of people, what would that be?

I'd like to encourage the growing number of cancer survivors to get involved and support newly diagnosed patients through a mentorship experience. Even though there are wonderful programs at local cancer centers that handle diagnosis, there aren't enough programs that address life after cancer or the emotional side of cancer survivorship and its direct impact on long-term health outcomes and survivability. I want to bring this conversation full circle by simply saying that there is healing power in human connection. If we engage the growing group of cancer survivors and thrivers through a mentorship experience, together, we can improve the quality of life of those who hear the words, "You have cancer." We at Cancer Kinship offer a peer mentor program called Cancer Connections, and I want to encourage both newly diagnosed patients and survivors to reach out and learn how you can participate.

We are very blessed that some very prominent names in Business, VC funding, Sports, and Entertainment read this column. Is there a person in the world, or in the US with whom you would love to have a private breakfast or lunch, and why?

I'd love an opportunity to meet with Glenn Stearns from Stearns Lending and the star of Discovery Channel's *Undercover Billionaire*. He was diagnosed with cancer twice and had such an incredible life story of resiliency. His belief that everyone has the potential to turn their life around and make their dreams come true align with my personal beliefs as well. Plus, he and his wife Mindy look like fun, down-to-earth people who have a thirst for life and love to laugh! We'd have a blast during private breakfast or lunch!

If I could personally thank a prominent individual who helped me indirectly during my cancer battle it would have to be Dr. Charles Stanley from In Touch Ministries. His Christ-centered and bible-based daily devotionals, as well as weekly church services, helped my sister and me during the darkest of times.

I'm also open to meeting with anyone who has been touched by cancer, understands the need for our programs, and is willing to roll up their sleeves to help us grow. We are a small organization with lots of passion and a focused mission and vision but have limited resources. So, I definitely would love to meet and explore a potential partnership to expand our mission reach. If you are interested in aligning your life's mission and purpose, or if you are a company leader and are interested in aligning your brand with our mission, let's talk!

How can our readers further follow your work online?

We have an online presence at www.cancerkinship.org

For real-time updates on all things Cancer Kinship, please follow us on Facebook and Instagram: @cancerkinship. Additional information can be found on our partner's website—such as UHSM Health Share: www.uhsm.com/resources/uhsm-community-brand-ambassadors

Connect with me on LinkedIn: @yolandaorigel

Author Request

If you enjoyed reading this book, may I ask you for a quick favor?

Will you take the time to leave me a thoughtful, but honest review on Amazon?

Reviews can make a huge difference in helping others discover this book.

You can refer to the link below or scan the QR code:

www.isurvivedcancer.co/review

www.ingramcontent.com/pod-product-compliance
Lightning Source LLC
Chambersburg PA
CBHW061835260326
41914CB00005B/1000

* 9 7 9 8 9 8 5 7 5 9 5 0 1 *